Green Pharmacy

Welcome

GREEN PHARMACY

The History and Evolution
of Western Herbal Medicine

BARBARA GRIGGS

Healing Arts Press
Rochester, Vermont

Healing Arts Press
One Park Street
Rochester, Vermont 05767

ISBN 0-89281-427-6

Printed and bound in the United States

10 9 8 7 6 5 4 3 2

Healing Arts Press is a division of Inner Traditions International, Ltd.

Distributed to the book trade in the United States by American International Distribution Corporation (AIDC)

Distributed to the book trade in Canada by Book Center, Inc., Montreal, Quebec

Distributed to the Health Food trade in Canada by Alive Books, Toronto and Vancouver

Note to the reader: This book is intended as an informational guide. The remedies, approaches, and techniques described herein are meant to supplement, and not to be a substitute for, professional medical care or treatment. They should not be used to treat a serious ailment without prior consultation with a qualified healthcare professional.

Contents

For my mother

Foreword

by Norman R. Farnsworth, Professor of Pharmacognosy at the College of Pharmacy, University of Illinois, Medical Center, Chicago.

One of the most talked about and debated issues pertaining to human health concerns the safety and efficacy of plants (herbs) as drugs. This is not a recent topic of interest; indeed, it has occupied the minds of humankind for millennia. Since we have depended on plants as a source of food, for shelter, for recreational purposes (e.g. marihuana) and for drugs over this period of time, it is amazing that there is anything left to be said on the subject.

It is well known, based on survey data from the United States, that 25 per cent of all prescriptions dispensed from community pharmacies during the period 1962 to 1973 contained at least one active constituent still extracted from plant sources (not synthesized). In 1973, these prescriptions cost the American consumer in excess of $3 billion; perhaps $4.0–4.5 billion in 1980. Yet, not a single pharmaceutical firm in the United States is currently carrying out research to discover new drugs from higher (flowering) plants. When one considers that as many as 750,000 species of flowering plants exist on earth, and that only a handful have been thoroughly studied for their potential drug value, one has to ask the question "Why no interest?" Surely the greatest antagonist must admit the value of such plant-derived drugs as atropine, codeine, digitoxin, digoxin, ephedrine, leurocristine, morphine, pilocarpine, pseudoephedrine, quinidine, quinine, scopolamine, tubocurarine and vincaleukoblastine; indeed, they are prototype drugs that are discussed in all pharmacology textbooks.

But these are examples of drugs used primarily by the medical establishment. They are effective, highly potent, and must be used with caution. In recent years, the "Green Revolution", or the "Back to Nature" movements, have spurred peoples throughout the world to look for alternatives that may be perhaps less effective than standard drugs in current use, but which may have less or no side effects. Such interest is perhaps more prevalent in the developed countries of the world, than in the developing countries.

To illustrate the rising interest by the laity in the use of herbal teas, it is known that sales of these products from health-food stores in the United States during 1979 were in excess of $150 million; an increase of some 35 per cent over the previous year.

Thus, we find a unique situation in which there is little interest by pharmaceutical firms in the United States to consider plants as a source of new drugs, coupled with a skyrocketing interest by the laity in the use of herbal teas.

Industry claims "patent difficulties", "inability to control the source of raw material", "biological variation from batch to batch causes nothing but frustration", and other reasons for this lack of interest. Perhaps the real reason(s) will never be known for sure, but an understanding of the historical development of pharmacy and medicine provides a foundation on which one may draw fairly obvious conclusions.

These problems are not unique to the United States. They exist to the same extent, albeit in different forms, in almost every country of the world. The problems undergo a metamorphosis based on economics, social customs, geography, national pride, scientific attitudes, legal differences and even on politics. Recently the Director General of the World Health Organization (W.H.O.), after a worldwide study by two international health agencies, declared that if the health needs of the world are to be adequately met by the year 2000, Western methods cannot be employed to achieve the goal. The last three sessions of the World Health Assembly (each country of the world has representation in this group) endorsed this concept through resolutions that the Director General of W.H.O. should begin to work towards the goal of "Health for All by the year 2000", through utilization of Traditional Medical systems in all countries. It was suggested than an inventory be made of the system used in each country, that the best elements of each be retained and that the ineffective elements be removed. Traditional birth attendants should be utilized more, training and research programmes initiated, and all information important to achieving the stated goal should be collected and analyzed, said the Director General of W.H.O.

Since many Traditional Medicine systems in developing countries depend heavily on the use of plant drugs, one would think that there would be a great deal of support for any programme that placed the use of these drugs on a more scientific basis. On the contrary, it is generally acknowledged that even within W.H.O. there is a great deal of strong opposition to initiating programmes in the area of Traditional Medicine. The course of events in this area remains to be seen.

Thus, one can see that understanding the pros and cons of further utilization of plants as drugs throughout the world is not a simple issue.

In writing *Green Pharmacy*, Barbara Griggs has given us a perspective of this issue that has not existed previously. She has approached the problem from a historical point of view. Beginning with the finding that the Neanderthal man used several species of plants as medicines more than 60,000 years ago, she skilfully takes the reader on a journey through time, bringing the reader into contact with those events that have shaped the course of medicine and pharmacy, up to the present time. Highlighted, to mention only a few, are the significance of the Chinese contributions to medicine through the writings of the *Pen Ts' ao Chino* (*c.* 2800 B.C.), information from Arabic medicine as first recognized from carvings on the Karnak Temple (*c.* 1500 B.C.), through the trials and tribulations of the more historic medical figures such as Dioscorides, Hippocrates, Galen, Avicenna, and Paracelsus. Since the seventeenth century, the more familiar names of herbal medicine come into focus, such as Culpeper, Withering, Rush, Thomson, Hahnemann, Coffin, Bach and Hyde. She vividly demonstrates how the course of medical and pharmaceutical history was effected by events surrounding the Black Death of 1348 in Europe, by the discovery of the cause and cure of scurvy, problems associated with the syphilis epidemic in Europe in the early sixteenth century, and the impact of the use of mercury and arsenic preparations, purgatives, emetics and blood-letting, on medical practice. The positive events concerned with the discovery of synthetic drugs, such as the "Magic Bullet" and Prontosil, as well as the discovery of life-saving antibiotics in the early 1940s, are contrasted with the insidious events associated with thalidomide and the recognition of a new category of diseases caused by drugs, that is, iatrogenic diseases.

A clear picture evolves from Barbara Griggs's treatment of a complex and highly technical body of information. One can see that the rise and fall of movements to utilize herbal therapy, both inside and outside of the medical system in vogue at any point in time, are related to failures of organized medicine. That is, medicine has historically reached low points when the therapy used was probably more severe than the disease. It is at this point that alternative systems, e.g. naturopathy, homoeopathy, eclectic medicine, etc. emerge on the scene to challenge the allopathic system. Further, from Barbara Griggs's treatment of the subject matter it appears that we are entering an era where alternatives to our major westernized medical systems have an opportunity to once again come to the forefront.

Barbara Griggs has written an account that most probably will become a modern classic that can be consulted by all of those interested in gaining a keener insight into the trials and tribulations, pitfalls and rewards, and the history and future of drug therapy from nature.

NORMAN R. FARNSWORTH

"The art of Phisitians is very imperfect, for I doubt not, but for every disease there is in nature a severall symple, if they could find it out, so that if their compounds do rather show their ignorance than knowledge."

James I

Introduction

In the mid-1970s, when I began work on this book, there was already a widespread and genuine revival of public interest in that medicine which we call herbal because it is wholly derived from plants. Herbs became fashionable, herbal suppliers began to enjoy a new prosperity, bookshops abounded with herbals old and new, and the handful of herbal practitioners available found their appointment books filling up.

Yet oddly enough, this rise of interest in medicinal plants was not, it struck me, paralleled by any real appreciation of their potential – or of their incalculable value to the human race over hundreds of thousands of years. The associations called up by herbal medicine are still, far too often, with the witch-doctor, with medieval mumbo-jumbo or with the magical rituals of the primitive tribe. Many of the people who were kind enough to ask what subject I was working on, backed away when I told them. "But do you actually believe in herbal medicine?" they would enquire anxiously, as though I had confessed initiation into some secret and alarming cult. And nowhere is this mistrust and contempt more deeply rooted than in orthodox medical circles, although today it is slowly yielding to a more informed response.

I found all this puzzling. Up to four or five hundred years ago, the prescription written out by any professional doctor, anywhere in the world, was much more likely than not to be for a plant-based medicine, although animal and mineral ingredients also entered into his materia medica; while for those untold millions who lived their lives out without benefit of doctoring, plants have always been the chief source of medicine.

How did it happen that almost from one century to the next,

medicinal plants were officially consigned to near–oblivion?

What were the professional, or economic, or social forces that brought this about?

Do we enjoy a vastly superior medicine as a result?

Are the synthetic drugs that have ousted plant medicine demonstrably better?

Or could it be that we are neglecting a therapeutic resource of immense potential?

These were some of the questions that arose in my mind as I read my way into the subject: I have tried to answer them in this book.

I am aware that had I been a trained doctor, a qualified pharmacognosist and pharmacist, an anthropologist, a historian, and an expert practitioner of herbal medicine, this would have been a vastly better and more authoritative book, free of the shortcomings which may be found in it. I can only plead that if such multidisciplinary experts exist, they must be few and far between − and none of them has so far shown any inclination to tell a story which, it seems to me, urgently demands to be told.

I am also aware that this book risks being read as a wholesale attack on the medical profession, although this was far from my intention. Inevitably, however, the Stepmother cuts an unattractive figure in any version of the Cinderella story, however admirable or agreeable a woman she may have been in other respects. And it is, sadly, a darker side of the profession that emerges in these pages, which relate its failings rather than its many glorious achievements. I hope I shall be forgiven for dwelling on this negative aspect of a profession for which I have the greatest respect, and whose dedicated talents I have compelling personal reasons to honour.

Similarly, my account of the pharmaceutical industry dwells on its sins of omission and its shortcomings, rather than on the vast and undeniable contribution it has made to the sum of medical knowledge, and to the better health of millions, whatever the defects of some drugs may be.

No doubt Cinderella, too, had her faults; in my favourite version of the Cinderella story, the stepmother bravely admits the error of her ways, after the Royal Wedding, and thereafter all is amity and accord between them.

All mankind would benefit, if the history of herbal medicine could have a comparably happy outcome.

*   *   *

This book was made possible by the generous help and encouragement I have received from experts in the many fields it ranges over; many of them gave lavishly of their valuable time, and went out of their way to assist this novice in their specialized subject. I should like to record outstanding debts of gratitude to Dr. Norman Farnsworth, Professor of Pharmacognosy, Head of the Department of Pharmacognosy and Pharmacology in the University of Illinois, who provided treasures of information on the present state and the prospects of international medicinal plant research, offered much useful comment, criticism and suggestion, and made available to me many of his papers, published and unpublished; to Mrs. Ann Warren-Davis, member of the National Institute of Medical Herbalists who over five years has responded patiently to a barrage of questions on matters both medical and historical, and to Frederick Fletcher Hyde, President Emeritus of the National Institute of Medical Herbalists, who allowed me to tap his encyclopedic knowledge in the field of herbal medicine: both of them read through my manuscript and made constructive criticisms, corrections and suggestions; and to Dr. Peter Hylands, of the Department of Pharmacy, Chelsea College, who did his best to instruct me in questions of pharmacognosy and pharmacy, particularly in the chapter dealing with the new "Chemical" Medicine of the late sixteenth century. If, despite so much expert help, errors of fact have crept into the book, the fault is mine alone.

I should like particularly to thank the Librarian and Staff of the Wellcome Institute for the History of Medicine Library, in which happy haven of medical historians much of my research was done: Assistant Librarian H.J.M. Symons was particularly helpful; Douglas Matthews and the staff of the London Library; the Librarian and staffs of the British Library, the Botany Library of the British Museum (Natural History); the Francis Countway Library in Boston; the Libraries of the British Medical Association and the Pharmaceutical Society.

Special thanks to Michael van Straten M.B.N.O.A. for much help and encouragement; to Paul Lee of the Platonic Academy of Santa Cruz, California, who suggested numbers of useful leads for me to follow, and whose own thinking on the subject of herbal medicine has influenced me considerably; to Dr. Percy Brown who gave me the benefit of his long observation of medicine in China today; to Lipmann Kessel, Professor of Orthopædics in the University of London, for helpful suggestions and comment; to Hein Zeylstra of the National

Institute of Medical Herbalists; to Dr. Malcolm Stuart of the Economic and Medicinal Plants Research Association; and to James Hewlett-Parsons of the General Council and Register of Consultant Herbalists.

I should like to thank Chief Big Eagle of Golden Hill Reservation, Trumbull, Connecticut, Mrs. Gladys Tantaquidgeon, Mrs. Nora Thompson and Mrs. Beryl Schwab for first-hand information on American Indian medicine; K. Mulder of Biohorma in the Netherlands, David Hampson of Messrs Potter's, and Martin Viner of Weleda (UK) Ltd, for information on modern marketing of plant medicine, Ian Thomas of Culpeper House who let me see cuttings, catalogues and papers on the history of his firm; Friedrich Pestalozzi of Bio-Strath A.G.; and John D. Hyde, F.N.I.M.H., who allowed me to study a modern herbal practice in action.

Among many others who responded to pleas for information, I should like to thank Professor I.I. Brekhman of the Department of Marine Biology, Vladivostock; Koert T. van der Plaats; Dr. Dimiter Pamukov; Miss Leverton of the Research Library, the Boots Company Ltd; Peter Alsted Pederson; Signor Paolo Morgante; Dr. Thomas Rey; Professor Jerzy Lutomski, Poznan; Dr. Feliks Kaczmarek; Oliver Gillie, Medical Correspondent of the *Sunday Times*; Muriel Hellings; and Barbara Rapoport.

I am grateful to Beata Duncan, my delightful and indefatigable researcher, whose digging in the field of Paracesus and the sixteenth-century chemical revolution in medicine was particularly fruitful; she also made many valuable criticisms and textual suggestions. Thank you to Caroline Hobhouse, whose firm editorial hand has guided this book from the initial idea to publication. And a very special thank-you to Mrs. Jean Wood, who removed all the cares of my household from my mind for crucial months at a time.

Finally, without the initial enthusiasm, and unceasing encouragement of my husband Henri van der Zee, I should never have had the courage to persevere in what has seemed at times an impossible task. He read through the text at all its various stages, and his many criticisms and suggestions have been invaluable. To him, and to our daughters Bibi and Ninka, my grateful thanks for their love, understanding and support.

May, 1981   BARBARA GRIGGS

1
The
Medicine of Mankind

In the grave of Neanderthal man, in a cave in Iraq, grains of flower pollens were found thickly scattered in the soil surrounding his bones. The family and friends of the dead man, it became clear, had surrounded his body with clusters of flowers and branches at his summer-time funeral. Analysed some 60,000 years after the death of this unknown caveman, the pollens were identified as coming from eight different genera of flowering plants, all of which flourish in the surrounding woods and fields at Shanidar to this day.

Of these eight species, seven are still used for medicine in dozens of different ways by the local people. For example, the mucilaginous roots of the marsh mallow from the *Althæa* genus yield a soothing and healing remedy for irritated throats and disordered intestinal tracts; the deep dark-blue-flowered grape hyacinth of the *Muscari* genus is valued as a diuretic; yarrow from the *Achillæa* genus is used as a general tonic – as well as an insect-repellent; and from the shrub *Ephedra* comes a potent remedy for asthma and a cardiac stimulant – a usage confirmed by modern science when the nerve-stimulant ephedrine was extracted from it.[1]

Such plants may have been chosen to grace this primitive burial because they were the brightest and most appealing in flower at the time – we have no right and no reason to assume that Neanderthal man was a dull insensitive brute. But since there is virtually no people known to anthropology – however remote, isolated or primitive – in which some form of doctoring with plants was not practised, we may also reasonably guess that these healing plants, which between them exert a beneficial effect on every important part of the body, may have been carefully chosen to fortify the dead man in his journey to another world.

Herbal medicine is the oldest form of therapy practised by mankind, and much of this medicinal use of plants seems to have been based on a highly-developed "dowsing" instinct, which led the healer of the tribe to the right plant and taught him or her its use. To a modern mind the idea may seem bizarre, but wild animals certainly possess such an instinct, seeking out plants which will supply the nutrients they need and unerringly avoiding those which will poison them.[2] These dowsing powers would explain the astonishing continuity of medicinal plant usage in the days before there were written records, or in tribes who have never known them, since the chain of oral tradition must have been broken over and over again by death, or by the scattering or obliteration of the tribe.

Without postulating such an instinct, moreover, how are we to account for the astonishing degree to which the same plant is employed for the same purpose in cultures so widely separated in place or time that there can have been no communication between them? As an example, a hot-water extract of the lovely *Hibiscus rosa-sinensis* has been used for menstrual problems and for fertility regulation among primitive peoples in places thousands of miles apart, in Fiji, Papua-New Guinea, Samoa, India, Indonesia, Kuwait, East New Britain, New Caledonia, Trinidad, and Vietnam.[3] Even a sceptic would have to concede that this was, at the very least, inspired guesswork: experiments with animals have shown that the plant-extract has marked anti-œstrogenic activity.[4]

And how long would it take modern scientists, working with the most sophisticated equipment, screening thousands of plants and sacrificing hecatombs of experimental animals, to stumble on the one plant which could provide a simple and effective form of birth-control, such as many tribes have been known to practise? In the Colombian jungle a white woman, Nicola Maxwell, who won the confidence of the Witoto tribe, was shown one plant which was administered to girls reaching puberty: a single dose, she was told, made them sterile for six to eight years. Another plant, they told her, worked as a morning-after abortifacient. And showing her a sedge-like weed, an old woman explained: "you take a teaspoonful just once of the root . . . Never get child again . . .".[5]

Explorers like Nicola Maxwell can tell us far more about primitive herbal medicine than anthropologists, since such medicine is still the only therapy known to countless remote tribes and peoples living in the jungle, forest, marshland, prairie, or desert. Practices may vary widely, but certain traits are common to almost all.

Almost every tribe has its priest or priestess, its medicine-man or woman who is the living repository of their medical knowledge. This knowledge is jealously guarded, often only handed on to a successor under the strictest oaths of secrecy, when death is felt to be near.* And although certain useful plants which gave remedies for everyday problems like wounds, digestive upsets, or mild fevers were common knowledge throughout the tribe, other plants were so highly valued, or so potent in their activity, that their use was restricted to the priest or healer alone.

Stress must have been as familiar to Neanderthal man, or to an Indian in the rain-forests of Brazil today, as to any Fifth Avenue executive, and the mental disorders to which it gave rise – hysteria, depression, paranoia – were equally the province of the medicine-man, to be treated not only with herbal decoctions, but by the primitive version of modern psychiatric treatment – chants, spells, loud rhythmical music, and incantations to drive away the evil spirits who might be causing the trouble. Plants with a narcotic or hallucinogenic action such as henbane (*Hyoscyamus niger*), may have been part of this therapy, used to induce states ranging from slight giddiness to frenzied convulsions, from hallucinations to mania, from a mild stupor to deep narcotic trance to death. They certainly played a role in the tribal religious rituals, and they may also have been the tools with which primitive man sought to experience another dimension to his mental and spiritual world. Probably, they were also used by primitive man as his "fix," to help him escape from the cares and responsibilities of everyday life – like the tobacco, alcohol, and other addictive drugs to which Western man turns today.

A pronounced gift for healing and a highly developed herb-"dowsing" instinct probably governed the tribe's choice of "medicine-man" for the most trusted and important function in their community. According to one African writer, the medicine-man was also expected to be "trustworthy, upright morally, friendly, willing

* This secrecy, incidentally, explains why Western observers have so often been disdainful about the medical knowledge of a native tribe. Its most important remedies were seldom revealed even to sympathetic and trusted observers, while the hostile and the sceptical often learned nothing of them at all.

and ready to serve, able to discern people's needs and not be exorbitant in their charges."[6] (This would have been a perfect description of the old-fashioned country doctor before the advent of the giant pharmaceutical companies and socialized medicine turned him into a harried and bureaucratized dispenser of pills).

As time passed, each tribe, each people and each growing civilization slowly built its herbal materia medica based on the local trees, shrubs, and flowering plants. Over the years there were certainly untold victims of this experimental plant therapy – the diagnosis was mistaken, the wrong plant was picked or the dose was excessive. It was not perhaps quite as hazardous as we might think, for those plants which can be fatal to man often flash built-in danger signals to the senses. Sometimes as with the tall feathery-leaved hemlock (*Conium maculatum*) they emit a fœtid, disagreeable smell – a smell that often becomes stronger when the plant is handled or bruised. Sometimes the smell alone is enough to induce giddiness or stupor, as with the leaves of the yellow-flowered henbane. Often the taste of these dangerous plants is so bitter and unpleasant that animals will not touch them – like the thorn-apple *Datura stramonium*. The fleshy branches of the violently irritant spurge (*Euphorbia resinifera*) leak a milky juice so acrid that it burns your fingers. Poison ivy (*Rhus toxicodendron*) can produce an instant tingling rash in the skin carelessly brushed against its leaves. And even if the berries of deadly nightshade (*Atropa belladonna*) are so tempting that countless children have died from eating them, the appearance of the plant itself is sinister in the extreme: lurking in dark sunless corners, it has dull deep green leaves, and produces a dingy purple flower before the shiny black berries are formed.

When these highly toxic plants were not used in psychotherapy or for religious rites, they served other useful purposes: smeared on the tips of spears, arrows and fish-hooks they made excellent hunting poisons, and were often the ordeal poisons of the tribe's judicial processes.

Much important information about medicinal plants was learned by observation. Tribesmen carefully noted which parts of the plant were the most active – leaf, root, flower, fruit or bark – and in which form it was most effectively administered – crushed and applied as salve or poultice, or steeped in cold water or fermented drinks or simmered in hot water to be swallowed. They learned, too, which season, what time of day, even which phase of the moon found the plant at its most active. And this knowledge, handed down through hundreds, perhaps thousands of years, eventually surfaced as part of the instructions in a medieval herbal: a plant was to be harvested at sunrise or dusk; in the new moon or when it was waning; at Lady Day (25 March – a feast that usefully marked early spring) or Michaelmas (late September).

Like everything else about traditional medicine, such observations attracted the merry scorn of modern doctors and pharmacists until, in one plant or another, it has been confirmed that the alkaloidal activity of a plant – which usually gives it its characteristic medicinal action – is often strongly influenced by the phases of the moon, and can vary not merely from season to season, but even between sun-up and sundown: findings which confirmed the accuracy of primitive practice much more often than not.

Many cultures have also believed in what has come to be known as The Doctrine of Signatures – the notion that plants have been signed by their Creator with visible clues to their usefulness: yellow plants would be effective against jaundice, plants with fruit shaped like genital organs might be effective in regulating or promoting fertility, a plant with fleshy lung-shaped leaves might be useful in respiratory ailments.

Traditional medicine was often unsuccessful. Often the cards were stacked against a tribe from the start. They had little idea how to cope with a disease carried by insects or parasites – like the malaria, schisto-somiasis, and sleeping-sickness which still ravage the Third World. In cases calling for major surgery, they were usually helpless. Their resistance to disease was often lowered by the innate hostility of their environment – jungle, desert or swampy marsh country – while their food supplies were threatened by warfare, drought, or flooding. Moreover, first contact with outsiders – settlers, explorers, mission-aries – often brought infectious diseases which were killers to a tribe with no inherited resistance to influenza or smallpox. But, generally speaking, traditional medicine was reasonably effective – much more so, quite often, than that of the "civilized" white man who sneered at it. Thanks to the imaginative lead given by the World Health Organ-ization from 1974 onwards, we are now, belatedly, beginning to recognize the fact.

As settlements grew into cities and civilizations developed, the professional doctor emerged, and among the earliest written records that survive are the drug inventories – the materia medica – prepared for his use.

Many of the drugs included in those lists came from animals, metals, or insects as well as plants, and have continued to figure in folklore, or to be used in domestic medicine – another source of amusement to those writing the history of medicine. They should learn respectful caution: a rationale for several of these "absurd" remedies has been uncovered by modern research. The species of cricket which is crushed and administered to T.B. sufferers according to Russian folk medicine was tested against the tubercle bacillus at the Pasteur Institute in Paris and found dramatically effective;[7] bee-stings, a notorious if not popular folk-cure for rheumatism, have been found to contain a substance christened Peptide 401, which proved one hundred times more effective than cortisone against rheumatism in animal trials;[8] mouldy bread often crops up in folk-medicine as a dressing for ulcers or dirty wounds, although penicillin extracted from just such mould is a fairly recent discovery; and the cutaneous glands of a toad have been revealed by the Chinese to contain cortisone.[9] In Russia today, a drug called pantocrine prepared from the boiled, ground and refined antlers of a species of deer is highly valued and widely prescribed as an all-purpose tonic, rather like ginseng.[10]

Hormones were only discovered and studied this century – but urine from a young man, or a pregnant woman, or a specified animal, has been used medicinally for this or that ailment for centuries – long before the U.S. drug company Ayerst began reaping millions of dollars annually from the sales of their Premarin, used in hormone replacement therapy and made from the urine of pregnant mares.

Pride of place in every materia medica, however, was occupied by the plant world, and in many cultures the only medicine known was almost exclusively herbal.

The *Pen Ts'ao* of a Chinese herbalist, Shen Nung, recorded in 2800 B.C., lists 366 plant drugs, including the little bare-branched shrub *Ephedra Sinica* found in a Neanderthal grave. In the eighteenth century B.C., King Hammurabi of Babylon established his own Public Records Office, with important information carved in stone tablets. Deciphered, they proved to contain many references to healing plants – including henbane, still used today as a sedative; the fragrant garden mint (*Mentha viridis*), highly esteemed as an appetite-stimulant and digestive for centuries; and *Glycyrrhiza glabra*, the shrub whose roots yield sweet soothing liquorice.

By 1500 B.C. there was already a brisk drug trade between the Mediterranean and the Levant: ancient temple carvings at Karnak in Egypt show medicinal plants being brought back from as far away as

Syria by a royal expedition. Moreover, the drug inventories of the three great civilizations of Mesopotamia, Egypt and India show such remarkable similarities that there was obviously a continual exchange of discovery and information among the professionals. Materia medica records of all three included mineral substances such as sulphur, antimony, iron and powdered precious stones; and all three used animal or human matter – hair, fat, blood, fæces, urine – not simply as external plasters but for consumption by their luckless patients. And from the Nile to the Ganges, the same herbs turned up over and over again in any physician's prescriptions.

Among these plant favourites were the handsome castor-oil tree (*Ricinus communis*) whose seeds yield that vile-tasting oil familiar to thousands of regularly-dosed Victorian children; linseed (*Linum usitatissimum*), the delicate blue-flowered plant from whose seeds comes a gentler oil used in poultices and cough medicines since time immemorial; and the white poppy (*Papaver somniferum*) that gave the world its most important hypnotic and sedative drug, opium.

Many of the herbs that we think of today as purely culinary were highly prized for their medicinal qualities as well: juniper (*Juniperus communis*), fennel (*Fœniculum vulgare*), saffron (*Crocus sativus*), and garlic (*Allium sativum*). *Cannabis sativa* – known today principally as an illicit pleasure, though increasingly used in cancer therapy to counter the side-effects of standard anti-cancer drugs – was already being used as a pain-killer and tranquillizer, and early surgical operations may have been carried out on patients anæsthetized with doses of hemlock.

As doctoring developed into a recognized profession, a subordinate commerce developed alongside it – that of the supply of the herbs, dried or fresh, essential to the busy physician. In no time at all, the trade had acquired professional overtones itself, and the public began to go to the traders direct for medicinal herbs to treat their minor ailments, or if they could not afford the doctor's fee.

In Ancient Greece, these herb-suppliers were known as *rhizotomoki* or root-gatherers, and it was probably for them, as much as for physicians, that the first careful lists of medicinal herbs and their properties – what we know as herbals – came to be written at a time when oral tradition was no longer relied on. The earliest of these was probably the *Rhizotomika* of Diocles of Carystius, a pupil of Aristotle. Written sometime in the fourth century B.C. it listed medicinal plants, and gave notes about their specific effects on various parts of the body.

In the first century B.C. there appeared another herbal, written by Cratæus, who was personal physician to Mithridates V1 Eupator, King of Pontus. It may have been written at the monarch's suggestion, as Mithridates was fond of dabbling in herbal medicine himself, and agrimony (*Agrimonia eupatoria*), one of the most popular herbs in Greek medicine, is believed to have been named in his honour. Only fragments of Cratæus' work survive, but according to Pliny it included an interesting innovation: "painted likenesses of plants" appeared above the descriptions of their virtues.

Illustrated or not, however, it seems clear that Cratæus' work was a fairly slight contribution to medical literature, at a time when almost every year that passed must have added new imported herbs or fresh uses for familiar native herbs to the general pharmacopœia. And in the first century A.D. an army surgeon set himself the gigantic task of bringing together all the current medical information on plants and other drugs and setting it down in one clear informative work. Pedanius Dioscorides came from Anazarba in Asia Minor, and had travelled widely in Asia Minor with the far-ranging Roman armies of Nero. He was a practising doctor, and he had a precise, enquiring mind. His work *Peri hulas iatrikes, About medicinal trees*, better known by its Latin name *De Materia Medica*, was instantly acclaimed, an authoritative reference work that has been copied and quoted to the present day, the prototype herbal and the prototype pharmacopœia.

Dioscorides prefaced his great work with an explanation of why he had written it: there was no definitive herbal in existence, and those in circulation contained not only omissions but astonishing errors. Accurate information on drugs was indispensable to any practitioner of the healing art, and as time went on, it was constantly being added to. Dioscorides intended to establish a solid foundation on which future experience and experiment could build.

While some animal or mineral substances are described in the work it was the section on plants, many of them unknown previously, that made Dioscorides a household name.

Each section began with a little drawing, and a lively description from which even someone without much botanical training could recognize the plant. This is how he describes the fennel flower (*Nigella sativa*): ". . . a little bush with a thin, light stem, of two spans or more in height, having small leaves like . . . groundsel but much finer, and . . . a delicate seed capsule on top, small like a poppy, longish, with partitions on the inside in which there is a black seed, bitter, fragrant . . .". There followed a detailed account of the plant's medicinal qualities, the different ways in which it was to be prepared, some suggestions perhaps as to dosage, and possibly a warning of its toxicity. "They say also that it is fatal if too much is drunk".[11]

Much of Dioscorides' information about foreign drug plants no doubt came from the surgeons of the much-travelled Roman armies: it is certain that they were among his most avid readers. The Romans looked after their armies well, especially when they were posted to distant countries. The legions travelled with their own doctors and surgeons, and when good local doctors could be found, they too were consulted and often enlisted: if doctors served the armies well, provincial governors were empowered to confer Roman citizenship on them as a reward.

The regular army doctors took supplies of the most important drugs with them, including exotics like opium and ginger that had to be imported from the East. A surviving army manual, written for the Emperor Claudius' expedition to Britain in A.D. 43 by one of his military surgeons, Scribonius Largus, gives numbers of prescriptions for remedies based on herbs that could be found all over Europe, together with directions on how to pack and transport their drug supplies.[12]

The Roman armies thus helped spread the knowledge of Mediterranean healing plants around Europe. In some cases, they spread the actual plants too, since they often took along seeds and fresh plants with them, to ensure regular supplies in new settlements. "In this way" says Whittle in his account of The Plant Hunters, "the Madonna Lily spread from Roman camp to Roman camp right through Europe – as a wound herb for the surgeons' use".[13] Rudimentary physic gardens often sprang up near Roman camps. No Roman quartermaster, for instance, could have envisaged any campaign without huge supplies of garlic for his men: not simply as a staple of their diet, as for any Campagna peasant, but for its marvellous medicinal virtues, useful for warding off infections, for coping with coughs, colds and lung diseases, and as a highly effective antiseptic dressing for wounds.

Other multi-purpose herbs spread throughout Europe by the legionaries may have included mustard (Sinapis nigra), which the Romans loved for reasons both gastronomic (they ate it pounded and steeped in new wine) and medical – they used it as a warming poultice in obstinate cases of pneumonia or bronchitis, as an emetic in cases of poisoning or upset stomach, and as a reliable aperient.

The occupational vice of the professional physician is the conviction that he knows everything – or nearly everything. This is easier to understand and forgive when you realize that if a doctor's patients do not have confidence in him, it will be much harder for him to treat them effectively: it is considered vital that they regard him as an infallible oracle who knows exactly what is wrong with them, and how it ought to be treated.

The other besetting sin of doctors is an undue attachment to everything they learned in medical school: the blind confidence of their patients is mirrored in their own uncritical acceptance of medical dogma. If what they learned in medical school was the importance of careful observation, of attention to their patient's diet and mental condition, of considering him as a whole individual, not simply a collection of symptoms, so much the better. But *ars longa, vita brevis* is an elegant way of saying that doctors are constantly being pressured into making snap diagnoses before they have had time to study their patients properly. So rules of thumb, rational explanations or indeed any theory that tends to simplify the problems facing a doctor are particularly likely to be revered and valued, and eventually enthroned as dogma.

Thus it happened that although today we consider Hippocrates (468–377 B.C.) as much the most important and interesting medical thinker of early times, with his emphasis on a balanced, wholistic approach to doctoring, it was not Hippocrates who was eventually enthroned as the patron saint of the medieval medical school. It was an emigré doctor named Galen (A.D. 131–200), a native of Pergamom in Asia Minor, who had travelled to Alexandria to study at the famous school of medicine there, and stayed on to practise.

He soon became well known as a surgeon to the gladiators, and on the strength of this reputation, went to Rome, where he established such a successful practice that when the post of court physician fell vacant, Galen's name was among those put forward. He was eventually appointed personal physician to the Emperor Marcus Aurelius (A.D. 121–180) whom he served till death, and he filled the same post for the succession of Imperial nonentities that followed, growing richer, grander and more sure of himself until his own death, full of honours, in A.D. 200.

Like the great medical traditions of Ancient China, India and Egypt, Hippocratic medicine had stressed the idea of balance – mental, emotional and physical – as essential to health: disease was a disturbance of this balance, which it was the duty of the physician to restore, assisted by the patient's own natural powers of recuperation. In Hippocratic teaching, the healthy body was one in which the four "humours" of blood, bile, phlegm and choler were equally balanced, and medical practice derived from this theory is known as humoral.

Four centuries later, Galen learned these ideas with enthusiasm. He adopted the Hippocratic teaching of the four humours and made it the corner-stone of an elaborate and rigid system of medicine, which effectively paralysed European medical thinking for the next 1500 years: for centuries the mere words "Galen says . . ." were enough to halt any daring attempts at medical free thinking. Not until William Harvey proved in 1628 that contrary to what Galen taught, the blood of a human being circulated constantly round his body, did Galen's great authority begin to crumble. By that time, physicians had become so used to having a solid bedrock of theory under their feet that they adopted, one after another, a series of "systems" in medicine which were often far more disastrous for their patients than conservative Galen ever had been.

On drug plants, as on other aspects of the healing art, Galen was authoritative. He brought system, rules, and a complete classification to the herbal materia medica, imposing his own rigid order on the untidy plant kingdom. In his massive *Peri krateos kai dunameos ton naplon pharmakon*, all drug plants were now evaluated in terms of their reaction with a patient's humours. Once the physician had diagnosed the particular humoral imbalance that was making his patient sick, he had only to prescribe the proper drug to counteract it, and he had dozens of plants to choose from, their virtue measured on a scale of four: "hot and moist in the first degree . . . cold and dry . . . cold in the third degree . . .". From Galen's painstaking classification comes the word "simple": to him it meant a herb possessing a single quality, such as heat or moisture. By extension, it came to mean one of the plant constituents in a complex prescription.

If Galen had lived and written a couple of centuries earlier, no doubt other great and more original medical thinkers would have arisen to dispute his elaborate theories, and dilute his authority. But the century that followed his death saw the first crumbling of that Roman order which had ruled the Mediterranean and Western Europe for so long. The Roman Empire first split itself into East and West, then divided itself again. Alaric leading his Goths finally appeared at the gates of Rome. And soon, in all Europe, there was nobody left to disagree with Galen.

The teachings of Galen marked the beginning of a sharp division in Western Europe between the professional physician on the one hand, and the traditional healer on the other. In professional medicine, careful observation of a plant's specific action disappeared, and was replaced by Galen's theoretical approach which assigned every plant to its proper station in an orderly scheme. The generations of doctors who memorized Galen's near-numerical classifications soon learned to despise those simple healers who still used marsh mallow (*Althæa officinalis*) for a severe case of diarrhœa because it was usually successful in such cases, without having the faintest idea whether it was hot or cold or what, or whether the patient suffered from an excess of phlegm or a deficiency of bile. Eventually, "specific" came to be a dirty word, meaning the plant that was administered in this uninstructed manner, rather than according to the professional rules.

Another great divide opened between the "amateur" healer – the village wise-woman, the tribal medicine-man, or the housewife – and the trained professional doctor. The "amateur" expected his plants to do their work gently and thoroughly, but not necessarily quickly: every countryman knows that you cannot hurry nature. The professional doctor, on the other hand, confident in his superior knowledge, was also confident that he could hurry nature as much as he wished to, with the most excellent results. Interventions in the bodily processes became the professional order of the day, as they have remained.

The most aggressive of these interventions were purging and blood-letting, and soon they became the most popular with physicians. The doctrine of the four humours provides an excellent rationale for both – as indeed, for any kind of "evacuation", in the form of urine, fæces, blood, vomit, or perspiration. Since time immemorial, purging their patients has been a favourite sport of doctors, for obvious reasons: it was sometimes effective therapy, and it was always brisk impressive medicine.* For centuries after Galen, two of the most popular purges were the various species of hellebore and the deadly hemlock.

Bloodletting seems to be almost as old as medicine itself. Primitive

---

* This was still true as recently as 1913, when the American John Uri Lloyd sent a list of the best-known cathartics then in current use to a representative number of American doctors, requesting that they cross off any that they felt could be safely dropped. To his astonishment, almost every doctor wrote back to say that far from being anxious to cross any one of them off the list, they did not feel that there were nearly enough reliable cathartics available, and would be happy to learn of more.[14]

people, seeing blood pour from a wound which later healed, and noting that blood flowed monthly from every woman without apparent injury to her health, may have reasoned that the release of blood had in itself some value, carrying off diseased or baneful matter, and although in some cultures it is viewed with the utmost horror, in others it was routinely practised.

From the time of Hippocrates, bloodletting slowly grew in importance in Western medicine, as the diseases in which it was thought useful multiplied. Since it is an effective – if risky – way of lowering the blood pressure sharply, bloodletting often brings immediate relief of pain in areas where tissue is badly inflamed, and there are still conditions in which it is thought useful, such as certain types of heart-failure.

In yet another direction, Galen's influence was to last for centuries: he favoured elaborate, costly medicines compounded of dozens of different ingredients, rather than simple infusions of two or three herbs. The most notorious example of these was Theriac, a complex antidote to all imaginable poisons and ills, invented a century before Galen, refined by him, and rechristened Galene in his honour. Into Galene went chunks of viper's flesh, dozens of different herbs, many of which were separately compounded beforehand, squills, certain mineral substances, wine, and honey. Galen insisted on the finest Falernian wine, the sweetest Hymettus honey, and had baskets of fresh herbs sent to him from all round the Mediterranean – crocus from Cilicia, dittany and scordium from Crete, bitumen from Judea, iris from Illyria, opium from Asia Minor. The pounding and stirring and mixing and brewing of this potent stuff went on for at least forty days, and the best Theriac continued to mature, like malt whisky, for at least a dozen years before it was thought to have reached its prime.[15]

With Galen's tremendous prestige behind it, Theriac in one form or another survived in European medicine almost as long as his reputation: the diarist John Evelyn watched it being publicly brewed with impressive ceremony in Venice during his visit in 1645. Following Galen, doctors came to feel that the more elaborate and complex a remedy, and the more ingredients piled into it, the better it was bound to be.

2

Medicine
in Transition

When the last Roman legions withdrew from Britain in A.D. 407, they left behind a frontier-town imitation of Roman culture – cities connected by an excellent network of ruler-straight roads, luxury villas, forums, public baths, at least the nucleus of a library here and there – and perhaps a handful of native healers to whom the names Hippocrates and Dioscorides were familiar. The villas eventually crumbled, the roads broke up, the towns fell into decay, and as the Angles, the Saxons and the Danes overran the country, the last vestiges of this Roman culture died out.

The plants that had emigrated to Britain in the Roman army baggage convoys flourished and spread, however, and some of the Mediterranean fund of knowledge of their particular healing powers must have lingered on as well, handed on from one generation to the next, jumping in a leisurely way from a small village to the next settlement over the downs, and perpetuating itself in a familiar nickname.

But long before the Romans came to Britain, traditional knowledge of the native healing plants was extensive. In Wales, medicine was a highly-regarded skill, considered by this small trading nation as one of the three civil arts, together with commerce and navigation. They may have learned something of Greek and Alexandrian medicine from the Phœnician merchants whose galleys toiled northwards to their ports from the Mediterranean. The traditions of their own priest-healers, however, were more venerable still, dating back to a thousand years before Christ.

The Druid priest-healers studied astrology and theology, and were adepts at divination, having a deep reverence for the moon which they believed had a powerful influence on both man and plant in her monthly cycle. They were also skilled in the use of medicinal herbs, and among these the mistletoe had a special place – the most sacred and magical of plants.

Alongside the priest-healers, an independent school of physicians with a rational rather than a priestly approach to their profession had developed at Myddfai by the sixth century A.D. The name of Hippocrates was familiar to them, his works were highly thought of among them, and his influence is obvious in their teaching.

Welsh influence is evident in Anglo-Saxon medicine. Some of the herbs used by the Druids, and at Myddfai, later came to be highly valued across the border in England. Among them was wood betony (*Stachys betonica*) prized by both Greeks and Romans as a panacea for all ills, particularly those of the head; feverwort, from the *Centaurea* genus which had once graced a Neanderthal burial, a small lilac-flowered roadside plant (*Erythræa centaurium*) thought useful in intermittent fevers, and an excellent tonic. Vervain (*Verbena officinalis*) was used to stimulate jaded appetites, though it is more familiar to us today as the distinctive taste in vermouth.

One way and another, it seems at least possible that Welsh practice may have influenced local medicine over the border in Anglo-Saxon times: is it coincidence that the mistletoe is particularly common in Hereford and Worcestershire, counties adjoining the Welsh border?

In A.D. 597 Christianity arrived in England, bringing with it the vigorous new traditions of monastic medicine – which over the next century were returned with interest to war-ravaged Europe by the Benedictine monks of England and Ireland. Throughout Europe in the Dark Ages, these monasteries maintained that network of communication without which medicine, like other civilized arts, can neither thrive nor develop. They wrote to each other, to Rome, to Jerusalem; some of the monks were enthusiastic travellers and most received a steady stream of visitors, among them educated and informed men able to keep up to date on the latest developments in theology, science, and medicine. Few of the major Greek and Roman medical texts were available in their entirety, circulating in the form of scrappy abridgements and compilations, but the monasteries made the best of that little, which they borrowed, annotated, copied out, and passed on. The demand always outran the supply: Boniface received letters from England asking him to send them more books on simples.

There was nothing academic about the monastic desire for more medical information. Benedict had laid down in the early sixth century

A.D. that it was the duty of monks to care for the sick, and to do so as skilfully and intelligently as possible. Cassiodorus (487–583) urged the same responsibility on his monks: ". . . study with care the nature of herbs and the compoundings of drugs. If you have no knowledge of Greek, you have at hand the *Herbarium* of Dioscorides, who fully described the flowers of the fields and illustrated them with drawings. After that read Hippocrates and Galen . . . and other books dealing with the art of medicine, all of which I have left you on the shelves of the library . . .".

As well as their own sick, the monks looked after the poor who came to their gates, the local people who had no other doctor, and passing strangers. Every monastery had its own physic garden, in which the common and most often needed medicinal herbs were grown.

These doctoring monks were, in a sense, amateurs. Working for love not money, they felt no need either to impress their patients or try and attract new ones; they simply dealt as best they knew how with the patients who came their way. But over the years of study and clinical experience, some of them developed considerable skill. Eventually, they were not only training the next generation of monks to take over in the Infirmary; they were also taking in pupils from outside the monasteries and turning them into a new class of professional practitioner. Until the first universities were established in the eleventh and twelfth centuries, there was no other training for the physician.

This development was actively encouraged by King Alfred (870–899). In the fourteen peaceful years that remained of his reign, after he broke the invading Danes, and drove them out of England, Alfred dedicated himself to the task of creating a civilized nation, importing scholars and establishing schools and monasteries. Like every educated layman of his time, he had a keen amateur interest in medicine, corresponding with the Patriarch of Jerusalem about prescriptions and new developments in drug therapy, and sending abroad for supplies of exotic drugs that could not be procured in England. He was anxious that his people should have the best possible medical care, and he arranged for some of the more important medical texts to be translated into English, so that they should have a wider circulation.

This was unusual: no other country in Europe at this time was bothering to turn standard works, like the fifth-century *Herbarium* of Apuleius Platonicus, into the vernacular, since monks were bound to be fluent in Latin, and it was generally assumed that medical practitioners would be equally so. The fact that numbers of these translations were produced in England over the next decades up to the conquest – no less than four different manuscripts of Apuleius have survived, for instance – suggests that there was a much wider demand there than on the Continent, possibly from mistresses of households, whose Latin was likely to be shaky, as well as from the leeches – as doctors were called – themselves.

Certainly the interest was greater: the Anglo-Saxons seem to have been far more knowledgeable about medicinal plants than anyone on the Continent. The popular *Herbarium* of Apuleius Platonicus, padded with borrowings from Dioscorides and Pliny, mentions fewer than 200 plants, but it has been computed that the English had names and uses for perhaps 500 different plants.[2]

Medically, England may have been ahead of the Continent. The earliest surviving Anglo-Saxon medical text, the *Leech Book of Bald*, written in the early tenth century, is a compilation from some of the best Greek and Roman medical literature available in Europe at the time, and a careful reading makes it plain that even by modern standards Bald – and the colleagues Dun and Oxa that he mentions – must have been excellent doctors.

In the best Greek – or monastic – tradition, Bald had a kindly, thoughtful approach to his patients that makes pleasant reading. If the sick man was to be let blood, he must be taken to a warm place first, and the doctor must be very careful not to overdo it; ". . . if thou lettest him too much blood, there will be no hope of his life".[3] The patient's diet must be carefully supervised: in a case of "sore side" it must be light but tempting and nourishing: "light meats and juicy broths, and juicy peas, and beaten eggs, and bread broken in hot water".[4]

The doctor or leech, according to Bald, must be a carefully trained observer: the symptoms of an acute chest infection are meticulously and vividly detailed. "There is also cold all through their fingers and powerlessness of their knees, their eyes are red, and red is their hue, and their discharge is foamy . . . the breathing is sorelike, the face twitched, and there is a dewy wetting of the breast, as if it sweated, a delirium of the mind . . .".[5]

There were also remedies for more trivial ailments, such as loss of appetite, sleeplessness, fatigue, a hangover – cases for the family medicine-chest rather than the doctor, suggesting that Bald was writing for a wide audience. Throughout, the remedies prescribed were largely herbal, and it is clear that Bald and his colleagues knew their physic gardens well enough to make the best possible therapeutic use of them. It was probably another leech who translated the *Herbarium* of Apuleius into English in the next century: when he came to the section on herbs, he felt confident enough to make several additions of his own to the text.

If Bald's patients were quite skilfully cared for by the standards of the time, those of the physicians of Myddfai were better off still – a trained Myddfai doctor would have an extremely prosperous "alternative" practice today. For over a thousand years, until the eighteenth century, an unbroken tradition of skilled doctoring was handed down in one Myddfai family, who served as personal physicians to the Princes of South Wales. At the beginning of the thirteenth century Thys Gryg – a sensible man – urged them to write it all down – "as a record of their skill, lest no one should be found with the requisite knowledge as they were" and thus we can study it in detail today.[6]

The medicine they practised must have been the best of its time in Europe: rational, humane, and Hippocratic in its emphasis on the patient's own responsibility for his health. They quoted with approval the classic philosophers: "whosoever shall eat or drink more or less than he should, or shall sleep more or less, or shall labour more or less from idleness or from hardship (being obliged to over exert himself), or who, used to being bled, refrains from doing so, without doubt he will not escape sickness . . .".[7]

The Myddfai physicians were holistic in their approach, looking for the causes of a disease as well as attempting to alleviate its local symptoms. For scrofula and other eruptive skin troubles, for instance, they prescribed a strong infusion of clivers (*Galium aparine*) – a little sticky-hooked hedge-plant – explaining that this was to dispel the "eruptive poison" from the blood which had caused the disorder in the first place.[8] Clivers is still used as a powerful diuretic in herbal medicine today, and for centuries it was one of the ingredients in rural "spring drinks" – those green brews with which country people, instinctively dosing themselves with vitamin C, drank away a lingering winter tendency to scurvy.

Myddfai use of medicinal herbs was obviously based on repeated observation in practice. They specified parts of the herb and quantity where they felt this was necessary, and were fussy about the cleanliness of the water used in their preparation.

Like the Anglo-Saxon leeches, the Myddfai physicians used herbs in plain country style, brewed up in infusions, or crushed and mixed with lard to make a poultice. As peasants do, they used them singly, although occasionally they combined one with two or three others. Although they drew on what has been estimated as a range of 175 herbs, and must have needed specially cultivated supplies, the ones they used most often were the simples which grew freely in the countryside, or could be cultivated with ease in a peasant's plot: garlic, pounded and boiled in milk, or eaten freely for a troublesome cough – a remedy found the world over; elecampane (*Inula helenium*), bruised with mallow in honey for suspected consumption*; lily roots pounded with egg-white to dress a burn; an infusion of white horehound (*Marrubium vulgare*) to be drunk warmed and sweetened with honey for a case of pneumonia.[9]

Here, brilliantly studied and used by experts, was the traditional green pharmacy of the peasant, part of that "vast lore of self-medication" without which, as Eric Maple eloquently reminds us, "they, the toilers, and the society which rested upon their backs, could never have survived".[10]

Hundreds of miles away from Myddfai, in the small Southern Italian town of Salerno, the works of Hippocrates were also studied and honoured. Here in the tenth century a guild of physicians had been established, and a Medical School founded to which students as well as patients flocked. Over the next centuries, the name Salerno became familiar throughout Europe as the origin of a charming and sensible manual of preventive medicine and hygiene, set out in verse: this *Regimen Sanitatis* is pure Hippocrates, preaching moderation in diet, sufficient sleep, the importance of fresh air and exercise. Highly popular, it circulated in dozens of manuscript copies, and once printing was invented, it appeared in over 300 different editions, in every European language. The first physician of Myddfai might have written it: the later ones may have drawn on it.

Myddfai and Salerno between them offered the best professional health-care available in early medieval Europe – holistic, sensible, humane, demanding high standards of professional concern and attention. Centuries would pass before anyone improved on it.

---

* In 1885 it was shown that the active, bitter principle of elecampane is such a powerful antiseptic and bactericide that a few drops of a solution of 1 part in 10000 immediately kills ordinary bacterial organisms, and is particularly destructive to the tubercle bacillus.

But for the physicians and students of Salerno, it soon came to seem merely a beginning. Salerno was the bridgehead of Arab culture in Southern Europe, and it was to the Arabs that everyone who was interested in the future of medicine looked.

When in the seventh century A.D. the Arabs overran North Africa and asserted Muslim supremacy over the Mediterranean world, a treasury of Greek and Roman medical texts, many of them unstudied in Europe, fell into Arab hands, and were collected and stored in "The House of Wisdom" in Baghdad. Under the Abbasid Caliphs in the ninth century A.D. the major works of Dioscorides, Galen, and Hippocrates, among others, were all translated into Arabic by Hunayn bin Ishaw al-Ibadi (809–873), and the Arab mind – alert, inquisitive, receptive – came to grips with the best of Græco-Roman medicine.

The Arabs had until this time produced few great doctors, but from the late ninth century, fertilized by this explosive cultural encounter, Arab medicine knew a long and brilliant flowering, producing physicians like Mesue, Rhazes and Avicenna who would leave their mark on the history of medicine.

At first, it was the writings of the Hippocratic school which had the greatest impact on the Muslim mind, and in the first decades of its development, this was the foundation upon which Arab medicine was raised. The Arabs set up marvellous teaching hospitals, devoted considerable thought and attention to environmental factors in illness, and concentrated on what today we call "clinical medicine" – the investigation of disease at the sickbed rather than in the lecture hall. Studies in Public Health and preventive medicine were eagerly pursued. Rhazes – as the West came to know Ar-Razi (865–925) – emphasized the importance of diet and hygiene rather than over-drugging: "where a cure can be obtained by diet," he said, "use no drugs, and avoid complex remedies where simple ones will suffice". In the following century Ibn Butlan (died 1068), wrote a treatise on the preservation and restoration of good health, the *Taquim as-Sihhah* in which he preached the importance of clean air, moderate diet, rest and work, the evacuation of superfluities, and emotional states. If all these were kept in balance, he maintained, health resulted: when they were out of harmony, sickness occurred.

But after this promising start, it was Galen and not Hippocrates who in the end prevailed. The Arab physician whose influence on the course of Western medicine was to be decisive – Ibn Said, known in the West as Avicenna (980–1037) – was himself a devoted disciple of the prodigy from Pergamom.

A phenomenally gifted youth, who had memorized the whole of the Koran by the age of ten, Avicenna was already a well-known, successful and highly respected practitioner in the city of Baghdad by the time he was seventeen years old. As well as remarkable mental powers, however, Avicenna – like Galen – gave evidence of a certain inflexibility of mind, and a passion for order and system, for facts tidily arranged and phenomena neatly classified. He took over where Galen left off. His great million-word *As-Qanum*, the *Canon of Medicine*, has been described by a modern historian as "the final codification of Græco-Arabic medicine, so closely interwoven than no single item could be subtracted without damaging the whole. . . . To contemporary medical science it gave the appearance of almost mathematical accuracy, and this it was that made the medieval world regard the *Canon* as an oracle from which it was impossible to dissent. . . ."[12]

The Arabs were experts in astrology, which they had developed to a precise science, and they believed firmly in the influence of the stars on human health and destiny. Avicenna explained how a knowledge of astrology was essential to the doctor, since both the patient and the medicinal plant which might be prescribed for him were subject to astrological influences. But it was in the field of materia medica that the Arab contribution was most striking.

The Muslim faith taught that God in his wisdom has provided medicines for all man's ailments, to be drawn from natural sources wherever they were needed. This belief encouraged active investigation of drug plants, and the Arabs threw themselves into the work with enthusiasm, using Dioscorides and his methodical approach as their model, and adding to their materia medica hundreds of medicinal plants already known in pre-Islamic Arabia, or imported from Persia, India and the Far East along the great trade routes.

The action of these medicinal plants was carefully studied, often by cautious experimentation on human beings, and the resulting observations on potency, dosage and possible toxicity recorded in collections of case-histories that were studied in medical schools.

By A.D. 800, pharmacy – the preparation of drugs – was already a separate and independent profession among the Muslims, practised by carefully-trained specialists. According to a modern historian, "the first privately-owned and managed pharmacy shops were opened in the early ninth century in Baghdad, the Abbasid capital, where drugs and spices from Asia and Africa were readily available and where the proximity of military installations increased the need for medications. Within a short period of time, pharmacy shops sprang up in other large cities of the Islamic world".[13]

For centuries Europe remained ignorant of these developments in medical science; but from the tenth century the teachings of Hippo-crates, as developed by earlier Arab physicians such as Rhazes, began to filter slowly north by way of the school at Salerno. By the twelfth century, Salerno was considered the leading medical school of Europe, and this reputation was more than earned when Constantine the African (died 1087) arrived there in the mid-eleventh century, and performed for Europe the vital service that Hunayn-al-Ibadi had rendered the Arabs: the translation of key medical texts. For the first time the West had available to it in Latin the early Greek works in their entirety, instead of isolated fragments, as well as the exciting new contribution of the Arabs.

The Europe that began to absorb this treasure of learning in the twelfth century was more than ready for intellectual expansion. For the first time in centuries, there was something like peace and order. Trade was bringing prosperity and leisure to the cities, and the first universities were taking shape. In the wake of the Crusades and their land-grabbing entrepreneurs, lines of communication were opening with the whole Arab world and its culture. The age of the Norman robber barons was also the age of Abelard, Thomas Aquinas and Albertus Magnus, and the scholars of this first Renaissance redis-covered Græco-Roman learning preserved and enriched by centuries of Arab thinking.

"An implicit faith in the opinions of teachers, an attachment to systems and established forms. . . will always operate upon those who follow Medicine as a trade. . . ." observed Dr William Buchan in the late eighteenth century.[14] This was not less true of the medieval European physician, and although Hippocrates and Rhazes were attentively studied, the best-known and most highly-respected name at European universities was soon to be that of Avicenna, whose passion for order and system struck a responsive chord in the dog-matic and authoritarian medieval mind.

Through Avicenna, Galen was confirmed as the supreme authority. And it was Galen and Avicenna who, between them, produced the typical university-trained medieval physician, armed with his astro-logical ready-reckoner and his chart of the twenty-four different ail-ments that the hue of a patient's urine might indicate. (Appropriately, this highly-theoretical physician came to be known as a "mouthing-doctor", as distinct from the surgeon who was known as a "wound-doctor".)

Salerno, with its fresh introduction of the Hippocratic tradition, might have brought about a revolution in Western medicine. As it happened, however, by far the most significant contribution made by the Arabs was in the field of materia medica, because it was in the profitable making-up and compounding of medicines that they had come to excel. They evolved numbers of new presentations – ointments and electuaries, conserves, elixirs, pills, confections, tinctures, suppositories and inhalations – instructions for preparing which were carefully detailed in a number of special formularies.

Soon Arab pharmacy was having an enormous influence on the prescribing habits of Europe's physicians – and on the commercial prospects of its apothecaries. Some of the Arabs' drugs and formulae were taken back to Europe by the wound-surgeons who picked up a smattering of Arab medicine while on active service with the Crusades. Many more were soon filtering steadily north through Salerno: compilations like the *Antidotarium Magnum* of Nicolaus of Byzantium, full of directions for preparing the elaborate, often heavily-sweetened or spiced compounds dear to the Arab taste, were pillaged by European doctors and apothecaries for striking new medicines, and became standard throughout Europe.

Dozens of new drugs were introduced into Western practice by the Arabs, among them many that today we consider mainly as spices for cookery – nutmeg (*Myristica fragrans*), cloves (*Eugenia caryophyllata*), and saffron (*Crocus sativus*) – although they were all used medicinally at the time.

Foremost among the exotic newcomers were the purges, the cathartics and the laxatives so essential to medieval medicine, with its emphasis on the evacuation of excess humours. The most popular of these – an enduring favourite to this day – was senna (*Cassia acutifolia*). The senna plant is a low bush with small yellow flowers, greenish-yellow leaves and fat seed-pods. The leaves have an odd distinctive smell, and the infusion made from them has a particularly nauseating sweetish taste, which does in fact induce nausea when drunk on its own. The Arabs corrected both taste and effect by adding aromatic spices. Manna (*Fraxinus ornus*) and tamarind (*Tamarindus indicus*) were also introduced by the Arabs – safe, mild and reliable laxatives. Rather brisker in its section was rhubarb (*Rheum palmatum*) from Turkey which was particularly effective in cases of diarrhœa. Brisker still was Scammony (*Convolvulus scammonia*) already well-known in medieval Europe and the subject of heated debate, some physicians maintaining that its action was so violently irritant that it should never be used, others that they could not possibly do without such a marvellous purge. The Arab pharmacists, with their usual confidence, had come up with a reliable preparation which tempered some of the drug's ferocity; picking up a tip from Galen, they advised boiling it in a quince: the scammony was then thrown away, and the quince pulp mixed with the soothing, mucilaginous seeds of psyllium (*Plantago psyllium*). This preparation was known as Diagridium.

In addition to numbers of elaborate herbal compounds, the medieval pharmacopœia was stuffed with animal and mineral substances, some of them drawn from European traditions of folk-medicine, others borrowed from Egyptian and Babylonian medicine, and imported into European practice by Arabs. Among the ingredients an apothecary might be called on to provide at a moment's notice were viper's flesh, crushed deer antlers, crab's eyes, rhinoceros and unicorn horn, oil of earthworms, scorpions and swallows, powdered mummy, the moss from a dead man's skull, urine from a goat, a wild boar or a boy, and the much-prized bezoar stone, which was actually the curious concretion found in the gut of the wild Persian goat.

Some of these, as we have seen, had a distinctive therapeutic action, though it may be doubted whether the medieval physician knew enough to employ this successfully. But they were highly impressive to the medieval patient, Latin names and all, and since medicine – even a completely inert substance – will cure at least some patients of their disease,* they must have been effective sometimes.

They were certainly effective at enriching the European apothecaries, who from the twelfth century on were fast developing an independent profession. Their enthusiasm for such elaborate and

* This curious phenomenon, known as the *placebo* effect, was for years thought to be the result of simple auto-suggestion: the patient had faith in the drug, so he got better. Since it confused the result of straight clinical trials of new drugs, the double-blind trial was invented to circumvent it, in which some patients got the new drug, and others a *placebo* or dummy, and nobody, not even doctors and nurses, knew which was which till afterwards. It is now thought that the *placebo* effect may be the physiological action of mysterious substances called endorphins, whose release is triggered by the brain; methods to harness this useful action are being investigated. Professor Lipmann Kessel has another theory: the *placebo* effect simply mirrors the fact that many diseases go away of their own accord.

exotic animal, vegetable, and mineral medicines was understandable. They certainly could not have made the barest living by selling the simples that grew in their customers' gardens or flourished in the nearest patch of waste land. (When relations between the physicians and the pharmacists grew particularly acrimonious in France in the sixteenth century, the physicians craftily took to prescribing simples: the apothecaries climbed down almost immediately.)

The enthusiasm of the physicians was equally understandable. Doctors have always been anxious to convince the public that medicine, in any of its aspects, is far too complex and perilous a matter to be meddled with by laymen. The fourteenth-century university graduate certainly had not spent years mastering the complexities of Galen and Avicenna in order to prescribe a handful of betony, an infusion of horehound or some such wayside simple which any village wise-woman could brew up into a useful remedy. His patients expected more of him, and were happy to pay for it.

Thus it happened that the study of medicinal plants – the raw material of so much medicine – continued to languish in European professional circles, and the Arab work on medicinal plants which became most enduringly popular in Europe was that of Serapio, written around the eleventh century. What probably recommended it to the medieval reader was the thoroughness with which Serapio sorted and classified the hundreds of new plants the Arabs had introduced into the West, into recognizable Galenic categories: ". . . those that are hot and drie in the first degree; then those cold and drie in the same degree: after that, those hot and dry in the second degree, and . . .".[15] This was the kind of information about medicinal plants which Western doctors found genuinely useful and interesting.

It might have been thought that the confidence of the medieval doctor in this theoretical medicine would have suffered a crippling blow from the Black Death, which fell upon an unsuspecting Europe in 1348 and slew within months an estimated third of its population. The most gifted and highly-trained physician found himself as completely at a loss before this sudden and terrible visitation as the most unlettered peasant healer. Every therapy known to contemporary medicine was tried: flight or seclusion proved much the most useful, as Pope Clement VI found – on the advice of his surgeon, Gui de Chauliac, he spent the duration of the epidemic sweltering between two vast fires in his chambers in the Papal palace at Avignon. Other preventive measures against the plague included regular purging and bleeding, bland diet, careful personal hygiene, the burning of aromatic substances to destroy "the corruption of the air," and the consumption of herbs known to be useful in infection, such as rue or garlic, as well as expensive compounds like theriac. For treatment there was more bleeding, more purging, and even costlier potions containing ingredients like powdered pearls and ground emeralds, while the agonizing buboes or plague-sores might be lanced or treated with hot poultices.

But the very dreadfulness of the Black Death removed it, in the eyes of the medical profession, from the number of those ailments against which they might reasonably be expected to be effective: a visitation so uniquely terrible, which, in the words of Boccaccio "seemed to set at naught both the art of the physician and the virtue of physic"[16] could only be an incomprehensible act of God, preordained and written since time immemorial in the stars. When the learned physicians of the Medical Faculty in Paris looked for astrological confirmation of this theory, they found it: "On 20 March 1345, at 1 p.m., there occurred a conjunction of Saturn, Jupiter and Mars in the house of Aquarius. The conjunction of Saturn and Jupiter notoriously caused death and disaster while the conjunction of Mars and Jupiter spread pestilence in the air: Jupiter, being warm and humid, was calculated to draw up evil vapours from the earth and water, which Mars, hot and dry, then kindled into infective fire. Obviously, the conjunction of all three planets could only mean an epidemic of cataclysmic scale".[17]

In the lay mind, on the other hand, the Black Death must have confirmed a suspicion that in diseases which were not quite so direct a manifestation of divine displeasure, self-help might be almost as effective as the professional kind. Continuing the earlier traditions inspired by King Alfred, herbals were already having a steady circulation in manuscript form, many of them perhaps going into wealthy households where the lady of the manor was already being relied on to provide simple first aid and doctoring for her family and the village poor.

An astonishing number survive in England alone: they were treasured, much-copied, often handed down over more than a century to have later additions scribbled in their margins. In one thirteenth-century version of the ever-popular Apuleius preserved in the Bodleian Library at Oxford, a later hand has added the names of the herbs in English. In a fourteenth-century manuscript thought to have belonged to the Countess of Hainault, sixty-eight fine pen-and-ink drawings of English wild plants have been added. English equivalents and notes were often pencilled in the margins – and some herbals even had special spaces left for their owners to write notes in, rather like the blank pages left in a modern cookery book for the reader's favourite recipes.

Certainly these herbals can never have been cheap: "This is John Rice is boke, the which cost him xxv d" runs a note on the second page of a fifteenth-century herbal: at the time it was written, a country parson with an annual income of £10 was considered well off, and in those days there were 240 pence to the pound. Equally certainly, the demand far outstripped the supply. Beyond the doctor and the apothecary, there was a wide general public, eager and anxious for more information about their native medicinal plants.

3
The New Disease and the New Medicine

A century and a half – almost to the year – after the Black Death had devastated Europe, another dreadful disease – syphilis – made a sudden appearance and spread with appalling speed. Like the Black Death, syphilis made its entry through an Italian port; like the Black Death, it was thought to be due to a fatal conjunction of three planets, two years earlier; like the Black Death, it was seen as a punishment sent by God for human wickedness. And like the Black Death, it found physicians helpless before its inexorable progress.

At first, everybody called syphilis the *Morbus Gallicus* – the French Disease – since it was the soldiers of the French King Charles VII who had unwittingly carried it back into Europe in 1496, after the siege of Naples. It was equally certain that they had picked it up there from the town prostitutes, who in turn had caught it from the sailors, and in particular those of Christopher Columbus, newly returned from the West Indies. Although it was generally assumed to be a brand-new disease, whether it actually was or not was a bone of contention to doctors at the time, and has been a favourite puzzle to medical historians ever since.

To its victims, of course, the question of whether or not it was a "new" disease must have been academic, to put it mildly. For on one thing everybody was agreed: no more virulent and painful form of syphilis has ever been seen.

Syphilis is a contagious venereal disease caused – though centuries would elapse before this was known – by a microbe known as a spirochæte because of its odd corkscrew shape. The first symptom is a small hard swelling, near the point of infection, that may break out into an ulcer: this usually disappears even without treatment. Weeks, even months later, the disease flares up again as the spirochætes multiply throughout the bloodstream, causing a variety of symptoms that may range from mild rash to sores on the genital organs, and racking pains in the bones and joints. This stage, too, often clears up of its own accord, but the truce is temporary: months, sometimes years, later, the disease again emerges, to attack its victim with renewed fury, manifesting itself in a dozen different forms, striking at heart or brain or nervous system, to cause paralysis or dementia and finally death.

Even today, when penicillin is an effective cure, nobody could learn without horror that they had contracted syphilis, and the desperation that its fifteenth-century victims must have felt is painful to imagine. Their physical sufferings were bad enough – contemporary writers speak of disfiguring ulcers that ate away the flesh to the bone, and gave off a dreadful stench – but the disease ate into the heart of the family and threatened dynasties too. Men who thought they were cured often continued to transmit the disease to wives or mistresses, babies were born deformed or congenitally idiot, and passed on the infection to their wet-nurses – who carried it off to other luckless homes. The highest families in the land were no more immune to it than the common soldier's sweetheart, and soon noblemen, kings, even popes were begging their doctors to do something. Anything.

It was an urgent medical problem and a considerable puzzle for the physicians, who could find nothing about it in Galen, or any of the great medical authorities on whom they relied. Many of them refused to handle cases at all, either because the disease was morally objectionable, or because the ulcers suggested it was a case for the surgeons. But it must have been hard for them to resist the desperate appeals of their patients, many of whom, like the great Borgia family, were both wealthy and important: "In Rome this kind of illness is very partial to the priests, and especially to the richest of them," wrote Benvenuto Cellini drily.

Initially, physicians began by treating their patients along classic, humoral lines. If possible, they isolated them from their families – sensibly – by sending them away to a dry, sunny climate. Lots of strenuous exercise, a bland diet, frequent bleeding, and repeated and thorough purging were among the measures to which they resorted. Patients were filled with expensive decoctions of aromatics and bitter herbs. And for the ulcers, physicians prescribed soothing ointments made of goose grease, mastic (*Pistacia lentiscus*) – an aromatic gum – linseed, honey, and the roots of daffodils (*Narcissus pseudo-narcissus*) – a plant under the dominion of Mars, appropriately, and thought by Galen to be a particularly good astringent.

Some patients may have been cured of mild cases by such treatments, others were delighted to find all their symptoms disappearing – only to have a relapse later. Even today, with modern methods of diagnosis, syphilis in its unpredictable course, and in its numberless forms, can baffle the most experienced doctor. To the medieval doctor and his patients, it was a nightmare, since nobody could be sure which, if any, treatment worked; whether a patient was truly cured or not; or even if he actually had the disease. Many patients must have endured long courses of tedious treatment by their physician, only to find at the end that the loathsome disease was with them still.

Unlike the Black Death, however, syphilis gave both sufferers and physicians plenty of time to experiment with different treatments, and it soon became clear that the surgeons, alone, were having some success. They were using unguents containing mercury – a remedy they had learned from the Arabs, who had developed it themselves in the course of their alchemical experiments.

Alchemy, that strange cross between philosophy and chemistry, "swept like a fever over thirteenth-century Europe" as Sherwood Taylor writes, "and it remained for at least three centuries the chief preoccupation of those inclined to the discovery of nature's secrets."[1] The goal of the alchemist was to penetrate the very deepest of nature's secrets, and of the universe itself, and so attain perfection, although the means by which this was to be achieved were shrouded in the most impenetrable secrecy – part of alchemy's great fascination.

But it was not simply another philosophy, and if the goal of the alchemist was spiritual, his tools were chemical. The secrets of nature could be probed in a laboratory; wisdom might be hidden in a metal, philosophy literally locked inside a stone. This philosopher's stone could even transmute a common metal into gold – a sensational notion that summed up alchemy for the man in the street, although true believers knew that only fools and charlatans would put it to such low use.

The Arabs, from whom Europe absorbed this heady new science, were expert alchemists, and as a result had developed chemical techniques far in advance of anything known at the time in Europe. Many of their leading physicians, Rhazes and Avicenna among them, were also alchemists – a combination which became quite common in Europe too – and had worked with some of the minerals used in medicine to see if they could achieve better compounds or more easily assimilated forms.

Mercury, or quicksilver, was an obvious choice for experiment. In the alchemical order of things, mercury occupied a special place, much the most suggestive and mysterious of all metals. This strange ever-moving substance, silvery to the eye, eerily responsive to changes in temperature, simultaneously light and heavy, was identified by the alchemist with the planet Mercury, the god Hermes, the soul itself. In Hindu the very word for alchemy – *rasassiddhi* – means knowledge-of-mercury.

As early as Roman times, quicksilver was known to be poisonous. The Romans had banned its mining in Italy on environmental grounds, because it not only destroyed fields, vineyards, and olive-groves, but also polluted streams and killed the fishes in them. (They thus anticipated the modern tragedy of Minamata in the early 1950s, when hundreds of Japanese died or were ruined in health for life after eating fish caught in waters into which mercurial industrial waste had been discharged.) Dioscorides described the unpleasant consequences of swallowing the metal or inhaling its vapours, and Galen thought it so poisonous it should never be used in medicine.

But some of the most potent plant poisons known to man also yielded some of his most effective remedies when cautiously administered and properly prepared: scammony and henbane, for example. If this were equally true of minerals, reasoned the Arabs, mercury was worth investigating. So Rhazes – in one of the earliest recorded animal trials of a drug – fed neat quicksilver to an ape, observed that the ape seemed none the worse for it, and concluded that taken in this form at least, mercury seemed to be free from side-effects. One day he heated a mixture of mercury, vitriol and salt, generating hydrochloric acid which reacted with the mercury to form mercuric chloride which sublimed to yield a substance which was first called sublimate. At some moment, some luckless Arab patient (or possibly another ape) must have had this interesting new compound tried on him: he suffered agonising stomach cramps, bloody diarrhœa and suppression of urine . . . and the compound was rechristened corrosive sublimate.

Undeterred, the Arabs continued to experiment with mercury, tried it in various combinations, and came to the conclusion that it could be quite useful in certain obstinate skin diseases. By the eleventh century quicksilver was being regularly used by Salerno physicians for such treatment this way, beaten into an ointment and applied locally to the skin.

They also found it extremely effective for getting rid of scabies, lice, and the itch, those irritating little consequences of the cramped and unhygienic conditions in which medieval Europeans lived; the thirteenth-century physician John of St. Amand, in his *Areola* or compendium of currently popular drugs, mentions several prescriptions of this kind. Used in very small quantities, combined with other medicines, he thought mercury could be quite harmless. He warned, though, that caution was necessary in its use, since merely inhaling its vapours could bring on bad breath, tremors, paralysis, and the loss of both sight and hearing.

Soon the surgeons – the chief users of mercury, since they dealt with sores, ulcers and other skin-diseases – began to notice something else about it: even when it was only applied externally, in an ointment, and there was no risk of the patient inhaling its vapours, it could have some disconcerting side-effects. Gui de Chauliac (died 1368) a particularly careful and observant surgeon, warned that it could be injurious to the mucous membranes, the gums and teeth.* When it had to be used, he suggested special gargles to counteract this effect. He was noting its use in yet another application: many of the Crusaders were coming back from the Holy Land with a form of what was thought to be leprosy, and an ointment known as *Unguentum Saracenum* – Saracens' Salve, almost certainly copied from Arab use – had proved remarkably effective in clearing up some of the horrible sores. In this ointment, quicksilver was mixed in a base of pig's fat with two violently irritant herbs: one of the many varieties of spurge (*Euphorbia*) and the expressed oil of stavesacre (*Delphinium staphisagria*). Juice from the leaves of the spurge was long used in medicine as a blistering plaster – beggars have often used it to produce loathsome sores for public exhibition and the seeds of stavesacre – commonly known as lousewort – are extremely poisonous, killing vermin and parasites when applied externally.

Saracens' Salve would thus have been highly effective in curing any disease caused by parasitic agents. Applied in a blistering plaster, much of the quicksilver would have been absorbed cutaneously, to give the familiar energetic action on the mucous membranes.

When the surgeons applied their salve to the hard chancres and

---

*Mercury in the form of quicksilver is relatively harmless and large doses of it have been swallowed without apparent ill-effect. But broken down by the intensive friction needed to turn it into an ointment it is easily absorbed into the bloodstream, and becomes acutely toxic.

abscesses of syphilis, they were giving their patients a dose of mercury, absorbed through the skin. Since mercury salts are highly poisonous to bacteria, mercury sometimes cured even quite desperate cases of syphilis. In no time at all, the quacks were following suit – again with apparent success – and soon numbers of them were in business as specialists in this one disease: like back-street abortionists, they offered a risky solution to a problem which many people were ashamed to take to their family doctor.

Finally the physicians, too, were forced to learn from the surgeons they despised, and use the remedy that Galen had warned against, since mercury alone seemed to be making an impact on the disease.

At first, the physicians were cautious, using ointments containing only tiny amounts of mercury. Such salves may have produced some of the characteristic side-effects, but they were certainly not powerful enough to cure a disease that was, as everybody agreed, "long in duration, stubborn, subject to relapses and rebellious to mild medication".

By this time the quacks were using mercury with reckless abandon, not merely the relatively harmless metallic form but corrosive sublimate as well, with results that can be imagined. They certainly killed numbers of patients, but they apparently cured a great many, too, and since syphilis was often a killer anyway, its victims may have felt that they had little to lose in such a gamble. Mercury became generally accepted as the one effective cure, but nobody pretended that it was anything but unpleasant.

One of the dozens of books written about syphilis in the first decades was actually a long and elegant poem by an eminent Italian physician, Hieronimo Fracastor (1478–1553). In it he described how the ordeal of the mercury cure by inunction – the rubbing-on of an ointment – was to be carried out. The mercury was mixed in a grease base with other powerful herbal ingredients. "Without hesitation, spread this mixture on your body and cover with it your entire skin, with the exception of the head and the precordial region [over the heart]. Then carefully wrap yourself with bed-covering and thus await until a sweat bathes your limbs with an impure dew. Ten days in succession renew this treatment, for ten entire days you are to undergo this cruel trial . . . very soon, an infallible presage will announce to you the hour of your freedom. Very soon you will feel the ferments of the disease dissolve themselves in your mouth in a disgusting flow of saliva. . . ."[2]

Sometimes the wretched choking patients crouched for days over their gruesome little dishes, the saliva pouring out of their mouths in a steady fetid flow, pints of it in a single day. For years the great object of mercury treatment was to raise exactly this "salivation" which was thought the most effective of all the ways by which the body could rid itself of the poison. "Verily we must so long use frictions and inunctions, until the virulent humours be perfectly evacuated, by spitting and salivation, by stools, urine, sweat or insensible perspiration," wrote the famous sixteenth-century French surgeon Ambroise Paré (1510–1590), never a man to put his patients to unnecessary suffering.[3]

But the sweating, the confinement, and the endless ignominious spitting were not even the worst of the mercury cure. It nearly always affected the patient's mouth: the tongue and gums swelled and became incredibly sensitive, the teeth were loosened, turned black or fell out, terrible sores formed on the tongue and palate, often whole portions of the jaw became ulcerated and sloughed away, leaving the victim grotesquely disfigured. Other patients developed all the symptoms of generalized mercury poisoning – the tremors, the paralysis.

These appalling consequences often followed even careful professional treatment, since individual responses to mercury are notoriously unpredictable. In the hands of reckless charlatans they were so common, and the fatality rate so high, that the inunction treatment acquired a bad name: "the common people, perceiving so manie to be spoiled and killed with Quicksilver would not willinglie be cured therewith".[4] Other quacks disguised the mercury with sweet smells and fumigated their patients, others washed them in mercury solutions, and others simply sold them ferocious purges.

Thus when it was first rumoured that there was a marvellous new herbal cure being practised by the Indian women in the West Indies, much milder, completely efficacious, and with no disagreeable side-effects, a great sigh of relief went up from Europe. The Spanish living in the Caribbean had soon realized that the natives suffered from what looked exactly like European syphilis – it was probably yaws – and when one of them caught it from an Indian woman, he went to one of their doctors who, Gerome Benzoni reported, "gave him a decoction of Guaiacum to drink, which removed the symptoms in a short time, and perfectly restored him to health."[5]

Other Spaniards followed his example, and soon syphilitics who could spare the time and money flocked across to the Caribbean to be cured. The cure turned out not to be quite as simple and trouble-free as

the Spanish account suggested, and two distinguished young French-
men, who had tried various European cures in vain and travelled to
Puerto Rico to try out guaiacum gave a more accurate account of how
it was done.

Their cure had been undertaken by one of the native women in her
own hut. She had collected twigs from the handsome, blue-flowered
guaiac trees (*Guaiacum officinale*) chewed them, then simmered them in
a covered earthenware pot. Every morning she made them drink a big
tumblerful of this decoction, then sent them out walking or fencing, or
else to work hard in a goldmine for two hours. ". . . then they came
back sweating to the house and changed only their shirt; then she gave
them dinner, drinking only rainwater. . . .

"At three o'clock in the afternoon they drank as much guaiac as in
the morning, and did the same exercise; and without any other ceremony or remedy, they were completely cured in six weeks. . . . The
chancres on their backs disappeared, the night pains went in a fortnight, their appetites returned . . . and they came back safe and sound
. . . to Paris."[6]

Realizing that guaiac was potentially big business, the Spanish
began importing it into Europe: one Gonsalvo Ferand shipped the first
supplies in 1508, and soon it was being widely used. Nicolaus Poll,
personal physician to the Emperor Charles V of Spain, claimed that by
1517 three thousand Spanish syphilitics, desperate cases, had been
cured by the use of guaiac alone.[7] Its fame spread.

One of the most widely-publicized cases of syphilis of the time was
that of the famous German patriot, humanist and satirist, Ulrich von
Hutten (1488–1523). He had contracted what was believed to be
syphilis at the age of twenty, and for nine years had suffered all the
horrors of mercurial treatment without success: he had been salivated
eleven times and still the racking pains and the obstinate sores persisted. On hearing about guaiac he put himself through a severely-
regulated cure – forty days of confinement to a warm room, drinking
vast quantities of the decoction of guaiac, sweating for hours at a time,
living on biscuits and raisins for the first fortnight, and even then only
adding a little broth or chicken to his diet. To his delight, all the
symptoms of his nine-year-long disease vanished, and von Hutten
wrote a pamphlet in 1519 lauding guaiac as vastly superior to mercury.

If it had not been before, guaiac now became very big business, and
as such it attracted the attention of the Fugger family. The Fuggers
were the leading banking dynasty of Europe, enormously wealthy and

powerful, with commercial interests that stretched across Europe and along the trade routes of the world. They had interests in half the East–West spice and drug trade, and now, as one of the conditions for yet another loan to prop up the Spanish throne, they asked for and got the monopoly of guaiac, no doubt congratulating themselves on a brilliant coup.

But as with many much publicized new miracle-drugs, the high hopes raised by guaiac were not fulfilled, and the earliest cures remained the most spectacular. Properly used under close medical supervision, with the hot Caribbean sun or blazing log fires in a closed room to help raise the temperature and induce copious sweating, accompanied by a long and strict dietetic regime, the guaiac treatment was often extremely effective. (It was shown in 1932 that raising a patient's temperature to 42°C was partially successful in destroying the syphilis spirochæte.) But it was widely used by quacks and charlatans, who, even if they had wished to do so, could hardly have insisted on the prolonged sweating treatment, or supervised its administration properly. Instead they vaunted it as an instant cure-all, selling hundreds of packets, probably to sufferers who imagined that a couple of doses would cure them.

Even among those taking guaiac under medical supervision, plenty of syphilitics found the forty-day course of near-fasting, confinement, no wine and no women so insufferable that they abandoned it as soon as their symptoms disappeared, before the cure was complete – like modern patients who seldom finish a prescription of antibiotics. Other cases failed to respond to guaiac at all, and Ulrich von Hutten, who had done more than anyone to promote the sacred wood, had a relapse – which this time guaiac failed to arrest. His death in 1523 was the worst publicity for the cure.

Most people believed that syphilis had come to Europe from the West Indies with Columbus' sailors, and since there was a general belief that whatever disease was native to a country might be cured by the medicinal herbs growing there, it seemed reasonable to think that other plants from the Spanish colonies might be effective against syphilis.

Accordingly since the great guaiac boom of the early sixteenth century, the Spanish had been studying the materia medica of trad-itional healers in their Caribbean and South American colonies with the keenest commercial interest. The galleons that ploughed back across the Atlantic carrying Peruvian silver to Spanish ports often had a small cargo of interesting drug-plants too. It soon became known to their captains that Nicholas Monardes (died 1578), a wealthy Seville doctor with a most fashionable practice (no doubt it included many cases of *Morbus Gallicus*), was an enthusiast for the new drugs, and delighted to try them on his patients.

In 1574, half a century after the death of von Hutten, and after years of what we now call "clinical trials," Monardes published a comprehensive account of these new drugs which was almost immediately translated into English and published as *Joyful Newes out of the Newe Founde Worlde*.

Among the exotics Monardes described were tobacco, sassafras, a most effective new purge called jalap (*Ipomœa purga*) from Mexico, and various balsams. But it was three plants in particular which had astonished the Seville physician with their powers, and of which he gave the fullest account. All three were effective, he claimed, against syphilis. One was guaiac – of whose efficacy Monardes was completely convinced. The others were the China root (*Smilax china*) and sarsaparilla (*Smilax aristolochia*), both species of *Smilax*.

Monardes' account of these drugs is particularly notable for the exactness with which he specifies types, soundness and quantity of the drug-plant in each case, and the scrupulously strict regime that he insisted his patients follow: in the sarsaparilla cure, for instance, his patients were confined to a warm room for thirty days, and for the following forty days they were to abstain from both wine and sexual intercourse.

As with guaiac it is thus easy to see why sarsaparilla, after a brief vogue, also sank in favour. Then as now, few patients were willing, even if they could afford the time, to lock themselves away from family, friends and jobs for weeks on end, to follow a regime of monastic severity. Soon physicians, surgeons, quacks and patients alike were turning once more to the unpleasant but effective remedy, mercury.

It is possible to believe today that "the use of mercury in the treatment of syphilis may have been the most colossal hoax ever perpetrated" in the history of medicine.[8] Certainly during the four and a half centuries of its continued use, there were always doctors who were violently opposed to it because of its frightful side-effects, or firmly convinced of the value of other discarded cures, such as guaiac or sarsaparilla, which they felt had never been given a fair trial.

During military operations in Portugal in 1812, a British Inspector General of Hospitals for the Portuguese noted that the Portuguese soldiers suffering from syphilis who were never treated with mercury but dosed with sarsaparilla instead, recovered much faster and more completely than the British, who were always given extensive courses of it. This finding was borne out in this century when some 2000 syphilis patients in Oslo were studied over twenty years, while receiving no mercury. Between sixty and seventy per cent appeared to have escaped the tertiary stage of the disease, and suffered no ill effects of their earlier infection.

Today, however, we have the security of penicillin, so we can afford to consider the matter dispassionately. To sufferers before this century – and to society at large – the central question was not so much whether the symptoms of syphilis had been successfully relieved, but whether or not patients were actually cured, and no longer capable of transmitting the disease to their sexual partners or their unborn children: a certainty for which almost no price seemed too high to pay.

Mercury certainly appeared to cure numbers of cases. Perhaps, too, the very unpleasantness of the cure may have confirmed it in general belief as the most effective one. There must have been a general feeling that the cure for such a particularly frightful disease needed itself to be correspondingly terrible: mercury may have been penance as well as remedy in the minds of those enduring it.

For all these reasons, mercury rapidly established itself in general and medical opinion throughout Western Europe, as the one foolproof remedy for syphilis. And once so established, social considerations soon outlawed any alternative therapy. It was the first triumph of a new kind of medicine, formulated and prepared in a laboratory and using the new techniques of chemistry – a potent and seductive rival for that older medicine, which since the dawn of time had relied chiefly on plants for its remedies.

4

The Revolutionary

"The physician's duty is to heal the sick, not to enrich the apothecary", wrote an angry young Swiss-German doctor in the early sixteenth century.[1] His name was Philippus Theophrastus Bombastus von Hohenheim (1493–1541), although he was more often known as Paracelsus. He was a child of the great revolutionary age that produced Calvin (1509–1564), Luther (1482–1546), and Zwingli (1484–1531), and just as these contemporaries castigated the abuses and corruptness of the medieval church, so Paracelsus devoted much of his enormous, restless energies to thundering against the follies and glaring abuses of medicine in his time.

His background was humble and unusual. Born at Einsiedeln near Zurich, in Canton Schwys, he was the only son of the local physician, a quiet and serious man who seems not to have been very successful as a doctor. The family was not well off – Paracelsus was brought up used to rough food, coarse peasant clothes, plenty of fresh air – but his interest in medicine began early. On long walks in the lovely Alpine countryside, his father would point out the medicinal plants, explaining how the local peasants used them to treat their ailments. He was pleased by his son's evident interest, and began to give him some of the proper grounding for a physician – little discourses on the teachings of the great Greek and Latin masters, some Latin, basic astrology, hints at the mysteries of alchemy.

Much of his father's income probably went for books. He was passionately interested in alchemy, and had a large library filled with works of the famous alchemists like Albertus Magnus, the Arab Geber, Villanova, Lullius, and Trimethius, through which the solitary and precocious child browsed.

When Paracelsus was nine years old, his father's reputation for chemical expertise earned him a new job – that of teacher in the mining school at Villach, in Karinthia, with which was combined the function of town physician.

Karinthia is mining country, its mountains – as Paracelsus wrote later – "like a strong box which when opened with a key reveals great treasure." Iron ore, zinc, cinnabar, even gold were among the minerals being mined locally, and at nearby Bleiberg, they mined "a wonderful lead ore which provides Germany, Pannonia, Turkey and Italy with lead".[2]

The Bleiberg mines were owned by the Fuggers, who had also founded the Villach mining school to train technicians in metallurgical processes. Paracelsus attended the school where his father gave classes in analytical chemistry and the treatment of minerals – and seems to have been instantly fascinated. He mastered the elementary techniques of chemistry, learned how to build a small furnace, handled retorts and alembics, and watched acids reacting and interreacting with metals. Chemistry burst on him like a revelation, at once an irresistible hobby and a sublime new science. At home, in his father's consulting room, he studied another aspect of mining: the human cost of the Fugger fortunes in the shape of men wasted by the special occupational diseases of lead–mining. This was an interaction of another kind, of man with metal.

Paracelsus' early interest in alchemy was reinforced by such studies, and – probably with the enthusiastic encouragement of his father – he seems to have spent some time formally studying this secret science with a well-known alchemist, the Abbot Trimethius. Paracelsus' fascination with alchemy was more than purely speculative, however; he had already determined to devote his life to medicine, and he had seen enough of contemporary doctoring, with its theoretical approach and costly apothecary compounds, to be convinced of its utter uselessness. Might not alchemy, with its insights and techniques, make possible the fresh start that was so urgently needed?

Probably his father could not have undertaken the financial burden of a conventional medical training, with its years–long course of elaborate studies. Thus it was very likely by deliberate choice that Paracelsus, instead, spent years of his young life endlessly zigzagging across Europe working as an army surgeon – into Italy, Portugal, Prussia, Holland, Belgium, and even further afield in Scandinavia, Asia Minor, and Tartary where his bizarre experiences may have included initiation into the Buddhist faith.

At Idria, in Slovenia, he visited the newly–opened cinnabar mines where the ore mercuric sulphide was obtained, and saw miners suffering the classic symptoms of mercury poisoning: tremors of the hands and feet, frightening grimaces, debility, loss of teeth. Even the rats and mice who entered the mine developed the same symptoms, and died in convulsions.

Paracelsus noticed such details – he had an extremely observant eye – and his years of practical medical work in the field – what we should now call "clinical experience" – combined with a natural gift for healing, not only gave him a thorough–going contempt for doctors trained exclusively out of books, but turned him into a first-class doctor who impressed patients with his instinctive understanding of their cases. Very few of his colleagues can have had such wide-ranging experience of chronic or occupational disease, epidemics, field surgery and syphilis, as well as more everyday afflictions. "I have not borrowed from Hippocrates or Galen or anyone else", he could later claim, "having acquired my knowledge from the best teacher, that is, by experience and hard work".[3]

One of his few friends, a gentle Greek scholar and former pupil named Johannes Oporinus, has left us a vivid picture of this forceful and unconventional personality. Paracelsus, he said, was not in the least scholarly or pious, making rude remarks about the Pope, about Luther, about all theologians. He spent most of the day busied with his furnace and his chemical equipment: nobody knew what he was up to, but his assistant was once completely knocked out by the violent fumes from a flask which Paracelsus made him sniff. He seemed to have plenty of money to spend on good meals and expensive new clothes, but he wore the clothes till they were so filthy they fell off him, and he never seemed to care where he slept, flinging himself down fully–dressed on a bed only to spring up again three hours later: his energy was phenomenal. So was his capacity for alcohol: he could drink solid peasants under the table, and then late at night sit down and dictate for hours, apparently almost senseless with drink – but what he had dictated read like the work of a perfectly sober man. His most successful cures were of ulcer cases: instead of restricting his patients to low, bland diets he would sit feasting with them all evening – seemingly with the same results.[4]

By the time Paracelsus settled in Strasbourg in 1526, to practise, to take on a few pupils, and to produce some of his vast flood of writing, he had a growing reputation both for his unconventional views on medicine, and for his professional skill. His fame had even reached Basel, where the important publisher Frobenius faced death from a gangrenous leg that the surgeons were totally unable to cure. As a last hope, he sent for the extraordinary physician at Strasbourg.

Paracelsus arrived, took charge, dismissed the surgeons, and saved Frobenius' leg. The humanist Erasmus of Rotterdam happened to be with Frobenius at the time, and was so much impressed by these medical talents – "you have recalled Frobenius from the under-world"[5] – that he consulted Paracelsus later, by post from Rotterdam, about his own problems – debility and pain in the liver and kidneys, for which his doctors had prescribed violent purges, both vegetable and mineral. Paracelsus advised other remedies – "you do not need evacuations" – prescribing strengthening medicine instead.[6]

The city of Basel at this time needed a municipal physician – a post that carried with it the right to lecture at Basel University. Probably at Frobenius' urging, the city fathers offered the post to Paracelsus, who accepted it. On 5 June 1527 he stood for the first time before the University's medical students. "I have been called here to Basel by the city fathers, with the incentive of a large salary," he told his delighted audience – not in the customary Latin but in their own German. The programme he outlined was bold, imaginative – and strongly abusive of current medical practice, with its emphasis on theory and tradition. "Who does not know" demanded Paracelsus, "that many doctors in this time have ignominiously failed their patients? Because they ad-hered too anxiously to the sayings of Hippocrates, Galen, Avicenna and others. . . . With these authorities they could become splendid university doctors . . . but never real physicians."

Titles, eloquence and book-learning were equally unimportant, Paracelsus continued: what mattered was a thorough familiarity with the causes and symptoms of disease, and the ability to prescribe successfully for them. He himself would not be teaching the students the work of these old authors, but rather his own experience, recorded in a number of his books. In his lectures there would be none of the usual insistence on the four humours and the complexions and all their sub-dividions – "the ancients wrongly attributed all disease to them", and contemporary physicians in consequence were so distracted by theory that none of them, "or very few, have attained exact knowl-edge of diseases, their causes and the critical days."[7]

His audience loved it. Soon his lectures were the talk of the University, and even the barber-surgeons, who usually made a point of despising academic studies, flocked to hear them. His popularity with his classes probably reached its zenith when, during the students' midsummer festival, Paracelsus tossed the fine fat volume of Avicenna's works onto a bonfire.

But the faculty seethed with indignation. They refused Paracelsus the use of the lecture-hall, denied his right to send forward candidates for the doctorate, and questioned his qualifications. They were soon joined in active hostilities by Basel's apothecaries, whose shops had been inspected by Paracelsus who exercised his duties as town physician with a dismaying thoroughness. (Paracelsus was always particularly rude about apothecaries – "their shops are nothing but foul sculleries, from which comes nothing but foul broths".[8])

As relations between Paracelsus and the faculty went from bad to worse, his pupils began to drift away, afraid of compromising their chances of a degree, and when his influential friend Frobenius died in October, Paracelsus was obliged to leave Basel. For the thirteen years that remained of his life, he travelled from town to town, sometimes working as healer and lay-preacher among the poorest of the Swiss peasants, occasionally settling in cities for another feverish spell of writing and chemical experimentation, before yet another angry outburst would antagonize yet another influential acquaintance or wealthy patient, or the local doctors and apothecaries – outraged by his success and by his scorn – joined forces to manoeuvre him out of town. He died in Salzburg in 1541, possibly from a tumour of the liver – or perhaps from systemic mercurial poisoning, the result of working for long years in the laboratory with this dangerous mineral.

Like the modern critic of drug therapy, Paracelsus inevitably found himself up against the vested interests of big business. Just as cancer today has been called an "industry" since it keeps so many thousands employed in the pharmaceutical companies, so in the early sixteenth century there were plenty of merchants and quacks making what could literally be called a killing out of the prevalent plague of syphilis. The Fuggers of Augsburg, for instance, had made fortunes from the guaiac boom. Paracelsus, who was anyway doubtful of guaiac's ability to cure syphilis, and strongly critical of such methods, had written a pamphlet denouncing guaiac, and sales had suffered in consequence. But the Fuggers had already hedged their bet. Scenting the impending collapse of the guaiac market, they had adroitly moved into mercury. In exchange for their underwriting of Charles V's election expenses as

Emperor, they had secured an interest in the important Spanish cinnabar mines at Almaden. Many practitioners had never stopped using
mercury, and since it was still the favourite remedy of the quacks, sales
were rising steadily.

The Fuggers might close their eyes to the general reckless abuse of
mercurial syphilis cures, but Paracelsus could not and did not. In his
travels and in his army experience he had seen too many needless
agonies inflicted by a course of mercury, and too much lasting damage
from mercury absorbed into the body's tissues. ". . . it runs together
again from the bodily heat and lies in the hollow places of the body . . .
with what damage . . . is evident at Idria: all those who live there, are
deformed and lame, easily out of breath, easily chilled, and never in
good health. . . ."[9]

Both guaiac and mercury, he thought, could be used to cure syphilis
– but in small, carefully calculated doses, and in chemically treated
formulations, together with a great deal of supportive treatment. In
1529 Paracelsus proposed to publish these opinions in a major work on
syphilis. The prospect so alarmed the Fuggers that they persuaded
their old friend Heinrich Stromer, Dean of the Medical Faculty at
Leipzig, to issue a decree banning publication. Stromer was happy to
oblige the Fuggers, who had cut him in on the guaiac boom, and
although Paracelsus had an edition of the first three chapters rushed
through the presses in defiance of this decree, he was obliged to leave
town before the work could be completed or published in its entirety.

The unholy alliance of medicine with commerce at the patient's
expense always made Paracelsus angry, and he repeatedly denounced
it. He found it ridiculous that German patients should be paying vast
sums of money for plants imported from remote countries, when
"there are many more and better medicines here than in Arabia,
Chaldea, Persia, and Greece."[10] Moreover, the practice of resorting to
exotic, imported drugs led to fraud on a grand scale: "he who brings
this to the German nation and takes advantage of those who buy it, is a
fraud. Such merchandise . . . is rotten and useless when he gives it to
the sick."[11]

But if patients who were too poor to go to the doctor or the
apothecary looked for reliable guidance to doctoring their own complaints with local herbs, they looked in vain, according to Paracelsus:
the herbals they turned to were so much waste paper. The earliest
herbals to be printed, only a few years before Paracelsus' birth, were
the medieval compilations with a long and solid history of popular

appeal, like the rhyming herbal of Macer Floridus, and the sixth century Herbarium of Apuleius Platonicus, which plenty of readers probably knew by heart. These and other works were at first printed in Latin, but the eagerness of the response had taken publishers by surprise: obviously there was a huge lay public, avid for information about native medicinal plants for domestic use. Following the lead of Peter Schoeffer of Mainz, who in 1485 published a German herbal, the *Gart der Gezundheit* (*Garden of Health*), printers all over Europe began bringing out herbals in the vernacular.

These herbals dealt chiefly with homegrown medicinal plants – "what may be found in the grounds of private gardens, in the woods and in the fields. . . . By their efficacy a sick person or one who is not perfectly healthy may be brought back to a state of health". They all followed orthodox medical teaching, many of them carrying little discourses on the humoral theory and the importance of astrology for the benefit of their readers, but the information they contained was largely anecdotal, and almost never original. This was hardly surprising, since all compilers were drawing on the same sources – Galen, Dioscorides, Avicenna, and Serapio – each editor borrowing texts and systems of classification and even illustrations from the other without acknowledgement. Despite these limitations, new editions, copies, pirated editions and translations continued to pour off the printing presses in Europe in a steady stream, constituting a publishing boom which even a century later had scarcely begun to slacken.

Paracelsus denounced these works with bitter scorn: ". . . scraped together from histories, poets and old women . . . useless except to book-publishers who in this way become rich and healthy in the kitchen. . . ."[12] Of the German *Herbarius*, the first "new" herbal to be printed, in 1484, he pronounced: "He who put together this book understood nothing . . . he has patched together rumours which are fun to read and tell of great feats . . . if it were all true, nobody could be sick or die . . . he has no knowledge of diseases or the herbs for them . . . it is a work to empty the peasant's pockets".[13]

So much emphasis has been placed on Paracelsus' advocacy of chemical medicine and of drugs prepared from minerals, that it comes as a shock to discover the degree to which his thinking was influenced by the traditions of Swiss-German folk medicine. In the first place, he saw clearly that herbs used according to elaborate humoral theory were a blunted weapon: ". . . with time the humorists have arisen, who do not heed the natural mysteries, but only their unfounded theory without recognition of the natural, correct properties . . ."[14] In their authoritative *History of Pharmacy*, Kremers and Urdang point out that Paracelsus "stressed the need for a treatment that would be specific for that particular disease. The action of a remedy, he felt, did not depend upon its qualities such as moistness, but on its *specific* healing virtue, which was determined by its chemical properties".[15] This approach – far from being original – is that which comes naturally to the folk healer, who although happily ignorant of the four humours, is well aware that lesser celandine is useful for piles, while a dose of male fern may get rid of a nasty case of tapeworm.

Again, Paracelsus' advocacy of mineral poisons like mercury and antimony, which has been seen as one of his most distinctive contributions to the evolution of medicine, is in fact based on a belief common in Swiss–German folk-medicine at the time – and three centuries later to become famous as homoeopathy – that like is cured by like, the effects of a poison remedied by doses of another poison: "It depends only upon the dose whether a poison is poison or not."[16]

Yet another strongly-held belief of folk medicine, to which Paracelsus subscribed, was that medicinal plants grew where they were needed, and that there was no need to travel far to find the remedy for a disease: ". . . They want medicaments from overseas, and better things grow in their own garden."[17]

Paracelsus was also a firm believer in the doctrine of signatures, and in illustration of it explained every single part of St. John's wort (*Hypericum perforatum*) in terms of this belief. ". . . the holes in the leaves mean that this herb helps all inner and outer orifices of the skin . . . the blooms rot in the form of blood, a sign that it is good for wounds and should be used where flesh has to be treated. . . ."[18]

If the inaccuracies of herbals, the frauds of herb-importers and the uselessness of apothecary confections made Paracelsus angry, it was because, as a result, herbs were seldom properly used, while their real virtues remained undervalued or unknown by foolish men who thought they could improve on nature. "To what purpose do you superadde vinegar to the root of Comfrey," he asked surgeons, "or bole, or suchlike balefull additaments, while God hath compos'd this simple sufficient to cure the fracture of the bones?"[19] And writing of the healing powers of St. John's wort, he adds that the simple balsam prepared from it "puts to shame all recipes and doctors, they may yell as they wish, they will only break their teeth."[20]

It is clear both from his writings and from the assurance with which he speaks of them that Paracelsus used herbs knowledgeably and confidently in his own practice – which may account for some of the successes which made other doctors so envious. Among his most neglected works is the rough outline of a new authoritative herbal "of herbs and roots or seed and leaves as much as I have so far experienced and known."[21]

Just as Paracelsus never assumed that the learned knew everything, he never imagined either that the unschooled were ignorant – a truth he tried hard to impress on his pupils. "A Physitian", he told them, "ought not to rest only in that bare knowledge which their Schools teach, but to learn of old women, Egyptians, and such-like persons; for they have greater experience in such things than all the Academians".[22] Few doctors before the time of Paracelsus – and even fewer since – have bothered to try tapping this fund of inherited knowledge of plant remedies. But during his long wandering apprenticeship as a surgeon, and throughout his life, Paracelsus went out of his way to cultivate these country healers and gypsies, and to study their methods of treating the sick.

All revolutions need a figurehead, and by the end of the sixteenth century, the name Paracelsan had been firmly linked to the medical revolution that was bringing chemically prepared mineral medicines into the apothecary's shop, and calling in question the value of the old Galenicals. Paracelsus must have seemed the obvious choice for this role, since his name was identified by everybody with opposition to the entrenched bastions of medical conservatism. ". . . an epitome and rallying-point of the diverse forces rising against the old authority in medicine".[23] For all his personal idiosyncrasies and absurdities, no other medical thinker of the time had a tenth of Paracelsus' driving energy and authority, and certainly nobody else had written so entrancingly and imaginatively of the application of alchemy to medicine.

Moreover, among the hundreds of thousands of words – some in German, some Latin, others in a strange mongrel language of his own – that he had dashed onto paper, could be traced the cloudy, suggestive outline of an apologia for the new chemical medicine that was all the more impressive for being only moderately comprehensible. "I must confess" admitted the English Paracelsan surgeon Clowes "his Doctrine hath a more pregnant sense, than my wit or reach is able to construe."[24] As with the Bible, it is possible to prove almost anything by Paracelsus' writings. Many of the Paracelsans of the sixteenth century had not even read his works. It was not until

1598 – nearly half a century after his death – that his papers were finally collected by Johann Huser, and printed in Basel (delightful irony) in ten substantial volumes. Another fourteen years passed before the first comprehensive Latin edition appeared, although various works or fragments had been translated into different European languages before that time.

The sheer volume of his prose output is daunting – the complete Sudhoff edition of his medical writings, published in 1929–33 runs to fourteen fat volumes. To make matters worse his prose style – intricate, turgid, maddeningly obscure – is no help to anyone trying to work out what he actually meant. Some scholars, in desperation, have suggested that as a practising alchemist himself, Paracelsus was deliberately writing to be understood only by other alchemists.

But neither the inaccessibility nor the obscurity of his writings prevented the "chemists" of the time from claiming him as their patron, and attributing to him their own violently anti-Galenic views. It came to be assumed that he depended much more on metallic medicines than on those of vegetable origin, and by the twentieth century, he was firmly established as "the founder of chemical pharmacology," the patron saint of the drug companies, the man who flung open the windows to let in a new scientific age, and pointed medicine firmly down the path to the pharmaceutical laboratory.

Whether Paracelsus would have found himself in entire sympathy with the revolution that has been credited to him is open to question. Far from being in a hurry to discard the simples used in traditional medicine in favour of powerful new chemical preparations, Paracelsus argued that alchemy offered new possibilities for penetrating the medicinal secrets of these plants, and using them more effectively.

He believed what we now know to be true, that the specific medicinal action of each plant often depends on a single chemical constituent – the "active principle" of the plant.

He believed equally strongly something which we have learned by disastrous experiment not to be true – that the active principle extracted from the plant and used in isolation will be even more effective, even more powerful medicine, while remaining as safe as in its original form. This was the tempting delusion that danced before the eyes of the medical alchemists, and Paracelsus believed in it as implicitly as any of them: "what the eye perceives in herbs or stone or trees is not yet a remedy; the eye sees only the dross. The remedy must be cleansed from the dross, then it is there. This is alchemy. . . ."[25]

Since alchemy had not yet turned this vision into fact, Paracelsus continued to use plants as he found them compounded by God – and to exercise the utmost caution when he treated patients with the perilous new preparations of mercury and other dangerous minerals. Iatrogenic disease – the sickness that ignorant doctors visit on their patients – always seemed to him the worst of felonies. And even Paracelsus might have been lost for words to express his indignation at the reckless slaughter for which, over the next three centuries, the new chemical medicine was to be responsible.

5

The Quacks' Charter

"Take violet leaves, night shade, of eche ij. handfull, chamomell flowres, one handfull, mallowes ij. handfull, rose leaves one handfull, swete appuls iiij, a manchett, Boyle all thse to guether in swete mylke tyll they be tendre . . ." begins the recipe for Henry VIII's poultice, "devised by the Kinges Matie at hampton courte".[1]

Like many a monarch before him, Henry VIII (1491–1547) had a keen amateur interest in medicine: he was "a great dabbler in physic and offered medical advice on all occasions which presented themselves. . . ."[2] He found the actual preparation and compounding of the plasters and ointments particularly fascinating, and no doubt had his own Royal set of apothecary's equipment which went with him on his travels.

A manuscript preserved in the British Museum, written in beautiful Tudor script, records a Royal collection of 114 favourite recipes for "plastres" and "cataplasmes", for "balmes . . . waters, lotions and decoctions". Thirty-two of these are noted as being of "the Kinges Maties devise," and there seems no reason to doubt that they were composed by the King himself, sending his servants scurrying for two ounces of finely-powdered red coral or another pint of rose-water, and consulting his personal Apothecary Thomas Babham on a fine professional point from time to time, while he pored over his Herbals and his Antidotaries.

Many of the medicaments devised by Henry must have been for his personal use. His leg with its obstinate ulcerous sore began to bother him fairly early in his reign, and he experimented with a plaster which, the manuscript note claims, "resolves humoures which there is swellynge in the legges", and another one intended "to ease the payne and swelling abowt the ankles". There were others designed perhaps for the same trouble: "a grane oyntement devised by the Kinges highnes to take awaye heat and Indurations", and others "to resolve and ease payne", "to heal ulcers without pain", and "to cool inflammation."[3]

His strenuous sexual life appears to have brought its own problems: the "King's Grace's oyntement" was invented at St. James's, "to coole and dry and comfort the Member", and another soothing ointment "to dry excoriations and comforte the membre" was devised at Cawood. ("Was not that an episcopal palace? How devoutly was the Head of the Church employed!" commented Horace Walpole waspishly, two centuries later.)[4]

The ingredients Henry used probably reflect fairly accurately the standard medical practice of his time. Most of them were herbal, plants and flowers known since Dioscorides for their soothing, cooling, healing and softening properties, such as plantain (*Plantago major*), linseed (*Linum usitatissimum*), fenugreek (*Trigonella fœnum-græcum*), and marguerite (*Chrysanthemum leucanthemum*). He used marsh mallow (*Althæa officinalis*), highly thought of by the Arab pharmacists as a poultice for inflammations, and the leaves of the sweet-scented violet (*Viola odorata*) which, as Gerard noted later, were commonly "used in cooling plasters, oyles and comfortable cataplasms or poultices."[5]

Henry also used the sweet yellow flowers of the tall weed melilot (*Melilotus officinalis*), which the country people called King's Clover. Tudor farmers hated it because it took over their pasturelands and ruined their corn, but country herbalists found it very useful: a poultice of melilot "boiled in sweet wine" with "the yolke of a rosted egge, linseed, marsh mallow and hog's greece" was the very thing, said Gerard, for assuaging inflammation.[6] Appropriately for a Tudor monarch, Henry also used plenty of "oyle of roses" and rose-water – probably as much for its sweet smell – perhaps concealing others less pleasant – as for its medicinal value.

As well as plants, he used lead and turpentine for his plasters; more exotic ingredients such as silver or powdered red coral – in which he seems to have had great faith; positively fabulous articles such as unicorn horn; and the occasional repellent animal substance – but carefully prepared for him – such as "the pouldre of long wormes well washed and dryed"; all of these were heated, stirred, and pounded together, and given the necessary body by contribution from the Royal kitchens such as manchet or fine wheat bread, freshly laid eggs, capon fat or veal suet.

There was nothing uncommon in this herbal expertise. Henry VIII was merely doing for fun, and in grand kingly style, what every housewife in his kingdom did from necessity. Shakespeare's plays are stuffed with knowledgeable allusions to herbs – "give me mandragora and let me sleep" – and it was part of every gentleman's breeding to be familiar with them. Every good library in the kingdom possessed one of the fine new Latin herbals then in print, and in 1526 – the year that Henry's eye first strayed to Anne Boleyn – the *Grete Herbal*, the first English one, was published with the object, like the French work from which it was translated, of "enformyng how men may be holpen with grene herbs of the gardyn and wedys of the feldys as well as by costly receptes of the potycaryes prepared."[7]

Not all the herbals published in this and the following century were intended for home consumption, however. On the contrary, the vast majority were the work of physicians, surgeons, or apothecaries, men professionally involved with medicinal plants, and anxious to have available in clear concise form all the most important information to be found in the works of Greek, Latin, or Arab authors.

Authoritative and complete texts of Dioscorides – as opposed to the scrappy and unreliable extracts the medieval doctor had had to rely on – were considered essential, and Latin translations of the West's first herbal, often running alongside the Greek original, were among the earliest works on medicinal herbs to be printed; other standard classic and Arab authors followed, while a French physician, John Ruellius, produced early in the sixteenth century the complete reference work, *De natura stirpium*, in three fat volumes, "wherein he hath accurately gathered all things out of sundrie writers, especially the Greekes and Latines."[8]

But as time went by, it became clear that the great task of clarifying and collating, so far from being nearly complete, was hardly begun; that confusion was if anything being made worse by so many different attempts to impose some kind of order; and that the world was full of plants which Dioscorides had never seen and about which he had not a word to say – a situation that at least one writer, Petrus Andreas Matthiolus, found so unnerving that he actually falsified the figures of some of these alien growths "to make them agree with Dioscori."[9]

We may suspect, too, that many of the physicians who wrote so happily and knowledgeably about medicinal plants were pursuing an academic hobby rather than adding to the general knowledge of their profession. Conrad Gesner (1516–1566), whose leisure for years was absorbed by "the great and general worke of plants" he planned, was professionally far more fascinated by the exciting possibilities of the new chemical medicine, and wrote a book strenuously advocating it as early at 1552.

Another well-known writer on plants, the youthful prodigy Valerius Cordus (1515–1544), spent much of his brief life collecting and improving pharmaceutical formulae. (When the Physicians of Nuremberg enquired if they might see the result of all his researches, they were so impressed that the Senate ordered a collection of his Aromatics and Opiates, Confections and Conserves, Cerates, Syrups and Electuaries to be printed as the first official pharmacopœia, and it caused a stir in medical circles throughout Europe. "Disgusting polypharmacal messes", comments a modern pharmicist. "If the physicians and Senate were so favorably impressed with the superiority of this work, one cannot but wonder what must have been the character of the formulae that had previously been used.")[10]

As for Master-Surgeon John Gerard (1545–1607), whose very name is almost synonymous with Herbal in England – who can doubt that if he had lived today, he would no more have thought of going in for medicine than of apprenticing himself to a plumber? He would have been a landscape gardener, a Peter Coats, a Harry Wheatcroft. Every line of his enchanting *Herbal or General Historie of Plantes*, published in 1597, betrays the keen eye, the skill, the patience and the enthusiasm of the born gardener. "Talke of perfect happinesse or pleasure, and what place was so fit for that as the garden place where *Adam* was set to be the Herbarist?"[11]

The fact was that apart from a few botanizing enthusiasts, most physicians in the sixteenth and seventeenth centuries were not interested in pursuing the study of medicinal plants other than on paper, in elegant herbals, and within the straitjacket confines of the humoral approach with its endless categories and subdivisions. It seems to have occurred to few of them to investigate for themselves the action of the abundant home-grown medicinal plants that were available in fresh, reliable form, to test them singly on patients instead of in the appalling combinations of dozens of herbs that doctors usually prescribed, and to make notes of the results.

Both indifference to and ignorance about their native medicinal plants seems to have been almost universal, confirming Paracelsus' angry conviction that physicians and apothecaries were only impressed by exotic imported herbs, while scorning those in the local hedgerow. In the preface to his 1542 work on medicinal plants, the German physician Leonhart Fuchs (1501–1566) took his colleagues severely to task: ". . . by immortal God, is it to be wondered at that kings and princes do not at all regard the . . . investigation of plants, when even the physicians of our time so shrink from it that it is scarcely possible to find one among a hundred who has an accurate knowledge of even . . . a few plants?"[12]

William Turner (1520–1568), himself a physician and a distinguished graduate of Cambridge, made the same point in his preface to the *Herbal* he published in 1551: in his student days, he said, he had found it impossible to learn the names – Greek, Latin, or English – "amongst the Phisicions of any herb or tre, suche was the ignorance in simples at that tyme."[13]

Professional snobbery is the most likely explanation of this attitude. Perhaps at no time in history had the physician's training been so completely theoretical, with its emphasis on classical studies. The full degree course at Oxford or Cambridge lasted up to fourteen years, (Thomas Linacre, Henry VIII's personal physician, was thirty-two by the time he graduated), and included a solid grounding in the classics. Many of the wealthy young men who took up medicine went abroad to take their degrees, rounding off their education in the widest possible sense at Paris, Montpellier, Salerno, or Basel. Linacre himself was a Padua man, and a meticulous classical scholar, who had delved in Italian libraries for obscure early Greek medical texts to add to the canons of received knowledge, and published his own recension and translation of them.

The sheer length of his training must have convinced the sixteenth-century physician that all available medical knowledge was now at his fingertips. To men like these – a well-bred and exclusively-educated elite – it was unthinkable that anyone less well-trained than themselves should dare to describe himself as a doctor. It was even more unthinkable that the homegrown simples used by amateurs and by vast numbers of illiterate quacks might possibly be more effective than the grand compounds taken from Avicenna or Mesue which they prescribed for their wealthy patients.

And in the reign of Henry VIII these quacks and amateurs represented real competition to the physicians. It was bad enough that, as a result of the flood of herbals, doctoring with simples had become a fashionable amateur pastime: "for now [say they] every man without any study of necessary artes unto the knowledge of Phisick will become a Phisician . . . every man nay every old wyfe will presume, not without the mordre of many, to practyse Phisick.''[14] But as well as these presumptuous amateurs, England – and London in particular – was running over with self-styled medical practitioners of every kind.

There were, first, the surgeons, who had been making rapid strides professionally, since the invention of printing began adding to their knowledge and resources. Theoretically, surgeons were supposed to stick to surgery and leave internal medicine to the physicians, but many of them had quietly been developing into general practitioners under the very noses of the physicians. The brand-new scourge of syphilis had brought them plenty of profitable business, as well as a new class of customer, since syphilis cases were commonly referred to them: "upon the cure of Venereal disease . . . alone," it was reckoned, "the subsistence of three parts in four of all Surgeons in town depended".[15]

Hard on the heels of the surgeons proper, who had neither Guild nor Charter, came the Barber-Surgeons, a proud and independent City Company who had obtained a Royal Charter in 1462; but they, in turn, were expected to confine themselves only to the lower reaches of surgery – cupping, bleeding and tooth-extraction, activities advertised to this day by the blood-red stripes of the barber's pole.

Next in actual importance came the Apothecaries, who learned their craft as apprentices. The English apothecaries fancied that they knew quite as much about simple and compound medicines as any grand physician. Many of them probably did, but in hard fact, they were a mere cog in the wheel of the great and powerful Grocers' Company, who had received their Royal Charter even earlier than the Barber-Surgeons.

The apothecaries were expected to keep on hand stocks of all the drugs commonly used in medicine, from agrimony to unicorn's horn. But since their most profitable lines – the sugar confections, spices, syrups and electuaries which kept for months – were always being creamed off their business by the grocers, leaving them with deteriorating supplies of costly perishable drugs, many had no choice financially but to do a little prescribing on the side, and drum up extra business in that way.

Below these ranks of skilled or semi-skilled practitioners there swarmed, according to the preamble in the Letters Patent which gave Linacre his College of Physicians, "a great multitude of ignorant persons, of whom the greater part had no insight into physic, nor in any other kind of learning; some could not even read the letter on the book, so far forth, that common artificers, smiths, weavers and women, boldly and accustomably took upon them great cures, to the high displeasure of God, great infamy of the faculty, and the grievous hurt, damage and destruction of many of the King's liege people".[16]

It was, one suspects, those illiterate smiths and weavers who particularly stuck in the Physicians' gullet. But all the same, there was an obvious need for some form of supervision or control over this seething mass of practitioners, many of them foreigners. And although everyone could see it was unrealistic to insist on over-rigid lines of distinction in the country at large – where people simply tended to call on whatever form of medical aid happened to be available – London was another matter altogether, and its exploding population, which climbed from 30,000 to 200,000 during this century, made it particularly vulnerable to exploitation by quacks.

So it was with the full backing of both Henry and his Minister Wolsey that the Physicians pressed for legislation which would give them authority to deal with these abuses, and in 1512 Parliament passed the first of a series of acts designed to regulate the practice of medicine in London and the provinces. This Act dealt chiefly with London, restricting the practice of medicine within a seven-mile radius of London in the future to graduates of either Oxford or Cambridge, unless they had been licensed by the Bishop of London on the recommendation of four physicians.

Six years later, in 1518, the College of Physicians was set up by Letters Patent, as the formal regulatory body which such legislation obviously called for; and in 1523 the existence and authority of the College were not merely confirmed by Parliament but actually extended – at least in theory – over the whole country.

Neither Wolsey nor Linacre can have supposed for a moment that this system of control, however sweeping in theory, could be made effective in practice. What it did, however, was set up administrative and legal machinery, lacking until then, by which the worst abuses mentioned in the first act – those practitioners threatening "grievous hurt, damage and destruction" to their victims – could be dealt with. And this appears to have been the intention of Parliament.

It was not, however, the first object of the physicians, who following the very first Act of 1512 had almost immediately set in motion the first of a series of demarcation disputes which eventually touched off a sort of domino effect throughout the medical hierarchy: the physicians suing the surgeons for practising medicine, the surgeons rounding on the barbers for practising surgery, and both of them occasionally falling on the apothecary.

In another attempt to straighten out medical matters, Parliament passed two more Acts in the early 1540s, the first of which reconfirmed the authority of the Physicians, and gave them control over both surgeons and apothecaries; and the second of which formally united the Surgeons and Barber-Surgeons into one grand new Company, and gave them control over surgical matters in an area extending one mile around the City. As a sop to the surgeons, however, the barbers were now strictly forbidden to practise surgery.

These Acts, far from keeping everybody happy, simply produced a fresh crop of victims, since the surgeons, smarting under their new subjection to the physicians, but at least secure in their own rights, fell mercilessly upon some of the simple, unlicensed practitioners they felt were poaching in their preserves – women who had been giving medicine "for helyng of womens papes" or "giving water to young children to heal cankers in their mouths", and a brewer named Margetson "for giving water to cleanse men's yeese [eyes]".[17] But it turned out that far from being the docile victims the surgeons had imagined, at least one of them – the brewer – had friends in high places, and the retribution of Parliament was swift and severe.

In an Act worded with biblical eloquence, it castigated the surgeons who "minding onely their own lucre, and nothing the profit or ease of the diseased or Patient, have sued, troubled, and vexed divers honest persons, as well men as women, whom God hath endued with the knowledge of nature, kind and operation of certain Herbs, Roots and Waters, and the using and ministring of them, to such as has been pained with customable diseases, as Womens Breasts being sore, a Pin and the Web in the Eye, Uncomes of hands, Scaldings, Burnings, Sore mouths, the Stone, Strangury, Saucelim and Morphew, and such other like diseases: and yet the said persons have not taken anything for their pains or cunning, but have ministered the same to poor people onely for neighbourhood and God's sake, and pity and charity."

This behaviour, the Act continued, was in contrast to that of the surgeons who allowed many to "rot and perish to death for lack of help" because they could not pay; furthermore, "the most part of the persons of the said Craft of Surgery have small cunning, yet they will take great sums of money and do little therefore, and by reason thereof they do oftentimes impair and hurt their patients."

Since the greed and ignorance of the surgeons left a void in medical care for the poor, therefore, the Act proceeded to legalise an entirely new class of practitioners: ". . . it shall be lawfull to every person being the King's subject, having knowledge and experience of the nature of Herbs, Roots and Waters, or of the operation of same, by speculation or practice within any part . . . of the King's dominions, to practise, use and minister in and to any outward sore, uncome, wound, apostemations, outward swelling or disease, any herb or herbs, oyntments, baths, pultes and amplaisters, according to their cunning, experience and knowledge in any of the diseases, sores and maladies before-said, and all other like to the same, or drinks for the Stone and Strangury, or Agues, without suit, vexation, trouble, penalty, or loss of their goods."

The final words of the Act were a warning to the physicians, in turn, that they could not invoke any powers granted to them under previous legislation to meddle with the newly legalized herbalists: ". . . the foresaid Statute in the foresaid third year of the King's most gracious Reign, or any other Act, Ordinance or Statute to the contrary hereof made in any wise notwithstanding".[18]

To schoolboys and doctors this Act has been known ever since as the Quacks' Charter. Modern herbalists, however, have called it the Herbalists' Charter, since the insolent greed of a handful of Tudor surgeons not only ensured the survival of their profession, but provided a flimsy legal roof under which it has sheltered and flourished to this day in Britain.

Three things are immediately remarkable about this Act. The first is its plain implication that outside the ranks of professional physicians, traditional medicine still flourished, and there were numbers of honest people – women as well as men – who were skilled and knowledgeable about herbs, and perfectly capable of providing a much-needed medical service for the poor.

The second is the quite astonishing range of diseases which these practitioners were to be allowed to treat – a range far wider than that of the surgeon, in fact, since not only could they supply dressings, plasters, and ointments for "outward sores" and other disagreeable skin afflictions, but they could also give drinks – which was internal medicine, the physician's province – for three diseases. Any one of these three ailments would be serious enough in our time, and two of them were in Tudor days life-threatening: the stone, strangury (or pain on urinating), and agues. Few remedies suggested by sixteenth-century physicians were effective against the agonies of the stone (literally, small calculi trapped in the kidney or bladder); patients who had been treated to no avail could choose either to continue suffering, or to undergo the surgical operation of lithotomy, or being cut for the stone – an ordeal which even two centuries later, when it had been developed into a highly skilled, swift and routine operation, the diarist Evelyn's brother died rather than undergo.

There are, however, highly effective plant remedies for the stone – an insignificant creeping plant called pellitory-of-the-wall (*Parietaria officinalis*), being one of them – and some of the City practitioners may have built a reputation for cures of the stone by using them.

Several herbs, usually with a marked diuretic action, have been found useful in urinary problems: the herbalists probably prescribed butcher's broom (*Ruscus aculeatus*), recommended by Dioscorides for such cases; horsetail (*Equisetum arvense*); or the tiny creeping scarlet pimpernel (*Anagallis arvensis*).

Ague in Tudor times was almost synonymous with malaria, which was then endemic in northern Europe. Although it was the milder of the two forms of malaria, caused by the parasite *Plasmodium vivax*, it was a debilitating disease, characterized by bouts of tertian, or recurrent, fever, which often led to chronic anæmia, and none of the classic treatments for it were very effective in the days before quinine. Plenty of country wise-women claimed to have a cure for it, though; the nineteenth-century Dr. Thornton in his Herbal tells the story of an old man who performed wonderful cures of ague and other diseases with the herb tormentil (*Potentilla tormentilla*), and became so cele-brated for them locally that Lord William Russell gave him a piece of land in which to cultivate his miracle herb.[19]

The third point, and perhaps the most striking, to be made about this Act is that it makes plain that however contemptuous physicians and surgeons may have been of the herbalists with their "simples", they had powerful friends in high places (Henry VIII included) who had a very considerable opinion of their skills, and thought that they deserved protection and encouragement – and possibly patronage too.

The offhand way in which Parliament, by this Act, legalized the practice of scores of illiterate nobodies shook the College to its foun-dations, and although the Act had seemed to be directed entirely against the surgeons, many of them actually took advantage of its deplorably vague phrasing to extend their practice.

What was threatened by the Act, moreover – as the doctors could see only too well – was the authority of the proud physicians: how could it be otherwise if any old woman with a glimmering of knowledge or skill should be allowed to take on diseases by which distinguished scholars and gentlemen, with years of training behind them, were defeated?

More than a century later Dr. Charles Goodall (1642–1712), a Fellow of what had by then been raised to the dignity of Royal College of Physicians, wrote a long account of its gallant struggles against "Empiricks and unlicensed Practisers." Largely an exercise in public relations, Goodall's book was intended to prove that the College had been devoting its energies for decades to the extermination of unscrupulous and restless quacks, even when these were protected by the highest in the land, as an extraordinary number of them in fact appear to have been; and some fairly horrific accounts of mercurial excesses and backstreet abortion rackets emerge from it.

What is also clear is how seriously the College took the challenge to their professional status represented by "the Quacks' " Charter, and how savagely they hounded down the modest practitioners of traditional herbal medicine.

In 1581, for instance, the College pounced on "one Margaret Kennix, an outlandish, ignorant, sorry woman", whose practice in ministering to her neighbours and charging for her services too was stopped by the College.[20] It turned out they had caught a tartar: this "sorry woman" boldly complained to no less a person than the Queen. Now Elizabeth, as it happened, was just as much interested in medicine as her father Henry VIII, and just as much given to dabbling in pharmacy, having once composed a tonic for heart and brain containing amber, musk, and civet dissolved in spirit of roses, which she sent to the Emperor Rudolf II.

Elizabeth may have felt an amateur's sympathy for another amateur, she may have suspected that the physicians were needlessly tiresome and overbearing, or she may simply have had a flicker of fellow-feeling for another woman struggling to keep her end up in a man's world. Whatever the reason, Elizabeth took a personal interest in this case, inquired carefully into the circumstances, and being satisfied that Margaret Kennix was no threat to her subjects' lives, directed Walsingham to write to the physicians.

It was, he duly wrote, "her Majesty's pleasure that the poore woman shoold be permitted by you quietly to practice and mynister to the curing of diseases and wounds, by the meanes of certain Simples, in the application whereof it seemeth God hath gieven her an especiall knowledge." There followed a courteous threat: "I shall therefore desire you . . . to take order amongst yourselves for the readmitting of her into the quiet exercise of her small talent, least by the renewing of her complaint to her Majesty through your hard dealing towards her, you procure further inconvenience thereby to your selfe."

The College was not inclined to take this lying down: they could not possibly reconcile it with their conscience, they wrote firmly back, to "allow either her [or any other person not qualified accordingly] to intrude themselves into so great and daungerous a Vocation . . . to the evident daunger of the life and health of such her Majesties most loving subjects, as shall be abused by their notorious and wilful ignorance."[21]

The College had their revenge on Walsingham for meddling when five years later, in 1586, he wrote again on behalf of an Empirick, asking them to have released from prison a man named Not, "forasmuch as both my self have heretofore used him, and divers other Gentlemen have also received good by him." In their reply, the College mentioned tongue in cheek that Not "protesteth openly (and that most infamously as we think and offensively to the credit and good name of such as admit him to their persons) that he dealeth with none but onely for the Pocks."[22]

By the end of the sixteenth century, however, the question of the unlicensed practitioner, though still a nagging preoccupation, was no longer foremost in the minds of the College physicians. The burning issue of the day – an issue which split the College itself into two violently opposed factions – was whether or not they could bring themselves to approve the new chemical medicine, which was rapidly making converts among professional physicians all over Europe.

6

"All Manner of Minerals"

At Christmas 1603, the small market-town of Exeter was rocked by a juicy medical scandal. Dr. John Woolton, a respectable physician, had sent a letter so highly offensive in its hints and accusations to Thomas Edwards, one of the town's most popular apothecaries, that Edwards intended to sue for libel. The case was to be heard in Star Chamber the following spring; over the next few months details of just what Woolton had said leaked out, and medical opinion began lining up on one side or the other.

On the face of it, it was a straight case of professional jealousy. Woolton was an Oxford man and one of the local gentry: his father had been Bishop of Exeter, and he seems to have been a physician of sound conservative views. But Edwards, although an apothecary, was no mere tradesman. His medical training had included a spell at Oxford, his business was highly successful – in 1602 his premises were taxed as highly as those of two physicians put together – and in 1600 he had been made Sheriff. He had only recently begun to practice medicine, but he was already so popular that many of the local gentry became his patients, attracted perhaps by the impressively up-to-date chemical medicines that he used.

To Woolton, however, Edwards typified the reckless upstarts who were ruining a decent old-fashioned profession, and the letter which finally goaded Edwards into legal action may have been the culmination of months of bitter professional attacks on him the physician. He taunted Edwards with his apothecary's training: "Mr. Trivett your master taught you not to go beyond your mortar and pestle;" accused him of dishonest dealings; and then came to what he must have felt was the most damning indictment of all – that Edwards used such

mineral drugs as "Stibium, Mercury crude, precipitate [and] sublimate, Turbith Mineral, Borax Crystalline, Ratsbane, Vitriol, Brim-
stone, Aqua Fortis."

C. S. Roberts, who exhumed the details of this fascinating case from
Star Chamber records, comments that "this rivalry was as much one
between the old and the new, as between a physician and an apothecary as such: Woolton ended his letter by telling Edwards to burn his
prescriptions and make salt of the ashes 'which you [I know] can do
being a perfect Paracelsan.' "[1]

Apart from any resentment he may have felt at Edwards's success,
Woolton clearly had the deepest distrust of the Paracelsian medicine
that Edwards practised. He accused the apothecary of aggravating the
illness of one patient, Sir William Courtenay – that Woolton had lost
to him – by excessive bleeding, and the administering of eight strong
purges and one vomit inside fourteen days. And he suggested that
many other patients of Edwards had "either miserably perished or
been greatly endangered of their lives".[2]

Woolton was found guilty of libel, heavily fined and ordered to pay
damages to Edwards, but to any doctor following the case, it must
have seemed that not one angry man but the new medicine itself had
been on trial in Exeter. In every sense, the new medicine had won, and
this country-town scandal mirrored a conflict which had been raging
in the ranks of the medical profession for the last twenty-five years: the
new "chemical" medicine as both its supporters and its critics called
it – or the old Galenic kind?

The first faint whiff of the new chemical approach to medicine had
drifted into England as early as 1527 with the publication of *The
Vertuose Boke of Distyllacion*, charmingly written by the German
Hieronymus Brunschwig, a manual of instructions on how to distil
different kinds of waters from herbs, bits of animal, and insects for
medical use. Brunschwig strongly expressed the alchemical view that
these distilled waters were superior medicine precisely because they
were distilled, which produced a "puryfyeing of the grosse from the
subtyll and the subtyll from the grosse." The resulting medicine
worked much faster than a Galenic medicine "mynystered with her
corpus or substance in the manner of electuaryes, confeccyons,
powders or syrops" which tended to weaken and enfeeble the body.[3]

Brunschwig's book was popular enough to run rapidly through
three editions, and the new idea of distilled medicines caught on with
apothecaries – the resulting waters were certainly prettier to look at

than the usual muddy infusions. Distillation was even more popular with housewives. By the end of the century every home that could afford one had its "still-room" (in its original meaning) and good housewives knew all about working a still. At the same time the idea that its products were both purer and more powerful germinated gently in the public mind, to be reinforced thirty years later when Conrad Gesner's *The Treasure of Euonymus* was published in England in 1559.

Gesner, whose name was probably familiar to many English physicians from his botanical works, set out to prove in his book that the use of chemistry in medicine was highly respectable and could be traced back to the Greeks. He gave details for preparing quintessences and oils from metals such as lead or antimony, and he restated emphatically the alchemical view that by such techniques "al the vertue . . . is separated from the substance of the medicine, so that . . . the more pure and subtil part of every remedy or medicine, maye be . . . drawn out from the grosse and erthy part".[4]

These fine theories were all very well: what the physicians saw in practice were the hordes of "Paracellis" quacks with their irresponsible and disastrous mercurial treatments for the pox: some of them were already being hauled before the College by this time.

And it was the progressive surgeons of England, rather than its conservative physicians, who first began to use the new chemical medicines they had read about in Continental works on surgery.

Men like William Clowes, John Banister, and George Baker were, it has been said, "the most enterprising and enlightened group of surgeons or indeed, medical practitioners of any kind, in England at that time".[5] They knew of Vesalius' work in Padua, which was making it clear that the great Galen could occasionally be wrong, and they took the sensible, open-minded view that if the new medicines worked they should be adopted without delay.

By the 1570s, there were at least three apothecaries in London preparing and selling them: "one mayster Kemech an Englishe man dwelling in Lothburie, another mayster Geffray, a French man dwelling in the Crouched friars, men of singular knowledge that way, another named John Hester dwelling on Powles wharfe. . . ."[6] It was the surgeon George Baker who publicized these progressive apothecaries in his writings, adding ". . . I . . . have . . . used of their medicines to the furtherance of my Pacients healthes".[7]

It was the surgeons, too, with the apothecaries hard on their heels, who were the first to familiarize themselves with the action of the new plant drugs – guaiacum, sarsaparilla, China root – thought to be effective in venereal disease, and to popularize their use. And it was the surgeons, once more, who in the 1570s and 80s began to pour out a steady stream of books in English, publicizing and extolling the new medicine.

Just what, exactly, was this "chemical" medicine which was giving rise to such burning debate all over Europe? In what way did it differ from the old Galenical kind? Its advocates – in England surgeons such as Baker and Clowes – did their best to explain.

The modern "chemical" practitioner continued to draw on the whole Galenic battery of medicinal plants, but he boldly added to his materia medica an arsenal of minerals, many of them active poisons such as arsenic and antimony, others known to be acutely toxic such as mercury or vitriol. He was able to do this, he claimed, because the chemical techniques by which these mineral medicines were prepared rendered them virtually harmless: "by Distillation are corrected the malignitie or venimous qualities thereof, as in oyles of Quicksilver, of oyle of Vitrioll, Antimonie. . . ."[8]

The tremendous and long-drawn out battering to which minerals were subjected in the laboratories did more, it was believed, than render them harmless: such techniques liberated their hidden therapeutic potential to act directly and powerfully upon the body of the patient. Banister's *Storehouse of Physicall and Philosophical Secrets* (1583) gave directions how to "prepare, calcine, sublime and dissolve all manner of Minerals, and how you shall draw forth their Oyles and Salts, which are most wonderfull in their operations, for the healthe of mans body. . . ."[9]

Plants and minerals alike were in need of this refinement, suggested the chemists, to purge them of undesirable side-effects, and unlock the "more pure and subtil part" of the medicine. And oils and distillations laboriously prepared from plants now took the place of the old haphazard Galenic compounds. Some of these must have taken days of painstaking brewing and careful watching: Clowes' Oil of Lilies, for instance, poetically called for fresh flowers to be steeped in oil, left in the sun for seven or eight days, simmered in a *bain-marie* for four or five hours and cooled; fresh flowers were then added, and the whole process repeated several times more, the last infusion to stand in the sun "a month or five weeks" before a final simmering and straining. But it was worth while going to so much trouble since "These unguents and Oiles", asserted Clowes, were "very profitable in these unctions wherein goeth quicksilver, whose mallice and force . . . may be killed sufficientlie to be used. . . ."[10]

It should be pointed out, indeed, that the "chemical" surgeons – far from abandoning plants, continued to rely heavily on them, often to counteract the irritant or corrosive action of the minerals they were using: plants with a proven cooling, or soothing, or antiseptic, or astringent, or healing action turn up again and again in the Antidotaries of men like Clowes and Banister, often quoted directly from Paracelsus. And the simple distilled waters of such healing plants as plantain (*Plantago major*), marigold (*Calendula officinalis*), St. John's Wort (*Hypericum perforatum*), and lady's mantle (*Alchemilla vulgaris*), must often have been responsible for the impressive success of the "new" medicine.

Chemical medicine certainly both looked and sounded more impressive than the old Galenical kind. And in the range of "outward" cases which were the special province of surgeons, they must often have seemed magically effective. Plasters of lead or copper sulphate were cooling and drying for "all foule Ulcerations and filthy sores";[11] antimony is a fast – if painful – way of scouring clean an open festering wound; arsenic and mercury salts were fatal to the parasites so often responsible for the "social" diseases often seen by surgeons – scabies, the itch and so on.

Unluckily for the patients, there was a hidden surcharge to their bills. Salts and powders prepared from minerals and poisons did not, as it was fondly supposed, lack the "malignitie" of the untreated substances – the reverse was very often true. And since toxic substances were readily absorbed into the bloodstream through the open wounds they were applied to, many of these apparently innocent and wonder-working cures must have left a trail of deadly side–effects in the form of systemic poisoning. Even mild lead poisoning, for instance, can cause gastro–intestinal problems, anorexia, and lowered resistance to infection; arsenic can damage heart, kidneys, and bone-marrow. Some of these side–effects might have taken years to show up, others manifesting themselves only as a general loss of vitality or energy.

Even the more acute and violent side–effects, however, were probably seldom ascribed to the surgeon's excellent cooling plaster. Even today, when all doctors are aware of the side–effects problem, it can take years for cause and effect to be associated: surgeons like Baker, Clowes, and the new generation of progressive surgeons were probably blissfully ignorant of the damage they were doing. And by the end of the sixteenth century, medical chemists all over Europe were feverishly experimenting with every metal or mineral known to man, reacting it with other chemicals, turning it into salts or oils, and then administering it to a patient. There were so many interesting things you could do to a metal or a mineral in a sixteenth-century chemical laboratory, but given the limited equipment of the time, there was not really very much that could be done to a plant. By the end of the century, extracts, distillates and alcoholic tinctures were commonplace, so popular with housewives that doctors disdained them. Apothecaries liked them too, finding these elegant new presentations highly marketable. Certainly they were likely to be better and simpler medicine than the long-stewed and complicated syrupy brews advocated in the old medieval antidotaries, if only because chemically prepared oils and tinctures were sterile as water-extracts were not.

But in attempting other chemical ways of "purifying" plants, or getting at their "quintessence" or "arcana" as Paracelsus would have called it, the chemists found themselves at a loss. It seems to have been generally assumed that every medicinal plant contained what we now call its active principle, which was responsible for its medicinal action, and that all the other parts of the plant were no more than the gross body to this ethereal soul, and the sooner discarded the better.

The chemists attempted to do this in various ways: by boiling down the tincture till only solids remained, by distillation or by incinerating the plant and preparing fixed salts from the ashes.

Since few plants are identical in their mode of action, some of the "quintessences" that resulted may have been completely inert, others quite effective medically – though not necessarily in the way that had been anticipated – and others again dangerously toxic. If you burn scurvy grass to ashes, for instance, the ashes will no longer contain the Vitamin C which made the plant effective against scurvy. When a tobacco leaf goes up in smoke, on the other hand, the alkaloid nicotine that it contains decomposes into a variety of lethal substances (including traces of hydrocyanic acid and carbon monoxide).

But the chemists were groping in the dark. They had never looked at a plant through the, as yet uninvented, microscope. They did not know that its healing powers might be due to a dozen different alkaloids or to one alone. They did not known that even should they succeed in isolating the "active principle" of the plant, it might be much weaker or even inert without the interaction of the "grosse" parts they had discarded – or that on its own it might be a powerful poison.

They did not know that a plant may consist of acids, sugars, alkaloids, glycosides, starch, gums, resins, volatile oil, tannin, mucilage, esters, steroids, vitamins, traces of minerals, traces of metals. They had no idea of the awe-inspiring chemical complexity that exists in one small plant, or that it lives, grows, breathes, transpires, has its own circulatory system, responds to stimuli, ages, and at last dies in so extraordinary a green mimicry of man himself that here, if anywhere in nature, is Paracelsus' microcosm of man to be found. The very lifeblood of the plant – its green chlorophyll – has a chemical formula almost identical to that of hæmoglobin, the red pigment in human blood which keeps oxygen circulating in our bodies.

The sixteenth-century chemist knew nothing of all this, and, understandably, it was metals that he found most interesting, and which seemed to hold out the most brilliant therapeutic promise. In Oswald Croll's *Basilica Chymica*, which the modern Paracelsan scholar Robert Multhauf has described as "perhaps the most clear and comprehensive statement of what the chemical remedies were," plants were already relegated to a subordinate place, although some of the more active were used chemically treated – scammony prepared with spirit of vitriol, for instance, or combined with mineral or metal ingredients.[12]

If the new Paracelsan medicines had arrived packaged together with the heretical anti-Galen theories of Paracelsus himself, most physicians of the time would have found it impossible to accept them, since the Galenic system of humours and elements was still the foundation of all medical training and practice. But even the most ardent of the Paracelsans tended to find that there yawned a curious gap between the alchemical speculations of Paracelsus and the medicine that was supposed to result from their application in practice.[13] And however much Galen himself might have frowned on some of the chemical poisons that patients were now being asked to swallow, they were still being given for the sound old Galenical purpose of adjusting the humours by "evacuation", as Multhauf points out. In other words, because they provoked sweating, vomiting, urine or bowel movements, and thus were thought to help the body expel disease in one of these four ways.[14]

What had specially struck Monardes about sarsaparilla was its diaphoretic powers – it worked miracles with agues, he thought, "by provokying of swet, in this it doth exceede all other Medicines."

Oswald Croll arranged his chemical medicines in these categories familiar to any physician – vomitives, purgatives, diuretics and diaphoretics, with a few cordials and sedatives for good measure.

The new chemical medicines certainly provoked these four kinds of evacuations even more impressively – and much more predictably and controllably – than galenicals, since the sweating and the vomiting, the bowel and the bladder activity that they induced were the body's way of expelling these inorganic poisons. And salts of mercury was the most impressive of them all since as we have seen, the human body, in its convulsive efforts to rid itself of this deadly substance, resorts to a fifth kind of evacuation – by the saliva.

It was thus perfectly possible for a doctor to have the deepest mistrust of Paracelsus and all his "exalted essences foolosophically extracted", as surgeon Clowes put it – and still welcome the Paracelsan medicine as useful additions to the pharmacopœia.[15] Clowes probably spoke for practical, moderate medical men all over Europe when he concluded: "If I finde (eyther by reason or experience) any thing that may be to the good of the Patients, and better increase of my knowledge and skil in the Arte of Chirurgery, be it eyther in Galen or Paracelsus; yes, Turks, Iewe, or any other infidell; I will not refuse it, but be thankful to God for the same".[16]

Clowes was writing in England in 1602, where Elizabeth had recently died after forty-five long and glorious years on the throne. A new century had opened with a new reign: appropriately, even the conservative College of Physicians was slowly coming round to the new medicine. As early as 1585, in fact, the College had planned a national pharmacopœia – the first of its kind in Europe – which was to include a whole section of extracts, salts, chemicals and metals, although the project had been dropped before it reached publication.

By contrast, the Medical Faculty of Paris was rabidly reactionary: diehard Galenists to the last man, and alert to the first sniff of heresy. They were disgusted when Henri IV actually appointed a young Swiss Paracelsan, Theodore Turquet de Mayerne (1573–1655), to be one of his personal physicians, and then continued to heap honours and appointments on him.

Mayerne had studied medicine at Montpellier (as progressive then as Paris was reactionary) and was deeply interested in the medical possibilities of chemistry – at the age of twelve, he was already sketching beautiful little stills in his school notebooks. When it became known that he was quite openly using mercury and other metals in his practice, one of the Paris Faculty published a scathing attack on this anti-Galenist.

Mayerne issued a dignified reply – in response to which another abusive pamphlet came hurtling back – and the Paris Faculty seized on this pretext to condemn his writings, forbade other physicians to consult with him, and advised Henri IV to remove him from his public posts. The King was deeply attached to his doctor, thought the world of him, and continued to employ and honour him, ignoring the shrill denunciations of the Faculty. But when his Royal patron was assassinated in May 1610, Mayerne must have realized that his career prospects in Paris had ceased to exist. Before he had time to wonder what to do next, a messenger arrived: King James I, who had met him and been deeply impressed by him, now invited him to London as his personal physician. Mayerne accepted.

Discreet, skilful and delightful, Mayerne seems to have been one of those rare and lucky mortals on whom honours fall as naturally as sunshine. He served three kings and their consorts, tended Prince Henry, the much-loved heir to the throne when he was fatally struck by typhoid at the age of seventeen – his father Charles I wrote a special certificate absolving Mayerne from all blame for his failure to save him – and counted some of the noblest and wealthiest families in London among his patients. In 1645 he was voted an unprecedented honour by Parliament which was not, at that time, disposed to look kindly on Royal favourites (they beheaded King Charles four years later). By a majority of three, they exempted Mayerne for life from all taxation, to mark their esteem for "a man whose extraordinary abilities would make him welcome in any part of Christendom".[17]

It was to be expected that such a personality, in a position of such eminence, should have a decisive influence in shaping the medical decisions of his day, and the mere fact that Mayerne habitually used chemical medicines in his own practice almost immediately conferred on them both prestige and respectability in English eyes.

He used them boldly and confidently: in syphilis cases, where Paracelsus would have suggested doses of a grain of mercury at a time, Mayerne prescribed pills made of Venice turpentine and gold leaf, each of which contained twenty grains of mercury – nearly one and a half grammes. For a case of eczema, he advised a solution of mercury – diluted with rose-water and an extract of plantain – as a soothing wash; for a case of worms in a twelve-year-old child his suggestion was a twelve-grain mercury purge which was, to put it mildly, drastic.[18]

In other respects, however, his prescriptions were completely orthodox, calling for plenty of the enormously elaborate galenical compounds which kept apothecaries prosperous, so the College took heart from his example. When in 1618 the first London Pharmacopœia was prepared for the press, it was to Mayerne that they entrusted the section containing those chemical medicines which almost everyone now agreed ought to be included. It was probably Mayerne, too, who composed the tactful and conciliating little note on these newcomers in the Preface: "we venerate the age-old learning of the ancients and for this reason we have placed their remedies at the beginning, but on the other hand, we neither reject nor spurn the new subsidiary medicines of the more recent chemists and we have conceded to them a place and corner in the rear so that they might be as a servant to the dogmatic medicine, and thus they might act as auxiliaries."[19]

Mayerne's copy of this 1618 pharmacopœia, with his own notes indicating the sources for each chemical, is preserved in the British Museum. He took *Mercurius Dulcis* from Croll's *Basilica Chymica*, where Croll describes the ingenious chemical process by which "there may be killed the destructive spirit of vitriol and salt in mercury sublimate," leaving behind only "a crystalline, completely tasteless powder."[20]

Croll was lyrical about the amazing properties of this innocuous-looking substance: "one of the most outstanding cathartics, by itself as well as combined with other drugs for internal medical use, it rapidly expels from the body anything harmful. This will not appear miraculous to those who know that mercury is nature's balsam, in which is the virtue of incarnation and regeneration mysteriously renewed and freed from all impurities."[21]

Mercurius Dulcis, eventually rechristened calomel, almost immediately became the most popular of all the mercurial preparations. The mysterious metal which Paracelsus had considered almost too dangerous for general use, even in syphilis cases, was now widely accepted as a useful all-purpose purge, and the way was now open for other poisonous metals and minerals – arsenic and antimony among them – to enter the lists against disease.

Medicines so very "active" were hardly likely to be considered mere auxiliaries for very long.

7

Galen
or Paracelsus?

"I never advance to the attack upon the diseases of Royalty without a crowd of Asclepiades fighting whole-heartedly by my side . . ." wrote Mayerne wryly to a friend in 1636.[1] On both sides of the Channel in the seventeenth century, royalty could be sure of plenty of doctoring, and of no monarch was this more true than of Louis XIV. Wherever the Sun King moved, a phalanx of physicians, surgeons, and apothecaries moved with him. A coachload of medical attendants followed closely behind the Royal carriage if he left Versailles; there were doctors waiting at his bedside when he awoke in the morning, doctors present when he retired for the night, doctors in anxious attendance as he sat at table.

In any illness, every smallest detail of his physical state down to the last drop of urine was monitored with a thoroughness we should find intolerable. And in a handsome bound volume, his personal physicians kept a day-to-day record of his health, illnesses, and medical treatment. Louis XIV, who was thoroughly conscious of his own significance, used to pick up the *Journal de la santé du roi* and read it attentively from time to time, so the doctors – under the twin inhibitions of being read by their patient and writing for posterity – were inclined to be both unctuous and evasive.

It seems fairly clear, for instance, that in the spring of 1655 the seventeen-year-old Louis contracted a venereal infection, probably gonorrhœa. His personal physician of the time, Antoine Vallot (1594–1671), was informed that the Royal shirts were so heavily stained by a thick greenish-yellow discharge from his penis, "that it was imposible to get out the marks either with washing-powder or with soap." This "incommodité", which lasted seven months, and caused Vallot great anxiety and embarrassment, was officially ascribed by him, in the *Journal*, to "a weakness of the spermatic vessels", combined with long hours on horseback and too much violent exercise. No question, wrote Vallot, of an unclean and dishonourable pollution, since the King lived "in pure and unexampled chastity".[2]

On the whole, Louis XIV submitted patiently to the attentions of his doctors, though on two points he was rebellious. He refused to consider cutting down on the gigantic meals which his doctors – no doubt rightly – considered the cause of some of his medical problems; and he loathed being bled, probably because he had been bled so much in his youth. After a bleeding in 1663 which was very nearly disastrous – "the blood came out with such violence that we had trouble stopping it", noted a shaken Vallot, his chief physician at the time – the King put his foot down and refused to be bled any more.[3]

Having taken this firm stand on bleeding, however, he was obliged to yield in another direction, since purging and bleeding were the twin props of seventeenth-century therapy. From that moment, the *bouillon purgatif*, usually concocted from fairly drastic ingredients such as scammony and jalap, figures prominently in the *Journal*. Fagon, his last doctor, was a particularly enthusiastic purger, and noted on one occasion that the wretched monarch had been purged to a bloody extreme – "a red stool . . . after thirteen prodigious stools", he noted happily.[4]

The importance of "evacuation" was one point on which all seventeenth-century French doctors could agree: how it was to be achieved and to what extent was matter for the most violent controversy. In Paris as in London, the debate could be summed up in three words: Galen or Paracelsus? There was never the slightest doubt whose side the Paris faculty was on, as Mayerne had discovered.

The conservatism of this stately 300-year-old closed shop was personified in the physician Gui Patin (1602–1672), for many years one of its most distinguished and outstanding members, twice its Dean, at all times its eloquent spokesman. The son of sound bourgeois parents, Gui had been sent to Paris to study philosophy, entered Paris University to study medicine at the age of twenty-one, and received his *licence* at the age of twenty-seven, becoming a member of that Faculty to which he was wholeheartedly and jealously devoted until his death in 1673.

The Paris medical school in the seventeenth century was a shrine to the memory of Galen and Hippocrates, along with some of the lesser medical lights of antiquity, and its teaching consisted almost entirely of endless studies, in both Greek and Latin, of the sacred texts. For Patin – unlike Paracelsus – this was a curriculum which could hardly be improved upon. He carried to his grave the conviction that Galen had been more often and more consistently right about medical matters than any other physician since, and he advised young medical students to stick to these masters, or else to sound orthodox commentators on them. "Read only Hippocrates, Galen, Aristotle, Fernel, Hollier . . . learn by heart, if you do not know them already all the 'Aphorisms' of Hippocrates. . . . There are three treatises by Galen which you should choose and read something frequently in them. . . . Do not lose your time reading many of the moderns who only make books of our art from lack of practice, and from having too much leisure", he advised a young medical student in 1646.[5]

For the Arabs, Patin had no time at all. Their one contribution to medicine, in his view, was that disgusting polypharmacy which was good for nothing but the enriching of apothecaries. "What good are all these compositions, all these sugared and honeyed alteratives? . . . We save more sick people with a good lancet and a pound of senna than the Arabians can with their syrups and opiates. . . . The great abuse of medicine is due to the multiplicity of useless remedies and the neglect of bloodletting."[6]

Patin himself was in no danger of neglecting bloodletting. "I had a bad toothache yesterday", he wrote to a friend at the age of sixty, "which obliged me to have myself bled. . . . The pain stopped all at once, as by a kind of enchantment. . . ."[7] For a bad cold, he once prescribed for himself seven bloodlettings, and he quoted with approval the case of Cousinot who as a young man contracted severe rheumatism: for the next eight months he was bled twice weekly on his father's instructions. Nobody, according to Patin, was too young or too old to be bled with profit: one of Patin's patients, a M. Merlet, was bled eighteen times for a malignant fever at the age of sixty-six; another patient, a seven-year-old boy, survived being bled thirteen times in a fortnight for pleurisy.

If Patin's patients seldom escaped a bleeding, they were at least spared the worst excesses of seventeenth-century pharmacy. The *Pharmacopœia* of Jean de Renou, published in 1608 and reissued in 1637, lists some of the more nauseating items an apothecary might be called upon to dispense: "One uses many entire animals, such as cantharides, centipedes, worms, lizards, ants, vipers, scorpions, frogs. . . . As to the parts of animals our physicians hold assuredly and truly that they are endowed with many and admirable virtues . . . the skull or the head of a man dead but not yet buried . . . the brain of antelopes . . . the intestines of the wolf . . . the genitalia of the deer . . . fat of man . . . human blood . . . the toe nails of an eland . . . pearls . . . the scales of many fishes. Finally, since the excrementes of the said animals have also their particular virtues, it is not unfitting for the pharmacist to keep them in his shop, especially the dung of the goat, hog, swan, peacock, pigeon, muskrat, civet. . . ."[8]

All these substances were routinely prescribed by doctors. Mayerne himself suggested white peacock's dung for a case of epilepsy; Louis XIV believed that ants were aphrodisiac; pearls were thought to be good for your heart; topaz was excellent for diarrhœa; gold was a wonderful all-round tonic, although silver often stained its takers a curious shade of blue – for life.

M. Antoine d'Aquin (1620?–1696), Louis' physician for more than twenty years, invented a startling remedy composed of pearls, hyacinths, corals, male peony root gathered during the waning of the moon, scrapings from the skull of a man who had died a violent death, and the nails of the eland. Mme. de Sévigné swore by essence of human urine – she took eight drops when she had the vapours, a seventeenth-century way of saying a fit of the blues.

If you suffered from pimples, you bribed a midwife to procure a human afterbirth for you to apply to your face – if it was still warm, so much the better. While mother's milk was not always thought good for babies – fashionable doctors often switched their tiny charges to *bouillie*, a mixture of cereal and cows' milk, instead – it was often recommended for those who had entered their second childhood: the great Duke of Alva had two wet-nurses in his old age.

As for the compounds prescribed by doctors, they must have taxed the integrity of even honest apothecaries, for how could the most searching of the twice-annual inspections to which they were supposed to submit establish that their *Eau de Vie de Dresde* contained just exactly the 118 different ingredients it was supposed to, all in good condition, and mixed in the correct proportions?

Patin thought that most of this was utter nonsense. He wrote to a friend in 1647 that he was preparing a grand exposé of "the bezoar, the cordial waters, the unicorn's horn, theriac, the confections of hyacinth and alkermes, the precious fragments and other arabesque bagatelles".[9] In his own practice he limited himself to the simplest and mildest of laxatives and purges – *pauca sed probata*, he was fond of saying: few but well-tried. His great favourite was senna, the perfect reliable purge, a drug he valued so highly that he could hardly bring himself to believe that it had reached the West via the despised Arabs. He also liked mild laxative syrups of pale roses or peach flowers, and sometimes cassia, rhubarb, or prune juice. Having given nature a good dig in the ribs with his lancet, Patin was happy to leave the rest to her.

In many ways he was well ahead of his time: he was very much opposed to the artificial feeding of babies – so common then in fashionable circles – and thought nothing could possibly be better for them than their natural food, breast-milk. Anticipating the discovery of antibodies by nearly three centuries, he was convinced from his own observation that artificially-fed babies were more susceptible to infectious diseases like smallpox and whooping-cough.

The great fortune that Patin amassed suggests that this mild Hippocratic practice was thoroughly popular with his patients: at the peak of his career, Patin had a large, handsome house in Paris with a library filled with well-bound books – he was an avid bibliophile – a well-stocked wine-cellar, and a country estate for which he had paid a small fortune.

But it·has to be admitted that the simple prescriptive habits of Gui Patin were not solely inspired by the desire to do good to his patients: a desire to do ill to the Paris apothecaries was at least as strong a motive. Relations between the Faculty and the apothecaries had been bitter for as long as anyone could remember – a running power struggle in which the physicians, as usual, tried to gain the upper hand, and the apothecaries, as usual, wanted independence and the right to practise medicine themselves.

The London physicians had sensibly arranged a truce with the apothecaries, helping them to establish themselves as an independent City Company in exchange for their agreement to accept the supervision of the College. The 1618 *Pharmacopœia*, crammed with the costly compounds so dear to the apothecary's heart, as well as the controversial chemicals, had sealed the bargain.

The Paris Faculty by contrast, far from attempting to improve the lot of "those arabesque cooks," as Patin had described them, had done its very best to grind their faces in the dust, even going so far as to publish edition after edition of a do-it-yourself medical guide, *Le médecin charitable*, which showed the poor how to make their own simple medicines for no more than a few sous, and even prepare and administer an enema. Patin exulted that with this work "we have ruined the apothecaries of Paris," and he lost no chance of being spiteful about them. In 1647 he published a violent attack on their profession in the form of a thesis. The long-suffering apothecaries had had enough: they brought an action against him in the court of the *Parlement de Paris*. Nothing could have delighted Patin more. The case was the talk of Paris, and hundreds jammed the courtroom to enjoy the fun. Patin conducted his own defence, delivered a witty and pointed attack on the apothecaries, was cheered resoundingly, and won his case.

Not all Patin's considerable reserves of spleen, however, were squandered on the apothecaries. He had another, much more significant target for his anger, and his fiercest professional criticisms were reserved for the Faculty of Montpellier, those reckless advocates of mineral poisons.

Montpellier was a medieval city of Provence, literally built on mercury: the English philosopher John Locke, who studied medicine there in 1675, remembered being told that running quicksilver was often to be seen when the cellars of old houses were dug up. The Medical School, raised on this untappable mine of mercury and situated on the frontiers of the Arab world, was devoted to the new chemical medicine. Where Paris was conservative, Montpellier was progressive and innovative; where Paris was for Galen, Montpellier vaunted Paracelsus. Where Paris used senna – Montpellier preferred antimony.

Antimony is a powerful irritant poison, with a record of medical use dating back thousands of years: but Dioscorides and Galen, Hippocrates and Pliny had reserved it for external use. It was the Arabs, once again, who had experimented with it for internal use, and the Paracelsans who had brought it into widespread practice, usually in the form of emetic wine – wine which had stood for some time in a cup made of antimony, and had absorbed some of the metal. Peter Severinus, the Danish Paracelsan, described antimony with enthusiasm as the Prince of Evacuants – and with reason: the human system reacted even to small doses so violently that it could drastically purge a patient, cause him to vomit, and bring out a heavy sweat almost in the same breath. When antimony was not expelled from the system in this way – when it was partially absorbed, or when the intestinal tract was in a particularly susceptible condition – it caused excruciating pain, nausea and vomiting, a burning sensation in the stomach and intestines, damage to liver and kidneys, convulsions, cramps, and even heart failure. Even today, when it is still sometimes prescribed in cases of schistosomiasis – a tropical disease caused by a minute burrowing parasite – its use has to be suspended in many cases because of the severity of the side-effects. In the hands of unscrupulous, ignorant quacks in sixteenth-century Paris, the mortality caused by it had been so devastating that the Faculty of Paris banned its use in 1566, classifying it as a dangerous poison, not fit to be prescribed.

In a legal tussle between the orthodox and empiric later that year, however, the French *Parlement* overruled the Faculty, and decreed that it should be legal for doctors – although not for anyone else – to use it, thus leaving the question open once more. And in 1604 the pros and cons of antimony therapy became the subject of heated public debate with the publication of an enthusiastic piece of propaganda, the *Triumphal Chariot of Antimony*, written by a chemiatrist named Johann Thöld under the pseudonym of a mythical German monk called Basil Valentine.

Antimony, Thöld claimed, was excellent for a host of illnesses, including syphilis, melancholy, chest pains, and the plague: it was particularly useful at the onset of fevers. Patients suffering from any of these complaints – and the spectrum was certainly broad – at once clamoured for this exciting new drug, and although the doctors of the Paris Faculty sternly refused to prescribe it, it was a source of infinite grief to them that there were plenty of Montpellier physicians in town who would – and who did.

In theory the Faculty of Paris – a private body – had a monopoly on the medical practice in Paris, and no graduate from another university might practise there without their special licence. But there was nothing to stop Montpellier doctors from accepting appointments to the Royal Family, and politicians as eminent as Cardinal Richelieu and Cardinal Mazarin naturally considered themselves entitled to choose their own physicians too. Thus for some time the Royal Family had been obstinately patronizing these southerners – who as a result had roaringly successful practices in Paris, too, and there was nothing much to be done about it.

The Royal Family and a few elder statesmen were not the only allies of Montpellier medicine in the capital. The apothecaries – snubbed and impoverished by the faculty – naturally sided with the Montpellier men, who in turn cultivated them assiduously, gave them plenty of business, and often laid on special courses in the new chemical medicine for their benefit. This alliance was forged into a weapon of war in 1630 by Theophraste Renaudot, a brilliant and politically able doctor who had graduated from Montpellier in 1605, at the age of nineteen. In 1612 Renaudot moved to Paris where his talents attracted the attention of Richelieu, from whom he obtained the office of Commissaire-General des Pauvres de France, an appointment confirmed by *arret du Parlement* in 1629. A year later he set up a weekly clinic for the poor of Paris, together with his Montpellier colleagues: treatment was free, and the patients came in droves to be seen and treated not only by doctors but also by surgeons, barbers, and apothecaries.

Renaudot courteously invited the great doctors of the Paris Faculty to associate themselves with this pious work of charity, but they indignantly declined – which was understandable but hardly good public relations. And Renaudot, in his *Gazette* – France's first political journal – made sure that these facts reached the public, using the columns of this journal for a relentless campaign in favour of progressive medicine – particularly the use of antimony. By taking medicine into the forum of public opinion, Renaudot certainly advanced the cause he championed, and there can be no doubt of the sincerity of his views, any more than we can doubt Patin's passionate conviction that such mineral medicine could be – and too often was – lethal to patients.

Unfortunately, the sheer virulence of the debate, the bitterness of personal feeling on one side or the other, and the glare of publicity in which the argument was conducted, hardly made for dispassionate consideration of the issues at stake, although it provided endless fun for the Parisian bystanders. In one typical exchange, the Montpellier Faculty addressed itself to "les soy–disants doyen, docteur et medecin en l'Eschole de Paris"; the Dean of the Paris Faculty addressed his reply to the "soy–disant professeur, dans ladicte pretendue Universite de Montpellier".[10] In such a climate of opinion, there was never a chance that antimony could be calmly and clinically evaluated, its virtues balanced against its terrible drawbacks. In the circumstances, antimony could only succeed.

It is a curious and depressing truth, demonstrated again and again in medical history, that the desire of the average physician to administer powerful and active drugs is only equalled by the desire of the average patient to have powerful and active drugs administered to him. This seems to have been just as true in the seventeenth century, when the dangers of such drugs were publicly trumpeted, as it is today when their side-effects – except in rare cases – are often merely noted in small type in the medical press.

The physicians who were so enthusiastic about antimony must have been perfectly well aware that it often caused severe pain to patients, that it occasionally aggravated rather than cured an illness, that it sometimes killed them. They presumably reasoned that pain and death might be the lot of a patient anyway if his serious illness was left untreated, and that antimony at least gave him a fighting chance of survival. At this stage, too, it was mainly being prescribed for illnesses to which Galenic medicine had virtually no answer – the plague, syphilis, and virulent infectious diseases. Since typhoid fever, the plague or smallpox very often killed people in the seventeenth century – and for centuries after, for that matter – and since patients given antimony very often got better, it was a natural – and human – assumption that medical skill and antimony had saved them. There was no pathology laboratory, to prove the case one way or the other by analysis of tissue from the dead man's body.

Inexorably, then, the tide of public opinion shifted in favour of antimony, and Patin found himself increasingly isolated in his insistence that a handful of cassia or senna, a little syrup of pale rose or peach or chicory, and a spot of rhubarb were almost all the drugs a good physician could possibly need. On these principles – allied to energetic and lucky use of the lancet – he had built a successful practice and a high position. But others of his colleagues may have been less lucky, and most of them were beginning to have second thoughts. Some of their patients had learned to do without doctors altogether, thanks to *Le médecin charitable*; others were flocking to the progressive doctors who were using the new wonder-drugs – and certainly getting the most impressive results; and the Court itself seemed indisposed ever to appoint a Paris-Galenic physician again. It was no longer merely their reputations that were at stake: it was their splendid fur-lined livelihoods too.

In the light of these harsh realities, the doctors who sat on the committee appointed in 1623 to draft the new French *Codex Pharmaceuticus* were not disposed to make an *a priori* decision against the controversial drug. Sure enough, when the *Codex* was finally published in 1638, the eager readers who raced through it to the emetic section found Antimonial Wine boldly listed there – included, said the committee, "après contestations faites de part et d'autre".[11] Its supporters on the Committee had been numerous, and more significantly, they included Harduyn de Saint Jacques, Dean of the Paris Faculty.

Patin was incensed by this betrayal, and when a few years later he became Dean, he briskly expelled another member, Jean Chartier, for advocating the drug in a published work without getting Faculty approval first. Chartier promptly sued him in the court of the *Parlement de Paris*, and this time, there were no sympathetic crowds to cheer on a triumphant Patin; instead, Chartier won his case and was reinstated, while Patin had to pay heavy costs. Thoroughly nervous by this time, sixty-one of the Faculty doctors banded together in 1652 to sign a document solemnly attesting the virtues of antimony: "grandement convenable à la guérison de quantité de maladies".[12]

Renaudot followed up this singular victory with an absolute paean of praise; "the human spirit must rejoice at the possession of this remedy which has never, among all the accumulated debris of antiquity, known an equal." The methods of Hippocrates and Galen were "scrupuleuse et timide"; the twin pillars of Hercules of modern medicine were antimony and laudanum.[13] Renaudot entitled his tract *"L'antimoine justifié et l'antimoine triomphant"*, and it illustrates another curious and persistent fact about medical treatment: once a powerful and potentially dangerous drug is accepted into practice on the grounds that extremely serious illness justifies its use, it tends to be increasingly prescribed for quite trivial ailments. (Modern antibiotics are an excellent example of this tendency.) Renaudot now declared that antimony was a sovereign cure for anything from asthma, catarrh, colic, fistulas, and ulcers to weaknesses of the stomach, and womens' complaints . . . for most of which it was, to put it mildly, unsuitable.

Patin spent much of his spare time assiduously collecting details of cases in which antimony had been fatal – he meant to publish it as *"La martyrologie de l'antimoine"*. His bias against both antimony in particular, and Montpellier doctors in general was so extreme that he can hardly be accepted as an impartial witness. Nonetheless, there must have been plenty of casualties similar to one he recounts, that of M. d'Avaux, one of the King's Surintendants de Finance, who in December 1650 fell ill with some pulmonary problem. He was getting perfectly acceptable medical treatment when a relative insisted that he should be seen by the King's physician, Vautier – who prescribed antimony, which he swallowed. "An hour afterwards he began to cry that he was burning and that he saw he had been poisoned, that he was sorry that they had allowed him to take the remedy, and that he regretted that he had not made his will. Then the poison having ravished his entrails, he died vomiting, three hours after having taken it".[14]

It was not so much the casualties of antimony therapy that tended to linger in people's minds, though: it was the successes. And the summer of 1658 brought the drug its most dazzling triumph yet.

On campaign in Flanders, the twenty-year-old Louis XIV fell dangerously ill. He had worn himself out day and night at the sieges of Dunkirk and Bergues, the weather was chilly and unpleasant, the countryside was marshy, and there was a constant reek of putrefying corpses in the air. On Saturday, 29 June he felt unwell – feverish, none of his usual vigour and appetite, a blinding headache. His personal doctor – the vigilant Antoine Vallot – would certainly have spotted these symptoms at once, and ordered him to bed.

Vallot, however, was absent – sent off by Louis to look after one of his generals – so the young monarch, anxious to get back to the siege of Bergues, said nothing, and Sunday found him in the same condition. By Sunday night, however, he felt so ill that he could keep up the pretence no longer. Mazarin at once took charge and ordered him to be conveyed to Calais where proper medical attendance could be given him, and messengers were sent flying for Vallot. The doctor arrived on Monday night, made a horrified examination of the King, and diagnosed typhoid fever. He at once ordered an enema, and a drastic bleeding – during both which heroic procedures, the King's condition worsened alarmingly. For the next four days his condition deteriorated rapidly: delerium, high fever, appalling pain, convulsions: "his thirst was great, his throat swollen, his tongue thickened and black . . . his body swollen as if he had been stung by a serpent or poisoned, his extremities chilled."[15]

A local doctor, Du Saussoy, had been summoned at once by Mazarin, Anne of Austria sent her personal physician Guenault, together with his colleague d'Aquin, post-haste from Paris, and this conclave desperately debated what was to be done, while the classic routine of drastic bleeding, enema, and blisters was followed, to no avail. Du Saussoy had immediately suggested antimony, and it might have been expected that Vallot, Guenault and d'Aquin – all Montpellier men and chemical doctors – would have agreed with enthusiasm. In a lesser patient, they would no doubt have had recourse to it at once.

But too much was at stake in the person of France's most important patient, and it was not until the following Monday, when it was clear that the King's condition was so desperate that almost anything might legitimately be tried, that Vallot finally made up his mind to administer antimony. Even then, Mazarin had to be appealed to to overrule the doubts and hesitations of the other doctors. It must have been with a hand that shook slightly that Vallot measured out three ounces of emetic wine that he had ready, added it to a bland laxative composed of senna, tamarind and manna, and made the King drink a third of the mixture.

For four or five hours the assembled doctors watched every pulse-beat, every laboured breath, every flicker of a muscle with agonized anxiety. Then the King stirred, vomited twice, and, wonder of wonders, was gently purged no less than twenty-two times. At once the fever began to abate; by the end of the week it was gone; and a month from the first day of his illness, Louis XIV was out hunting again.

The news of his astounding recovery burst like a clap of thunder on Paris, on France, on all Europe: antimony was the hero of the hour. Patin was furious: "absurd to claim that emetic wine saved the King's life, seeing that he took such a small amount of it he could hardly have taken less . . . what saved the King was his innocence, his strong and vigorous youth, nine good bleedings and the prayers of good people like ourselves".[16]

Renaudot exulted: the campaign for the legalization of antimony was at once renewed with vigour, and when in 1665 the Faculty of Paris was asked to give its formal views, only ten out of 102 doctors still opposed it. Versailles adopted antimony with its usual enthusiasm for all things royal. Mme. de Sévigné, who loved trying out new medicines, christened it "la poudre du bonhomme," and wrote to allay her daughter's anxieties: "why are you so worried about it? It has done absolute wonders for me".[17]

Henrietta Anne Stuart, adored sister of Charles II and wife of the Duc d'Orléans, was less fortunate. In the summer of 1670 she was seized by violent abdominal pains – probably from a perforated ulcer. Nothing would satisfy her but to have antimony: it was given her, and she died in agony. Patin, no doubt, added her to his *Martyrologie*.

8

The Seventeenth-Century Superwoman

No woman running a seventeenth-century home would have described herself as "just a housewife". Being a housewife three centuries ago was a full-time job which demanded a high degree of skill, training and devotion. And the larger the household, or the grander the estate, the more exacting the task became, so that the high-born and titled Lady of the Manor, far from sitting around doing a little light embroidery, was probably rushed off her feet from morning to night.

Even in cities, many of the amenities we take for granted – were not always conveniently to hand; and the country household, connected to the nearest town only by a tedious jolting coach-ride, had by sheer necessity to be self-sufficient.

Even if she, the housewife, had a house full of servants to make her life easier, she was still expected to be capable of supervising, if not performing herself, a variety of highly skilled domestic tasks such as baking, brewing, weaving, preserving, and concocting in her still-room – literally, distilling-room – the perfumes, the pomanders, the flowery lotions that sweetened daily life in houses without running water. But more important than any of these, she was also obliged to be the family doctor, since professional physicians were few and far between, and even the nearest apothecary might be a day's ride distant. Thus elementary doctoring – not to mention nursing – was "one of the most principal vertues which do belong to our English Housewife";[1] and it was considered an indispensable part of a well-brought-up young woman's education to acquire the beginnings of "a Physical kind of knowledge, how to administer any wholesome receipts or medicines for the good of their healths, as well to prevent the first occasion of sickness, as to take away the effects and evil of the same. . . ."[2]

When the housewife was also the vicar's wife, or the lady of the manor, her "practice" was assumed to include the whole village in times of sickness. Many women of the time, indulging a natural bent or an instinctive bossiness, seem to have flung themselves into this rôle – almost the only career open to them – with enthusiasm. One such was Lady Brown, who when her husband Sir Richard was appointed Ambassador to Paris, turned the Embassy into "an Asylum for her exiled country, and an hospital for the sick and needy"; another was Anne, Countess of Arundel who regularly supplied "medicines, salves, plasters and other remedies to all kinds of people".[3]

Just as women today will keep a scrapbook for recipes into which they paste newspaper cuttings, or copy recipes picked up from a friend or a favourite magazine, so the seventeenth-century housewife, in her time, collected useful medical tips from any number of sources. A good reliable herbal – like a sound basic cookery-book – was the first essential for the young housewife; and no herbal ever eclipsed in popularity and prestige that of Gerard. A copy of the 1633 version turned up nearly two centuries later in a second-hand bookshop in Wakefield, with the following inscription written on the back of the title-page: "This book was given me by my grandmother, Miss Judith Denton, of Barton, widdow of Matthew Denton Esq. in the year of our Lord God 1654 [signed] Amy Denton, Daughter of Nico. Denton Esq.,".

Half a lifetime later, having meanwhile married twice and borne at least one son, Amy wrote below the first inscription: "It is agreed between Madm. Amy Egleton, wife to Mr. Thos. Egleton, and Lyon Pilkington, her son, that whensoever it shall please God to take ye above-named Madm. Egleton out of this world, that she will then wholly bequeath this book unto ye above-named Lyon Pilkington, her son, as a gift or legacy given to him, and to ye ayres male of his body."[4]

Many other herbal cures must have been passed down by oral tradition in a family from one doctoring housewife to the next. In one collection two headache cures – anointing the head with "Oyl of Lillies", or "Rue steeped in vinegar", one with poppyseeds for insomnia, and the recommendation of celandine "for bleared Eyes" go straight back to the Leechbook of Bald. Recipes or cures from noble households had particular cachet: physicians sometimes graciously passed on a prescription; the local rector occasionally came up with something in the course of his reading that seemed worth a trial, after it had been checked with Gerard; and tips from a passing wise-woman, or tinker who seemed to know his herbs, were not to be despised. One fairly typical household collection, from the early eighteenth century, gives a written list of sources the compiler had drawn on most frequently. "Mrs. Mariamne Packer the Travelling Doctress. . . . Aunt Frances Major's Receipts. . . . Madam Sparks's Receipts a great Doctress in Pater Noster Row that kept her Coach and 6 Horses . . . Mary Burton a Traveller . . . The Rd. Mr. Isaac Taylor of Bosworth . . . Mr. Sherard Serjent's Receipts of Melton. . . . Rembert Dodoen's *History of Plants or Herbal*. . . ."[5]

As the century wore on, more and more specialized books aimed at this huge domestic market appeared. The most famous and popular of all was itself drawn largely from just such a private collection. Although Gervase Markham's *The English House-wife* first appeared in 1615, it went into edition after edition for the whole century that followed, the Mrs. Beeton of its time. Dedicating it to the "most excellent Lady, Frances, Countesse Dowager of Exeter", Markham admitted frankly that "much of it was a Manuscript which many yeeres agon belonged to an Honorable Countesse, one of the greatest Glories of our Kingdome, and were the opinions of the greatest Physitians which then lived."[6]

Like all best-sellers, *The English House-wife* had many imitators, and Markham's "Honorable Countesse" was followed into print by a number of other titled ladies, right up to Henrietta Maria herself (already in exile at the time), each of whom offered a similarly delightful variety of medical and culinary hints – the borderline between cookery and pharmacy was not always clearly drawn at this time.

Although the Western world may never again see a case of smallpox, the seventeenth century saw it all too often, a devastating killer-disease to which few families had not lost at least one of their number, while even those it spared, it often left cruelly disfigured. Plague was another occasional visitant, up to 1665, though rare in the country areas. Malaria or ague, the tertian or quartan fever – was endemic in many parts, and tuberculosis was common. Parents must have needed every last grain of Christian faith to steel them against the appalling mortality rate in their nurseries – often swept bare over and over again by baffling fevers, acute infectious diseases or by rhesus incompatability in the parents.

Christina Hole, in her account of the housewife of this age, quotes a mother's heartbreaking list of her dead babies: "Harrison, my eldest son, and Henry, my second son, Richard, my third son; Henry, my fourth; and Richard, my fifth, are all dead . . . my eldest daughter Anne lies buried in the Parish Church of Tankersley, in Yorkshire, where she died; Elisabeth . . . died of a fever at ten days old; my next daughter of her name lies buried . . . and my daughter Mary lies in my father's vault . . . with my first son, Henry".[7]

Most of these acute illnesses were beyond a housewife's competence, and professional help was called in. Markham does not even attempt to suggest a remedy for smallpox – though he does offer a prescription "to take away scarres of the Small-poxe".[8] But in most cases, the housewife was still the first line of medical defence: on her fell the burden of initial diagnosis, and the responsibility of seeing the patient through both illness and convalescence, since hospitals in those days were only for the destitute. Other great or trivial ailments she might have had to take in her stride included epilepsy (the "falling sickness"), jaundice, toothache, anæmia ("the green sickness"), gout, burns, constipation, diarrhœa, ruptures, and the stone.

Modern writers have had plenty of fun at the expense of the seventeenth-century domestic pharmacopœia: they giggle at the plague cure supposedly contributed by Henrietta Maria, which involved a series of cock chicks whose rumps were to be plucked bare and applied to the plague sore, "so long as any one do die"; when the final chick lived, the poison was all out.[9] They make fun of Dr. Stevens' Water, which almost every housewife copied into her personal collection: composed by adding an incredible and costly assortment of herbs and dried fruit and spices to a gallon of "good Gascoign Wine", and supposedly a "polychrest" or cure-all – whatever the ailment, Dr. Stevens' Water would do the trick. And almost everyone has heard of the Oyle of Swallows – made by pounding in a mortar twenty young live swallows, complete with guts and feathers, then boiling them with herbs in fresh butter.

But just as the modern housewife will pore happily over exotic and elaborate recipes in her spare time and then make Shepherd's Pie yet again, so her predecessor is likely to have passed by Dr. Stevens and the cock chicks to go straight for the simpler herbal recipes on which she knew she could rely. As Christina Hole says, "The mother of a large family and mistress of many servants could not afford to make too many mistakes, and every intelligent woman slowly acquired, if only by trial and error, a good deal of useful knowledge".[10]

The enduring popularity of Gervase Markham's book – like that of Mrs. Beeton in the nineteenth century or Elizabeth David today – can only have been based on one fact: his prescriptions and recipes worked. And what is striking about the majority of the remedies in Markham and in similar stillroom books is their relative simplicity, based – very often – on the known therapeutic effect of one or two herbs; although for the sake of making them palatable to her patients, the housewife often used them in concoctions of red wine, added spices to disguise the bitter earthy taste of a herbal infusion, and sugar or honey to sweeten it.

Here is a typical recipe from Markham to cure the cases of violent diarrhœa or dysentery common at that time: "To cure the worst bloody flux that may be, take a quart of red wine, and a spoonful of Cummin seed boyl them together untill half be consumed, then take knot-grass, and Shepherde-purse, and Plantane, and stamp them severall, and then strain them, and take of the juice of each . . . a good spoonful; and put them to the wine, and so seeth them again a little; then drink it lukewarm, half over night, and half the next morning."[11]

Knotgrass (*Polygonum aviculare*) has astringent qualities useful in cases of diarrhœa; and shepherd's purse (*Capsella bursa-pastoris*) is famous for its power to arrest bleeding or relieve dysentery, but its taste is distinctly disagreeable, so that the cumin seeds were probably there to disguise it – as well as being themselves nicely warming and anti-spasmodic. The red wine was not purely for fun: alcohol – and Aqua vitæ or brandy in particular – were thought to "draw out the sweetness, savour and vertues of all manner of spices, roots and herbs that are wet or layd therewith in," while the red wine itself had useful trace minerals such as iron and copper.[12]

In draughty, unheated seventeenth-century houses, coughs, colds and laryngitis were common. A recipe to cure laryngitis copied into her still-room book by Mary Fairfax in the early part of the century went as follows: "For them theyr speech faileth. Take a handfull of ye cropps of Rosemary, a handfull of sage and a handfull of Isop and boile them in Malmsey till it be soft, then put them into Lynen clothes and laye about the nape of the neck and the pulses of the armes as whott as it may be suffred daily . . . and it will help it by God's grace."[13] This hot aromatic poultice of stimulating and antiseptic herbs very probably did the trick – and reminds us that until only very recently, poultices and foot-baths were very common ways of applying medicine, not just because of their local heating or counter-irritant value, but because their virtues are absorbed through the skin. Mustard foot-baths – piping hot – have always been a popular remedy for coughs, colds and chestiness in my family – a folk-remedy of hundreds of years' standing which we have always found highly effective. Research by the German firm Madaus has recently revealed a rationale for this treatment: mustard seeds contain a powerful antibiotic, which is absorbed through the particularly sensitive skin of the feet.[14]

And in an anonymous stillroom book of this era somebody has copied the single cure "for such as are Franticke": it was to "Distill the flowers of Cowslips, and give thereof to the Patient morning and evening; put thereof in all his drinks".[15] Whether he was frantic with hysteria, or genuinely out of his wits, this would at least have made the patient easier to have around the house: the cowslip (*Primula veris*) is sedative and antispasmodic in its action, and cowslip wine has long been a favourite country remedy for restlessness, giddiness or insomnia. Other cures are frankly magical – or else designed to work by suggestion: "to stay bleeding at the nose . . . Take a dryed Toade, and hang it about the neck. . . ."[16]

But rational or magical, most of the remedies to be found in these stillroom collections were made from herbs which the housewife could grow in her own herb garden, or which grew wild and abundantly in the neighbouring countryside, and whose virtues she would teach to her own daughters in turn. Picked and used fresh, dried and hung in bunches in a cool place, distilled with brandy or steeped in oils and small beer, or turned into salves and ointments or waters ready for use, the herbs that made up this green pharmacopœia were the basis of domestic medicine.

Not for the housewife the exotic concoctions of powdered pearl, dried mummy, or stag's heart-bone, that a London physician might prescribe. And certainly not for her – with exceptions such as the famous Oyle of Swallows – the animal and "filth" pharmacopœia that still figured largely in the apothecary's shop, revolting remedies composed of animal excrement or human urine or mashed-up millipedes.

The explanation for their absence is surely very simple: the housewife-doctor who prescribed them also had to administer them – unlike the grand physician or the visiting apothecary. An early eighteenth-century housewife – dubiously noting a remedy for convulsions made from powdered dried moles, added "I dare say this is an approv'd Receipt, because I had it from a very choice Hand; but I should fear t'would be impossible to make a young child take so much of so loathsome a Thing as this Powder must needs be".[17]

Equally conspicuous by their absence from such books, at least in the earlier part of the century – were mineral and chemical remedies, although Markham suggests antimony for a vomit, and mercury in an ointment for the pox. In every such collection of medical recipes, it is easy to pick out the ones culled from professional physicians: long, complicated "blunderbuss" recipes, designed to give joy to the heart of an apothecary by the sheer number of their ingredients. In a collection written down by Lady Sedley in 1686, many of the cures were contributed by famous doctors of the time, including the great Sydenham. His "Prescription for the head" starts with Venice treacle – which itself contained seventy-two ingredients and was hideously expensive – to which Sydenham suggested adding Wormwood (*Artemisia absinthium*) – the expensive, imported Roman one, naturally – orange peel, angelica, and nutmeg; a quantity of this decoction no bigger than a nutmeg was to be taken in a diuretic draught of horseradish, elecampane, garden scurvy-grass, white horehound, tops of Roman wormwood, centaury, broom, chamomile flowers and juniper berries infused in five pints of sack.[18] There was nothing *stingy* about Sydenham's prescribing!

Stuart England was desperately short of trained doctors, but the wealthy members of the College of Physicians did their utmost to prevent the sacred secrets of medicine from leaking out even to apothecaries: every professional medical work, like the *London Pharmacopœia* itself was printed in Latin, a language of which few housewives and by no means all apothecaries had more than a smattering.

One apothecary who found this attitude both absurd and contemptible was Nicholas Culpeper (1616–1654). The son of a Surrey rector, he was handsomely educated at Cambridge University "where he continued some years, profited in all manner of learning, and gained the applause of the University whilst he remained there".[19] He might have gone on to become one of the grand doctors himself but before his studies were completed, he fell in love, planned a runaway marriage with the girl, and, having borrowed £200 from his mother, arranged to meet her near Lewes, where they were to be married.

On her way to meet him, a bizarre accident occurred: she was struck by lightning and killed. Shattered, Culpeper abandoned his studies, and eventually his grandfather paid £50 to have him apprenticed to a London apothecary, although he heartily disapproved of this inferior choice of vocation. Culpeper, having taught his master the Latin in which he himself was fluent, and studied physic for some years, set up his own shop in Spitalfields, a once-wealthy quarter of London already decaying into a slum, and filled with the desperately poor. To these people Culpeper inevitably became – like so many other apothecaries – their neighbourhood doctor. Culpeper – a dark-haired, keen-eyed young man, with a "gentle, pleasing and courteous" manner, "a despiser of the world", with a "sparkling ready Wit"[20] – was an unusual apothecary in more ways than one, not least in his passionate concern for his poor patients. Instead of conning them into the most expensive drugs on his shelves, he used to prescribe "cheap but wholesome Medicines . . . not sending them to the *East Indies* for Drugs, when they may fetch better out of their own Gardens. . . ."[21] Soon he was seeing forty and more patients in a morning although he often refused to take a fee: clinical experience in the use of the cheap, readily available English herbs which he was in the habit of prescribing was later proved invaluable.

Culpeper knew that apothecaries with his degree of skill and knowledge were rare – although for hundreds of thousands of Englishmen, an apothecary would always be the only doctor they could afford to consult – and single-handedly he campaigned to change his state of affairs by raising the general level of knowledge in the profession. He translated several major medical works of the day into English, and planned to make available in this way "the whole body of physick."

As a start, in 1649 he translated the *London Pharmacopœia* – previously only published in Latin – into English as the *Physicall Directory*, for the benefit of the many apothecaries whose Latin, he knew, was shaky or non-existent, yet who depended for their livelihood on being able to make sense of the *Pharmacopœia*. Throughout this translation he coolly criticized, amended where he thought necessary, and gave as much guidance as he could to the apothecary-doctors who would be reading the book.

The mere notion of their precious trade secrets being thus carelessly laid bare to the world was enough to give the College apoplexy, but there was worse: every page of Culpeper's translation reveals his scornful contempt for the "proud, insulting, domineering Doctors, whose wits were born above five hundred years before themselves".[22] He took them sharply to task for their callous indifference to the poor:

"Send for them to a poor man's house who is not able to give them their fee, then they will not come, and the poor Creature for whom Christ died must forfeit his life for want of money."[23]

He was worried by many of the strong purges they included, particularly scammony: "a desperate purge. . . . I would advise my countrymen to let it alone. It will gnaw their bodies as fast as doctors gnaw their purses."[24] And of the endless prescriptions calling for costly imported drugs: "Would it not make both a man's ears glow to hear a man affirm that God hath created no remedy for such a disease nearer than the East Indies?"[25]

He wondered even more why, when the College turned to English herbs – cheap and freely available – they listed neither their English names nor their virtues: "It seems the College hold a strange opinion 'that it would do an English man a mischief to know what the herbs in his garden are good for' " commented Culpeper with savage scorn.[26] This omission he made good himself, describing the various herbs and listing the parts of the body for which they were appropriate, before turning with renewed rage to consider the omissions of the College: "I would they would consider what infinite number of poor creatures perish daily who else might happily be preserved if they knew but what the Herbs in their own Gardens were good for."[27]

If Culpeper himself had not been a noble practising physician, the College would hardly have enjoyed his criticism. As it was he was everything they feared, resented, and despised: an upstart with enough Latin and learning to make their ignorance a laughing-stock, an apothecary who dared to practise medicine – and with huge success – in defiance of their statutes, and to crown everything, a self-confessed Puritan and Parliamentarian who had actually been wounded in the chest by a musket-ball while fighting in the rebel armies six years earlier.

Thus it was in a Cavalier broadsheet, the *Mercurius Pragmaticus*, that the physicians – courtiers and Establishment men, for the most part – spat out their shrill fury. After a vicious attack on Culpeper's morals and way of life ("he lived . . . meerely upon Couzenage and Cheating the poore People") the writer thus described the *Physicall Directory*: ". . . by two yeeres drunken Labour, [he] hath Gallimawfred the Apothecaries Booke into non-sense, mixing every Receipt therein with some Scruples, at least, of Rebelliom or Atheisme, besides the danger of poysoning Mens Bodies". They were even scathing about his appearance: his own friends admitted that Culpeper was careless in

his apparel, and the *Mercurius* writer describes him as "a most despic-
able, ragged-fellow" . . . in his "old hack-Cloake lined with Plum",
and his swarthy complexion that suggested that "he had been stued in
a Tan-pit".[28]

Culpeper was completely unmoved by these absurdities, and two
years later he produced the work which has made the name Culpeper
almost synonymous with the word "herbal" in English: his *English
Physician*, containing "a Compleat Method or Practice of Physic,
whereby a Man may preserve his Body in Health, or cure himself
when sick, with such things one-ly as grow in England, they being
most fit for English Bodies."[29]

Culpeper prefaced his herbal with an explanation of why, given the
works of Gerard, Parkinson and others, he thought another one was
necessary. It was, he explained, because these authors simply quoted
other authors: "Perhaps their authors knew a reason for what they
wrote, perhaps they did not; what is that to us? Do we know it?"
Culpeper claimed he knew because he had approached the subject in
the only possible way – astrologically. "He that would know the
reason of the operation of the Herbs, must look up as high as the
stars."[30] Like many learned men of his time – including many
physicians – Culpeper regarded himself as much an astrologer as a
doctor and claimed that he consulted the motions of the planets in
prescribing for his patients. He identified each herb with one of the
astrological houses, and thought the remedies for a disease would be
found either in herbs of the house opposite that which caused the
disease, or else by sympathy, with each house curing its own disease.

Whether or not you accept Culpeper's astrological rationalizations,
a long apprenticeship as an apothecary and twelve years of a crowded
and diverse herbal practice among the sick poor had given him a
confident knowledge of his subject. You didn't have to believe that
agrimony is "an herb under Jupiter, and the sign of Cancer . . .
and removes diseases . . . under Saturn, Mars and Mercury by
antipathy"[31] to be interested in his statement that "A draught of the
decoction taken warm before the fit, first removes, and in time rids
away the tertian or quartan agues."[32]

The English Physician was an instant and enormous success, as it has
been through the centuries. The British Library lists no less than
forty-one different editions, and as recently as 1979 an expensive
facsimile issue appeared, testifying to its enduring popularity. Its
contemporary success – like that of the work of another successful

seventeenth-century "quack" doctor, William Salmon – was based on Culpeper's own high reputation among his thousands of patients. Culpeper's herbal served to reinforce a strong English tradition of domestic herbal medicine at a time when professional physicians were beginning to learn contempt for such homely remedies. "Nowadays" grumbled Sydenham late in the century, "every house has its old woman, or practitioner, skilled in an art she has never learned, to the killing of mankind."[33]

9

Indian Physic

Tobacco first arrived on the London commodity market late in the reign of Queen Elizabeth I in the improbable guise of a useful medicinal plant. For decades the Spanish had been making fortunes shipping back across the Atlantic the exotic drug plants Monardes had described with so much enthusiasm. Sassafras, various gums and balsams, sarsaparilla, and guaiac were all now in steady professional demand, firmly established in Europe's pharmacopœias. So when Raleigh's men landed on Roanoke Island, off the coast of Virginia, in 1585, they studied the native use of medicinal plants attentively, hoping for equally lucrative discoveries.

They thus were delighted to find ". . . Sweete Gummes of divers kindes and many other apothecary drugges . . .", including the tobacco (*Nicotiana tabacum*) mentioned by Monardes. It was the free use of tobacco, they assured themselves, that preserved the local Indians from "many greevous diseases wherewithal we from England are sometimes afflicted."[1] The new colony of Virginia was soon shipping quantities of tobacco back to London, and over the next few years it was publicized in England as an exciting new wonder–drug, in language that would make any modern cigarette manufacturer sick with envy: "who hath ever found a more sovereign remedy against coughs, rheume in the stomacke, head and eyes?" demanded a promotional pamphlet in 1595.[2] *Unguentum nicotianae* duly found its way into the London pharmacopœia, and its medical reputation for one ailment or another survived until early this century, although the fortunes of the Virginia settlement soon came to depend on thousands of addicted smokers rather than doctors.

The English settlers further north, at Plymouth and Boston, were equally interested in the local medicinal plants – but for reasons more medical than commercial. These people had crossed the Atlantic as settlers rather than traders, and were determined to be self-sufficent as soon as possible. They were sure that there would turn out to be wonderful medicinal plants among the vegetable plenty of their new country. Certainly what they saw of the native Indians was an extremely good advertisement for the local green medicine, and early observers sent home accounts of a super-race.

In what was admittedly a piece of propaganda for New England, where he had stayed five years, William Wood wrote of the Indians in 1633: "I have beene in many places, yet did I never see one that was born . . . a monster, or any that sickness had deformed, or casualty made decrepid." They appeared free of such "health-wasting diseases . . . as Feavers, Pleurises, Callentures, Agues, Obstructions, Consumptions, Subfumigations, Convulsions, Apoplexies, Dropsies, Gout, Stones, Tooth-aches, Pox, Measles or the like." Instead, their physique told of the kind of vigorous good health that every modern jogger longs for: "straight bodies, strongly composed . . . broad shouldered . . . small waisted, lanke bellied, well thighed."[3] The Dutch in New Amsterdam recorded in 1624 ". . . it is somewhat strange that among these most barbarous people, there are few or none cross-eyed, blind, crippled, lame, hunch-backed, or limping men; all are well fashioned people, strong and sound of body, well fed, without blemish."[4]

The Indians who so impressed the first settlers belonged mainly to one of three centres of Indian culture in North America. There were the town civilizations of the Southwest. There were the Plains Indians, "so perfectly adapted to their environment" as Eric Stone has written, "that no change in their manner and customs had been necessary for centuries and where theology, myth and poetry had risen to peaks scarcely exceeded by any European literature."[5] And in the North there were the Iroquois based on Manhattan: hunters, warriors, and farmers, whose rude health would not have astonished a modern naturopath. They lived out of doors most of the year, and had plenty of strenuous exercise, while their diet consisted of fresh meat, plenty of raw fruit and vegetables, whole grains, and nuts. Their drink was fresh – and unpolluted – spring water and alcohol was almost unknown among them.

As with most primitive cultures, emetics and purges were strongly emphasized in their treatment of diseases. The Indians believed that all sickness was introduced via the digestive tract, and since many of their diseases must have been parasitic in origin, this was sound practical medicine. The sick man was thoroughly purged and vomited – early observers spoke of vomits strong enough to kill a horse – before a preparation of healing herbs was given to him. Then he was fasted before being put on a light diet of gruel made from grain and roots, until recovery was complete.

The Indians were a great deal cleaner than many Europeans of the time: from the north to the south, almost every tribe used a primitive form of sauna to sweat out illnesses or for a thorough cleansing. The Indian sat in a small, specially constructed cabin, while cold water – sometimes with medicinal herbs – was thrown on red-hot stones. An icy plunge in the nearest river followed, then a rest warmly wrapped in a bearskin.

Few generalizations can be made about the medical practice of a great race scattered over a vast continent and organized into hundreds of different tribes, but one can: that their materia medica was almost exclusively herbal.

Different tribes used the same plant for different diseases. For instance, the handsome blue flag (*Iris versicolor*) was cultivated by the Creek Indians as a cathartic; the Albany Indians used its root crushed as a poultice for leg-ulcers; the Meskwakis made a decoction of the roots for colds and lung problems; the Ojibwa considered it an emetic; and to the Penobscots it was a complete panacea, thought by some to be their most treasured medicine.

Other plants were used in much the same way by Indians every-where. Boneset (*Eupatorium perfoliatum*) was popular with all North American tribes, so widely used by them to break a fever or help sweat out a bad chill that the settlers were soon calling it "Indian sage", and using it as a tea in cases of malaria, typhoid and influenza, while for every cold it soon became the first remedy everybody turned to, the aspirin of the European settler.

These plant remedies were used singly, often as specific cures for a particular affliction: the Indians did not believe in complicated "messes of altogether", as Culpeper used to call them. The most widely-used form of preparation was a decoction, made by simmering the sub-stance in water in iron-hard birchwood kettles; other plants were steeped in cold water. Roots and the inner skins of barks were dried and pulverized between flat stones, boiled and crushed into soft poult-ices or made into ointments with animal fat, and the oil was extracted from nuts – acorns were highly thought of – by boiling them in a strong lye till the oil settled on the surface.

Virgil Vogel, in his encyclopedic work *American Indian Medicine*, concluded that "so complete . . . was the aboriginal knowledge of their native flora that Indian usage can be demonstrated for all but a bare half dozen, at most" of American vegetable drugs, not to mention the hundreds used in settler domestic medicine which have never been officially recognized by inclusion in American approved drug lists.[6]

The Indians were not simply brilliant herbalists, however, and Indian medicine was not "rational" in today's cool materialistic sense of the word. To the Indian, mind, body, and spirit were inseparable, and their view of nature was pantheistic: "every animal, plant, tree and every aspect of nature was invested with spiritual life".[7] A modern Indian, Big Thunder of the Wabnakis tribe, has movingly expressed this view: "The Great Spirit is our Father, but the Earth is our Mother. She nourishes us: that which we put into the ground she returns to us, and healing plants she gives us likewise."[8] Thus while external injuries might be treated by straightforward applications of herbs, internal diseases for which there was no obvious cause were treated holistically. The entire tribe might be assembled by the medicine-man to sing and pray over the patient, and to help drive away, by loud music, rattles and chanting, the evil spirits which had caused his sickness. This concern and involvement of the whole tribe was believed to impart special curative powers to the plants the medicine-man would use.

European observers were naturally full of scorn for these noisy ceremonies. Today, however, modern medical research increasingly demonstrates that the mind can make the body sick or well, and scorn is slowly changing into grudging admiration for what was demonstrably effective therapy. Of such medicine – "rational" or not – the first English settlers in the early seventeenth century were desperately in need. They arrived weakened by the long transatlantic voyage, often prostrated by fevers or scurvy, in an alien country where there were no roofs for shelter until they had built them, no crops for their food until they had planted and tilled and harvested. The winter crossings were so prolonged and terrible that ships soon took to starting out in the late spring to avoid the worst of the bad weather. The voyage was then shorter – a mere two months, perhaps – but as a result, the Plymouth and Boston settlers arrived too late in the summer to prepare and plant crops, with the long hard New England winter looming ahead.

During the first winter in Plymouth "halfe of their company dyed, espetialy in Jan: and February, being the depth of winter, and wanting houses and other comforts; being infected with the scurvie and other diseases, which this long voiage and their inacomadate condition had brought upon them; so as ther dyed some times 2 or 3 of a day".[9] Of the first hundred Plymouth colonists, more than fifty died; by 1625, barely a thousand were left of the original 7,500 Jamestown colonists.

The first years were the worst, and once they were used to the more rigorous climate and their new tough life, the Boston and Plymouth settlers found themselves in general more healthy than they had been in Europe. But for many the life was too hard, and all the colonies were subject to epidemic diseases which swept through them, carrying off hundreds. Malaria, rampant at Jamestown, was common enough in New England in the early years. Bacillary dysentery often decimated newcomers during the transatlantic voyage, before spreading like wildfire at their landing. The *Neptune* and the *Treasurer*, arriving in Virginia in 1618, "brought a most pestilent disease [called the Bloody flux] which infected the whole colony."[10] There were regular epidemics of it in New England; influenza was another occasional visitor, and a deadly one; and if the settlers thought they had left the smallpox behind them in Europe, they soon learned their mistake – the disease struck again and again.

The first serious epidemic in New England brought a major blow to the Plymouth settlers. It carried off Samuel Fuller, who had come over with them on the *Mayflower*: he was their "surgeon & Physition, and had been a great help and comforte unto them."[11] Such physicians, surgeons, even common apothecaries were rare in the colonies. Unless he had pressing personal reasons for emigrating, what established physician would give up eight years of costly training and a good practice to travel to a country where hardly a single patient could afford his fee? Nor was there much temptation, in the early days, for an apothecary to go West, since his profit consisted in selling drugs, and most of the drugs with which he was familiar – except sassafras – were not to be had for love or money in the New World.

Even the most competent of pioneer housewives, clutching the Gervase Markham she invariably packed, could hardly be expected to cope with major epidemics of acute infectious disease. But the colonists felt that marvellous medicinal plants *must* be growing all around, if only they knew how to identify them. "This country abounds naturally with store of roots of great variety and good to eat . . . divers excellent pot-herbs . . . also . . . divers physical herbs," wrote Francis Higginson from Boston in 1629, "also abundance of other sweet herbs delightful to the smell, whose names we know not".[12]

Adriaen van der Donck, in Manhattan, was frustrated by his ignorance: "it is not to be doubted that experts would be able to find many simples of great and different virtues, in which we have confidence, principally because the Indians know how to cure very dangerous and perilous wounds and sores by roots, leaves and other little things."[13]

The experts, however, were few and far between; and when they did come, they tended not to stay for very long. Lawrence Bohun was one of them: a physician carefully trained in the Netherlands, he arrived in the company of Lord Delaware in 1610, and investigated, during his stay, the medicinal properties of the local sassafras and a plant which he believed to be a sort of North American rhubarb. After a year, however, Lord Delaware succumbed to scurvy – plainly, Bohun's researches into the local plants had not been very fruitful – and when the physician suggested that nothing was better for the scurvy than a trip to the West Indies, Lord Delaware agreed at once.

Half a century later, in 1663, a much more enthusiastic observer, John Josselyn, came to New England. He stayed eight years and made it his business "to discover all along the Natural, physical, and Chirurgicall Rarities of this New-found World."[14] Having noted the abundance of potentially useful herbs, Josselyn observed Indian use of them, and in 1672 he published his findings in a book, *New Englands Rarities Discovered*, which is in effect a paean of praise for skilled Indian use of herbs.

He thought the fruit of the wild cherry (*Prunus virginiana*) an excellent remedy for the flux; was impressed by the efficacy of the turpentine the Indians extracted from the white pine (*Pinus strobus*), "for the curing of desperate wounds"; and noted that blue flag (*Iris versicolor*) – which he called Blew Flower-de-luce – was "excellent to provoke vomiting." He found that bearberries (*Arctostaphylos uva-ursi*), were "excellent against the scurvy," and he carefully studied the native treatment of the abscesses: the Indians brought them to a head and healed them with a poultice made by "boyling the inner Bark of young hemlock (*Tsuga canadensis*), very well, then knocking it betwixt two stones to a Playster and annointing or soaking it in Soyls Oil."[15]

Josselyn has been accused of excessive enthusiasm, but many of the remedies he noted eventually found their way into the American pharmacopœia, and he demonstrated forcefully what therapeutic riches grew green around them for anyone with some knowledge of the subject, keen eyes, and a patient willingness to learn from the Indians. Colonial housewives often made apt pupils, from sheer necessity. Many of these dauntless women had brought plants and seeds to make their own English physic-gardens in the New World – great mullein (*Verbascum thapsus*), plantain (*Plantago major*) and penny-royal (*Mentha pulegium*) were all introduced by settlers, although the Indians soon discovered their medicinal virtues for themselves – and Colonial housewives were pleasantly surprised to find other treasured herbs growing wild and free: clown's woundwart or all-heal (*Stachys palustris*), much valued in rural England to stop bleeding and heal wounds; the pretty little Maidenhair fern (*Adiantum capillus-veneris*) – so useful in chest troubles, and other important herbs – marjoram, yarrow, brooklime and comfrey – were also to be found. Ladies who were willing to pick the brains of "Mrs. Mariamne Packer the Travelling Doctress" were probably equally receptive to useful hints from the Indian Doctor, and gradually, over the years, a domestic pharmacopœia slowly evolved, to be handed down from one generation to the next.

At a professional level, however, there was only the slightest attempt to learn physic from the Indians. Tragically, the racial gulf that soon came to yawn between white man and native swallowed up all hope of such a dialogue. The Plymouth colonists would have perished to a man without the help of their Indian friend Squanto, but that first Thanksgiving, when whites and redskins feasted happily together, created no precedent for inter-racial accord, while Boston's relations with the indigenous population seldom rose above the level of uneasy truce, and towards the end of the century, flared into open war.

The Dutch on Manhattan had official instructions to treat the natives kindly, and they came close to a working relationship with the tribes in whose midst their settlement was planted. But this was shattered almost beyond repair by the crass ineptitude of their Governor Willem Kieft, who in 1643 successfully embroiled the Dutch in an inter-tribal war, and drew down upon New Netherland the savage reprisals of the Indians.

In the nature of things, warm accord between the settlers and the Indians was unlikely, since their interests were mutually exclusive. Even if there had been room and to spare for both, the appalling racial intolerance of the English would eventually have reduced the likelihood to zero. The Puritans of Boston regarded the Indians as "savage and Brutish", and their Governor Winthrop, writing of the smallpox epidemic which wiped out as many as ninety-nine per cent of the Indians in the decade before the arrival of the Pilgrims, commented coolly: "So the Lord hath cleared our title to what we possess".[16] Contempt on one side was matched by increasing resentment on the other: as Vogel puts it: "Not only the European unwillingness to learn, but also an aboriginal refusal to teach, marks those areas which seethed with racial antagonism".[17] So the Indians kept their herbal lore to themselves, and thousands of white settlers sickened and died, victims not simply of disease, but of their race's arrogant contempt for the natives.

What professional or semi-professional doctoring there was during the earlier years of the English colonies, reveals, instead, a continuing dependence on Europe.

The physician's place in New England was often supplied by the clergyman or the Governor, and the new colony of Connecticut thought itself singularly fortunate to have a man for Governor who was not only a brilliant and forceful personality, but a skilful amateur physician as well. John Winthrop, Jr. (1606–1676) had a lifelong interest in medicine, kept up as far as he could with contemporary developments in the subject, and doctored his settler patients with the very latest in European medicine.

A small paper, sent to "my worthy friend Mr. Winthrop" in 1643 listed "Receipts to cure Various Disorders", from a Dr. Edward Stafford in London. Winthrop had been in London two years earlier: possibly he had picked his medical friend's brains and this was an aide-memoire, prescriptions for seventeen different disorders, ranging from "Madnesse" through "Diseases of ye Bladder" to "ye Blooddie Flix", followed by some useful "Cautions in Phisick" such as an experienced doctor might think it advisable to address to a part-time amateur. He might well have added a caution against following his own suggestions too energetically: at least three of the purges he recommends – black hellebore (*Helleborus niger*), bryony (*Bryonia dioica*), and spurge (*Euphorbia resinifera*) – are violent irritant poisons, cathartics of such severity that their use has been abandoned, while jalap and scammony both needed shrewd judgment in their use. All of these would have had to be imported from Europe. Of the simples he suggests, only snakeroot (*Aristolochia serpentaria*), might perhaps have been borrowed from the North American Indians – one of Stafford's "Best Sudorificks". The dreadful "Black powder of toades" – made by charring live toads over charcoal in an earthen pot – seems uniquely European.[18]

In a paper read to the Massachusetts Historical Society, Oliver Wendell Holmes went into delightful detail about Winthrop's actual prescribing habits, culled from notes that the Governor carefully kept of all his cases. He "employed a number of the simples dear to ancient women – elecampane and elder and wormwood and anise and the rest, but . . . his great remedy, which he gave oftener than any other was *nitre* . . . One of the next remedies, in point of frequency, which he was in the habit of giving, was [probably diaphoretic] *antimony*; a mild form of that very active metal and which, mild as it was, left his patients very commonly with a pretty strong conviction that they had been eating *something* that did not exactly agree with them."[19] (Nitre, as potassium nitrate was called, was popular in European medicine at this time as a diuretic. As its side-effects, it sometimes caused gastro-enteritis with severe abdominal pain, vomiting, vertigo, and collapse. Nitre, too, must have disagreed with more than one patient.)

Winthrop's practice, in a word, was as impeccably European as he knew how to make it, and a similar dependence – not just on European thinking, but on actual drug supplies – was soon an established feature of colonial medical practice. In this respect at least, the dream of self-sufficiency was short-lived. The Ursuline nuns of Quebec wrote out a shopping-list for their hospital pharmacy in 1665 which consisted almost entirely of Old World drugs like senna, scammony, opium, corrosive sublimate, and various compounds. And when the English surgeon William Locke, serving with a Massachusetts army against the Indians in 1675, sent a list back to Boston of urgently-needed drugs and "Old Linnin as much as you can get", almost every item on his list was official in the 1650 *London Pharmacopœia*.[20] Most of them would have had to be imported – particularly the immensely costly compounds such as Mithridatum, which, properly made, contained no fewer than fifty ingredients.

Two years later, on 9 May 1677, Dr. Daniel de Hart of New York wrote out a huge order for medicines addressed to a London apothecary, Moses Rusden. The Third Anglo-Dutch war was well and truly over, New York was settling down in English hands once more; transatlantic shipping was back to normal, and sweet-smelling, costly, complicated European compounds were just what the doctor ordered for his Manhattan practice. In his flowing hand he listed the exotic precipitate of coral, and oil of yellow amber, the soothing syrups of roses and the outrageously expensive *Confectio Alkermes* which contained, among other things, raw silk, lapis lazuli, pearls, musk and gold leaf. He ordered the famous Dr. Stevens' water, the best Venice treacle, and the ruinous *Aqua Cælestis* which needed nearly a whole page to itself in the *Pharmacopœia* to list all the various ingredients that had to be steeped twelve days in spirit of wine, after which all sorts of elaborate compounds might be thrown in for good measure. Having added other necessities – aloes, myrrh, jalap, laudanum, rhubarb – Dr. De Hart added a note of persuasion: "My Harty Desire to you that you Lett me have of your Best and Fresh medicines. I hope it shall Engage me to send Every yeare for Sume of yor."[21]

Even the London quacks were now aware that there was a potential gold-mine to be tapped in the New World. Towards the end of the century the self-styled Doctor Trigg invented what he called his Golden Vatican Pills, composed of a number of spices, some mercury, an assortment of brisk purging drugs, and syrup of roses to sweeten them all. According to Trigg, there was no disease from scurvy to ague that his marvellous pills would not cure. Sold in tin boxes, sealed with the doctor's own seal, at 2 shillings for twenty, they had one further attraction: "They will keep their virtues many years, even the age of man. They may be conveyed to any plantation without the least danger of decay".[22]

10

"Horrid Electuaries"

"If you ayl anything", obseved Nicholas Culpeper, "everyone you meet, whether man or woman, will prescribe you a medicine for it."[1] At no time in history, perhaps, has medicine been a matter of such universal concern and interest as in the seventeenth century: from monarchs to maid-servants, everyone was involved. This was not simply because the times seemed cursed with particularly bad health, with plague and smallpox, the rickets that were becoming known as "The English disease", and the mysterious "sweat" epidemics, scurvy and malaria. Nor yet was it only because medicine still seemed to most people a matter of book-learning that any intelligent layman could master.

It was also because doctoring at this time had an appallingly bad reputation: if you could save a friend from falling into the clutches of the medical profession by passing on some tried and trusted family receipt for his disorder, you would be rendering him a service indeed.

Almost all the standard professional treatments for illness were at best unpleasant; at worst they meant agony. Most medicines tasted vile: "How much Physicians are reflected upon, for prescribing such large and unpleasant potions (fitter to bear the name of Drenches or Farryer-Physick) . . ." mused one critic of the profession.[2] Some remedies must have been almost too revolting to choke down. One for pleurisy, which continued to be prescribed until early in the eighteenth century in London hospitals, contained six ounces of "fresh horse-dung". The author of the *Dispensatory* in which it appeared noted "If the dose here mentioned be too noisome, it may be lessened, and repeated the oftener."[3] Another popular remedy in the reign of William and Mary, was "The Ashes of a whole burnt Owl Feathers and all . . . said to open the apostemation of the Quinsie to a wonder.''[4]

Revolting drugs were only the beginning of the patient's torments. In both London and Paris he could expect to be bled as a matter of course, whatever the illness. Harvey's discovery in 1628 of the circulation of the blood had only added weight to the argument in favour of bloodletting as therapy, and by the end of the seventeenth century, even Gui Patin would no longer have felt that the lancet was being neglected.

Mme. de Sévigné was convinced that it was excessive bleeding that had killed the brother of her son-in-law, rather than the smallpox for which the doctors were attending him. "They bled him barbarously", she wrote. "He was against the last one, which was the eleventh, but the doctors insisted and had their way: he told them that he was giving up all hope, and that they were determined to kill him for form's sake".[5] And in 1675, when she heard that her grandchild was to be bled, she wrote to protest: "I don't understand how it can be good for a child of three. In my day, bleeding a child was unheard of. I'm afraid that they're treating your child, by way of compliment, the same way as they treat the children of the King and M. le Duc."[6]

Her misgivings were prophetic: in the last years of Louis XIV's reign, four heirs to the throne died from sickness, one after the other in a matter of weeks. Three had been babies, all had been repeatedly bled, and if the Duchess of Ventadour had not locked herself up with the last survivor – who was to become Louis XVI – and refused to let the doctors come near him, the Bourbon line might well have become extinct.

Over the years a number of different reasons for letting blood were put forward by the medical profession. They claimed it reduced vascular pressure, evacuated peccant humours, diminished the violence of the arterial action, and eased distempered bodily organs. It was also thought to stimulate the body's natural defences, and to tone up the whole system generally – many people had a routine spring bloodletting even when they were in excellent health.

But most doctors and apothecaries bled patients because doctors had always done so, and patients expected it. Ingenious little gadgets evolved along with the lancet to help them do so efficiently. One of these was a small hollow box containing six sharp blades mounted on springs: you applied the box to the skin, pressed a catch, and the six blades swept down into the skin. Cupping – and then lancing the hot mound of flesh drawn up into the vacuum – was another method.

The death of Charles II, in 1684, shows seventeenth-century medicine at its most elaborate and worst. Charles probably died of inflammation of the kidneys, and the general systemic poisoning that followed: the first fatal symptom was a kind of seizure. His Chief Physician, Dr. C. Scarburgh, describes the treatment he received: "Precisely at eight o'clock his Most Serene Majesty. . . having just left his bed, was walking about quietly in his bed-chamber, when he felt some unusual disturbance in his brain, which was soon followed by loss of speech and convulsions of some violence. There happened to be present at the time two in all of the King's Physicians and they, so as promptly to forestall so serious a danger to this best of kings opened a vein in his right arm, and drew off about sixteen ounces of blood".[7]

The rest of the physicians were sent for urgently, came flocking, and offered suggestions on what was to be done. As a result "they prescribed three cupping-glasses to be applied to his shoulders, to be quickly followed by scarification . . . and in this manner about eight ounces of blood were withdrawn. Within a few moments after this, so as to free his stomach of all impurities . . . they administered an emetic, to wit half an ounce of Orange Infusion of the metals made in white wine."[8]

Since Charles only took a little of this antimony preparation, with no apparent effect, they gave him a little white vitriol to act more energetically, and then another purgative a little later, followed by an enema. Their efforts were in vain.

Growing desperate, "After one or two hours they repeated the Clyster, with the addition of 2 ounces of Syrup of Buckthorn, 4 ounces of emetic wine, and 2 drachms of Rock Salt. But as these were slow in operation they made still another effort to attain the same end with yet more purgatives."[9] Buckthorn (*Rhamnus frangula*) was a particularly violent cathartic, of which Dodoens had remarked that it was only "meat to be administered but to the young and lusty people of the country which do set more store of their money than their lives."[10])

Meanwhile, "so as to leave no stone unturned, Blistering agents were applied all over his head, after his hair had been shaved . . . and . . . Cephalic Plasters combined with Spurge and Burgundy Pitch, in equal parts were applied to the soles of his feet."[11]

Charles survived these tortures for three days, rather to the surprise of his doctors, but at last "all his natural strength was exhausted by the immensity of his sufferings", and he was allowed to die.[12]

Few seventeenth-century patients were unlucky enough to have eleven anxious and active physicians hovering around their sickbed, but simply sending for the doctor must often have required a degree of steely resolution: a sentence in Aubrey's *Brief Lives* is an epitaph to the luckless Lady Howland, one of William Harvey's last patients, whom he treated as a special favour. She "had a cancer in her breast, which he did cutt–off and seared, but at last she dyed of it".[13]

However unpleasant their attentions, physicians certainly were not cheap, and they charged handsomely for scarcity value: for the whole of London and its estimated 700,000 inhabitants in the year 1700, there were still only about 130 fully–trained physicians, the more successful of whom could expect to make £2,000 or £3,000 a year: the great Dr. Radcliffe, physician to Queen Anne, left an estate worth £140,000, well over £1,000,000 in today's money.

If doctors were scarce, there were plenty of apothecaries, and all the evidence suggests that they, too, were doing very nicely. A well-publicized row between the doctors and the apothecaries over who should actually finance and run the free medical service for the poor for which the City of London had asked, brought several unpalatable truths about apothecaries into the open, one of which was that their regular mark-up on drugs was around 300 per cent. It must often have been more.

There was, for instance, the case of William Rose, whom the College took to court for practising medicine illegally. He had, it transpired, been advising a patient for a year, to whom he had supplied drugs at a cost of £50; the patient then applied to the College Dispensary where drugs were sold to the poor at cost – and was cured in six weeks' time for a total outlay on drugs of under £2.

As in the United States today, sickness could be a financial catastrophe: Gideon Harvey – the author of *Family Physician*, one of the countless self-help medical handbooks which were still appearing – claimed that he had known "mean Families by a fit of sickness or two . . . unavoidably . . . ruined in Estate . . . I have often seen Bills of Apothecaries risen to twenty and sometimes thirty pounds in the time of a fortnight."[14]

He thoughtfully listed the going wholesale rates of the more commonly-prescribed medicines so that his readers could see for themselves what fat profits the apothecaries were making. *Mercurius Dulcis Subl.* 10d an ounce; *Vitrum Antimonii*, 2s a lb; jalap 3s 4d a lb; guaiac wood, 2d a pound; the best rhubarb (it came from Turkey) 14s a lb; Scammony 12s a lb; Opium 12s a lb; a dead man's skull, from 8s to

10s a lb. Herbs could be bought from the physical herb-women in Newgate Market or Covent Garden; scurvy-grass was sold by the basket, violets by the pint or quart – rather like mussels today; and for most fresh herbs "a halfpenny a handful is the usual rate," while "the common price of most English Roots among the Herb-women is a Groat for a Pound".[15]

Figures like these remind us of a harsh truth: that profit has nearly always been a more decisive factor than human misery in medical issues. No wonder Culpeper was angry as he passed by the physical herb-women offering their cheap wares, and then saw his fellow-apothecaries pressuring customers into buying extract of bezoar at £8 an ounce. At least on this one issue – the excessive profits made by some apothecaries – he and the College of Physicians saw eye to eye.

Given the prevailing system, such abuses were almost inevitable. Apothecaries were not allowed to charge for their advice, only for the drugs they sold. Most apothecaries were not saints, simply ordinary men trying to make a decent living and support their families. They would have been superhuman if they had made a habit of prescribing the simplest, cheapest drugs available to their poorer patients; if they had not occasionally sold to richer customers the high-priced compounds of which their stock was deteriorating; or if they had not singled out for their special commendation those doctors who made a habit of "writing well" – prescribing frequently and expensively. Culpeper on his deathbed is reported to have claimed "I never gave a Patient two medicines when one would serve the turn".[16] Few apothecaries could have said as much.

But the system that de facto turned the apothecary into a General Practitioner for the majority of the population, and then forbade him to consider himself as anything but a tradesman, hardly favoured the appearance of a Culpeper. Even after a vital test-case – that of the profiteering William Rose, in fact – went against the Royal College in the early eighteenth century, and compelled them to accept the practitioner-apothecary as a fact of life, the snobbish distinction was maintained: the apothecary could charge only for drugs, not for attendance or advice. Thus for centuries doctoring and drugging were synonymous in the British public mind, as they still are today.

Resentment between apothecary and physician often boiled over into highly public shouting matches, which did little to raise the public estimate of either profession. Their confidence must have been further eroded by the running fire of attack on Establishment medicine kept up almost to the end of the century by the advocates of the new chemical medicine.

It is true that the Galen-or-Paracelsus debate never knew in London the heights of a bitter acrimony it reached in Paris, since both sides were represented in the College itself, and by mid-century both mercury and antimony, as well as other Paracelsan remedies, were being freely prescribed by doctors and stocked by every apothecary. But this victory, while it robbed the "chemists" of their most telling debating-point, by no means silenced them. They remained the most outspoken and eloquent critics of Establishment medicine. And if the tone of some of their broadsides was so shrill as hardly to deserve serious attention, others must have given plenty of food for thought to laymen intelligent enough to see that all was not well with the healing art.

The "chemists" attacked College medicine on several grounds. It was, first of all, very nearly useless, in their view: "what . . . impotence to heal infirmities there is in their Preparations . . . is obvious to anyone that hath made a considerable progress in the Theory and Practice of Physick", declared George Thomson in his anti-College *Galeno-Pale* of 1665.[17]

They assailed it, equally, because so much of it was both unnecessarily painful, and risky for the patients, like the excessive bloodletting, the blistering, and the purges so violent that "our nature cannot without great prejudice endure [them]."[18]

Finally they attacked the College for its blinkered conservatism, its hidebound refusal to move with the scientific times. The Cromwellian Noah Biggs, assailing the College Fellows in 1651 in his *Mataeotechnica*, wondered when the public could expect to see regular courses in anatomy, an experimental attitude to the science of medicine, a critical appraisal of "the Old Experiments and Traditions, and wasting of the rubbish that has pestered the Temple of Knowledge?"[19]

But while the Montpellier faction in Paris at this time was first and foremost the advocate of mineral medicine, many of the English "chemists" insisted just as strongly that the potential of medicinal plants was being tragically ignored by orthodox physicians. ". . . in searching out and chusing simples . . . there hath bin no progress made," lamented Noah Biggs. ". . . the powers of simples . . . have remained unknown."[20] The English chemists were modest enough to believe that they could not necessarily improve upon nature: "there may be sometimes greater virtues in a Simple, such as Nature affords it, . . . than almost anything that the fire can separate from it", Robert Boyle stated.[21] Like other chemists, he found it hard to believe that the "ill-pleasing and distasteful slime of herbs"[22] produced by standard pharmacopœia procedures could still retain all the marvellous therapeutic powers of the plant. But the chemists, like the physicians, were groping in the dark.

All healing plants contain what is known as their "active principle" – the one or more constituents, out of the hundreds of thousands composing them, which are chiefly responsible for their characteristic therapeutic action. Although this may be balanced, reinforced, moderated, or diminished by other constituents, it is the business of modern pharmacognosy (the study of plant drugs, especially in their natural or untreated state) to determine and isolate chemically this active principle, examine its structure, and determine its mode of action.

What Biggs and the other "chemists" called for, in effect, was the establishment of such a science long before the tools and techniques which made it possible had been invented. Nearly two centuries were to elapse before this particular vision began to be realized.

Few people would have disagreed with another of the "chemists," Marchmont Needham, when he assailed the *London Pharmacopœia* in his *Medela Medicorum* (1665), for its "Horrid Electuaries . . . crude Drossie syrups, endless varieties of Unguents & Plasters, most of which are useless."[23] By contrast, the minute doses of chemical medicine, and their ease of administration – calomel was a tasteless white powder – must have been one of the most telling arguments in their favour for both doctors and patients. And their excellent keeping qualities warmly recommended them to apothecaries: those costly Electuaries and syrups had a nasty habit of going "stale".

But what could the "chemists" offer that physicians were not already prescribing? For all their criticisms, they could not claim to have made any striking advances in the field of materia medica. They could not as yet point to a single plant preparation demonstrably superior to anything already on offer. So their passionate arguments that plants deserved closer and more thorough investigation fell on deaf ears.

Their hopes had risen high when Charles II was restored to the throne in 1660, and turned out to be not merely an enthusiastic amateur dabbler in medicine – in the best Royal tradition – but an admiring patron of chemical medicine. He had his own laboratory, he ordered a Physic garden to be planted for his use, and he appointed Nicholas Le Fevre as his personal Royal Professor in Chymistry. Charles began experimenting with mercury shortly after his return from exile, and it has been suggested that exposure to mercury fumes over the years might have been at least partially responsible for the disease that finally killed him.

In England as in France, Royal patronage made chemical medicine fashionable. And just as in France the new medicine had stood trial in a blaze of publicity at the sick-bed of the young Louis XIV, so now in England, seventeen years later, there came a grand and public chance for the "chemists" to prove how infinitely superior their therapy was.

By the spring of 1665 it was ominously clear that the Plague which had emptied Amsterdam that winter had crossed the North Sea: already the weekly Bills of Mortality in London were swelling alarmingly from this one cause. The Court, the nobility, and all who could afford to fled London. Most of the physicians went with them – they would plead, later, that these were, after all, their patients. Meanwhile the College of Physicians, at the request of the Privy Council, drew up for the benefit of the abandoned Londoners a list of "Certain Necessary Directions as Well for the Cure of the Plague and for the Prevention of Infection" into which they threw everything they could think of, from "Garlick with butter, 2 or 3 cloves", through doses of London theriac (cheaper than the Venice kind), to fourteen different chemical remedies for "those that are delighted with Chymical Medicines only."[24] The garlic at least may have been some use: garlic has powerful antibiotic properties (it is in the official U.S.S.R. pharmacopœia) and it was the principal ingredient in the famous Four Thieves' Vinegar (so called after a quartet of thieves who during the great Plague in Marseilles in 1722 sprinkled themselves liberally with it before plundering the bodies of plague victims: they all survived).

But still the Plague raged, and the empty streets of the city echoed to the dismal sound of tolling bells. Earlier that year, the existence of a Society of Chymical Physicians, with many important ducal and ecclesiastic backers, had been announced by one of their number, Thomas O'Dowde, who hoped for nothing less than a Charter from Charles II to put them on an equal footing with the Royal College of Physicians. Broadsheets now appeared all over the stricken city announcing that in response to "his Majesties command", members of this Society had all consulted "about the preparation of such Medicines, both *Preservative* and *Curative* by Art *Chymical*, as are not borrowed out of former Authors, but agreeably devised and fitted to the nature of the present Pest" – a dig at the College's fourteen chemical remedies. The Society felt confident that with God's blessing these Remedies would "secure the sound, and save the sick from this devouring Maladie". It listed the names and addresses of eight doctors – including Needham and Thomson – who could supply them.[25]

Chemical pride went before a fall. Within the next year more than 26,000 people had died of the Plague, whether they had swallowed theriac, pressed the rump of a live chick to the swellings, or applied to one of the eight for their remedies – "their most admired Preparations proving altogether unsuccessful" as a trumphant physician wrote.[26] Among the plague victims was O'Dowde himself: a martyr to his sense of duty, no doubt, but hardly the best possible advertisement for chemical medicine.

So the grand dreams of a reformed science of healing came to nothing, and public confidence in the medical profession sank to near-zero. Physicians became a favourite butt of cartoonists and satirists – rather like politicians today. The seventeenth–century French playwright Molière knew how to amuse his polished Versailles audience: no less than three of his most successful comedies – *Le Médecin Malgré Lui, L'Amour Médecin* and *Le Malade Imaginaire* – made fun of physicians. Louis XIV, curious, once asked Molière how he got on with his own doctor. The playwright replied: "Sire, we chat; he prescribes remedies for me: I take no notice; and I get better".[27]

In the circumstances charlatans and quacks flourished, as did more serious forms of what we now call alternative medicine, and in every capital of Europe there was one disease which ensured their success. Martin Lister, physician to the Earl of Portland who visited Paris with him in 1698, wrote: "All the talk here is of the Pox, a sickness which in Paris as in London has gone a fair way towards ruining medicine. Secret treatments for it have set up a number of wretched little animals of every kind."[28]

The great hope held out by all the syphilis quacks was summed up in a handbill printed by the famous London charlatan, John Case: "Over against *Ludgate* Church, within *Black-Fryers* Gate-way . . . liveth your old Friend Dr. Case, who faithfully Cures the Geand P- with all its Symptoms, very Cheap, Private, and without the least Hindrance of Business."[29] Another quack declared that he made it his life's study to find out means "more effectual than the common ways" for coping with what he stylishly termed the *Affection Allamode* and by God's help had attained to "a most expeditious, safe and easie method."[30]

First-time victims were certain to fall for such specious promises. Old hands like the Earl of Rochester, Charles II's companion in debauchery, of whom it was said that "he was ever engaged in some amour or other, and frequently with women of the lowest order, and the vilest prostitutes of the town"[31] – soon learned better and took themselves gloomily off once more to Mrs. Fourcard's Baths in Leather Lane, Hatton Garden, for a cure that had only privacy and an exclusive clientele to recommend it. Rochester's friend Savile wrote to him in 1678 from Leather Lane: "I confess I wonder at myself, and that mass of mercury that has gone down my throat in seven months, but should wonder yet more was it not for Mrs. Roberts [the daughter of a clergyman and one of the King's mistresses], for behold a greater than I, she is in the same house, and we have met here from several corners as mad folks do in Bedlam. What she has endur'd would make a dam'd soul fall a laughing at his lesser pains, it is so far beyond description or belief."[32]

No doubt Paris, too, had its Mrs. Fourcards for those who could afford them. For those who could not – beggars, prostitutes, even the pathetic children of poor and syphilitic parents – there loomed the Dantesque horrors of the Bicêtre Hospital, and the "Grands Remèdes". After a drastic initial regime of near-fasting, purging, bleeding, and vegetable tisanes, the patient swallowed his mercury and was sent to the "salles au noir" to spend his days spitting. In the first stage of the cure, the object was to excite salivation, in the second to control it; it was judged satisfactory when the wretched victim was spitting out four to six pounds of saliva a day. So that no mercury should be wasted, patients changed neither their shirts nor their sheets, both blackened with mercury they sweated out, and since the windows were kept tightly sealed – fresh air might be fatal to those undergoing the cure – the heat and the fetid stench were beyond description.

As with Mrs. Fourcard's Baths, there was certainly nothing "expeditious" about the "Grands Remèdes" – patients could count on at least a month of its horrors; and by no stretch of the imagination could it be called "safe" or "easy." Patients routinely lost all their teeth, and those who succumbed neither to the disease nor to the cure – as many did – often had their health permanently impaired by mercury poisoning. Any doctor who could genuinely have found a less disagreeable cure would have won fame and fortune overnight.

Louis XIV himself, despite his troops of official doctors, had a perfectly open mind on the subject of medicine. He had installed at the Louvre, for instance, a little laboratory, where two Capuchin friars busily confected an early tranquillizer made from aromatic plants, for which they claimed to have found the recipe in Egypt. The *baume tranquille* soon became the rage of Versailles, and Mme. de Sévigné christened them "les Pères Esculapes". When the Sun King developed a peculiarly painful anal fistula, for which the only cure seemed to be surgery, numbers of quacks and charlatans flocked to Versailles offering secret "cures." On Louis' orders, all but the most patently ridiculous were solemnly tried on a series of human guinea-pigs suffering from the same affliction.

Many quacks' cures were perfectly useless, pills and potions offered by arrant rogues who were marvellous entertainers but low on medical skill, like the Dutch quacks of London who cashed in on their country's medical repute – Leiden was among the most esteemed universities in Europe – to make a quick profit. One of these claimed to have attended William III at The Hague, and now offered his "Incomparable Powder", which never failed "to restore bodies decay'd by consumptions, to remove the raging heat of violent Feavours, to restore decaying Nature and prop the trembling frame of weak mortality, and to procure health to all that have been sporting in the Garden of Venus."[33]

Some quacks were worse than ignorant, like the so-called *Médecin du Chesnay* called in by Mme. Durafort, one of the ladies-in-waiting at Versailles. He administered to her so violent a cathartic that the wretched woman was purged not only of bloody stools but of yards of her own intestines, and died.

But although most people could tell a horror story or two of this sort, and although both in Paris and London the medical establishments were loud in their denunciations of charlatans, the public – led by the highest in the land – continued to flock to them, and to go on hoping for a quick and safe solution to their medical problems. Once in a while, their faith was justified.

There was, for instance, the London quack who made a speciality of treating piles, for which he was extraordinarily successful. There was nothing complicated about his cure, it turned out: he had probably taken the trouble to look up his Culpeper, found under Lesser Celandine (*Ranunculus ficaria*), the comment that "the decoction of the leaves and roots doth wonderfully help piles and hæmorrhoids," and put it to work.[34] It is, in fact, a remarkably successful remedy in many such cases, and has been used as such for centuries by country people, from whence comes its popular name pilewort.

Then there was the cheerful Dutchman called Adrian Helvetius who arrived in Paris in 1684 and set up what soon became a successful and fashionable practice, though frowned on by the Faculty as an "empirique." A Paris merchant called Garnier had received a consignment of one hundred and fifty pounds of ipecac (*Cephælis ipecacuanha*), from South America, and brought it to Helvetius with the report that it was said to be good for dysentery, the endemic "bloody flux" of the times. Helvetius probably tried it on his next cases of flux. If he had taken the trouble to look into its history more thoroughly, he would have learned that in a late sixteenth–century account of Brazil, written by a Portuguese friar, three native remedies had been mentioned for the flux, one of which was "igpecaya" – almost certainly this root. Helvetius' cases of flux, at any rate, got better, and he hastened to patent a composition containing the bitter-tasting root.

A few years later the remedy achieved resounding fame when Helvetius cured the Dauphin of a bloody flux with it, and went on to become Europe's leading dysentery expert, even travelling to Madrid in post chaises specially provided by Louis XIV to attend the Spanish Queen. He died rich and famous, one of Louis XV's doctors – and ipecacuanha entered Europe's official pharmacopœias, where its derivative emetine remains a specific cure for amœbic dysentery to this day.

Most remarkable of all the remedies promoted by practitioners outside the ranks of the College or the Faculty was the Peruvian bark (*Cinchona succirubra*), containing quinine. In the seventeenth century, malaria was the world's number one killer disease, endemic throughout Europe as well as Asia. A missionary in Peru announced to his Order's chronicle, in 1633, that the natives seemed to have a cure for it: "A tree grows which they call the Fever tree in the country of Loxa, whose bark is the colour of cinnamon. When made into a powder amounting to the weight of two small silver coins and given as a beverage, it cures the fevers and tertians. It has produced miraculous cures in Lima."[35]

Nobody in Europe seems to have paid much attention at the time – there was beginning to be a general feeling that South American wonder–drugs had been distinctly over-rated – and not until a Jesuit brought some to Rome, a notoriously malarial spot, and successfully tried it, did its fame begin to spread around Europe. Soon the Jesuits were shipping it regularly to Rome, and pilgrims began to take home little packets of "Jesuits' bark" for malarial friends and relations.

Among those it cured was the ageing Cardinal de Lugo, who was so astonished by its wonderful powers that he set himself the task of seeing that it was correctly administered. Soon every sample of the bark carried a little leaflet with directions for its proper use "against quartan and tertian fevers accompanied by shivers". The patient was to take "two drams of finely ground and sifted bark mixed in a glass of strong white wine three hours before fever is due. When first symptoms are noted, the patient is made to drink the whole infusion . . . and . . . put to bed . . . bark can be administered . . . when fever has persisted many days. . . . It must be used only on the advice of the physician who may consider whether it is timely to administer it."[36]

For one reason or another, the medical profession in Europe was curiously cool towards quinine, perhaps because it found no mention in Galen, possibly because – as a contemporary cynically surmised – "physicians and apothecaries resented the cure of a disease which had been for so long an unmixed financial blessing."[37] Its religious associations – with Rome and the feared and detested Jesuits – were certainly against it, too.

Unluckily, two eminent physicians who tried it both made well-publicized mistakes about its action. In 1652 the Archduke Leopold of Austria had it successfully administered to him by his doctor, Jean-Jacob Chiflet – who failed to give him another dose for the next attack. The Archduke died and Chiflet – disconcerted, enraged and embarrassed – thundered into print with a denunciation of "the Febrifuge Powder", claiming that it had a disastrous drying effect on the internal organs of patients. A decade later came another blast, this time from an English physician, the famous Thomas Sydenham, who announced gravely that the bark could endanger patients' lives, since by lowering their temperatures it stopped the process of "fermentation" by which the corrupt humours of the malaria patient were destroyed.

Two years later a young apothecary's apprentice called Robert Talbor arrived in London and set himself up as a "pyretiatro" or fever specialist, selling vast quantities of a secret remedy which had a huge success. He soon built the most lucrative practice in London, successfully cured Charles II of a bout of malaria, was knighted, appointed court physician, and sent to Paris when the Dauphin contracted malaria to cure him too. All this while, Talbor solemnly warned his patients and the public to "Beware of all palliative Cures and especially of that known by the name of Jesuits Powder . . . for I have seen most dangerous effects follow the taking of that medicine," thus cornering himself a lucrative monopoly of both the patients and the remedy.[38] Among those he cured were the Prince de Condé, the Duc de Rochefoucauld, and the Queen of Spain. (One of the nicest gestures a king could make at that time to an ailing royal friend was to dispatch his own physician to him with a successful remedy.)

Talbor was paid 3,000 gold crowns, a large pension and a title by Louis XIV, who promised not to reveal his secret until after the miracle-worker's death. The Sun-King – who may well have enjoyed this splendid joke on the medical profession – kept his word, and only after Talbor's death in 1681 was his secret formula revealed: it contained rose leaves, lemon juice, wine – and a strong infusion of Peruvian bark. One way and another, the public concluded, it was wisest to give the quacks a chance. You never knew your luck.

11

"Systematic Slaughter"

". . . The Arabians, Gentiles, Barbarians, Savages and Indians do more diligently observe their simples and things growing among them than all the European world besides" sadly noted Noah Biggs in 1651.[1]

There was perfect justice in this comment. Virtually all the new plant–drugs that excited the medical world of the sixteenth and seventeenth centuries were exotics: from 1602 when England at last signed a peace treaty with Spain, imports of these plants from the Spanish colonies had been increasing by leaps and bounds. By mid–century guaiac and sarsaparilla, balsam of Tolu and Peru, contrayerva and sassafras were all standard items on any European apothecary's shelves. And from the 1620s, these supplies were augmented by exports from Virginia, which had added to physicians' resources another new drug-plant– the snakeroot (*Aristolochia serpentaria*), a useful tonic and diaphoretic.

By the beginning of the eighteenth century, it was estimated that seventy per cent of the plant–drugs stocked by a European apothecary were imported, mainly from the Far East and the Americas. All these new drugs had been slotted neatly into the humoral approach to therapy: they purged, raised a sweat, were tonic or aromatic, and, as such, the seventeenth-century physician welcomed them with open arms.

The exotic origin of these drugs gave them the respectability of distance, as well as the appeal of novelty – always a powerful factor in medicine – while the apothecaries were naturally well–disposed towards costly imported drugs. Yet as it was pointed out a century later, "those celebrated medicines we import from the Indies at a considerable annual expense" were nothing more nor less than the local folk-medicine – "remedies by long experience approved among the common people in the countries from which we purchase them."[2]

The folk-medicine traditions of Europe itself were still rich and vigorous at this time, as we know from a number of sources. And there were certainly as many interesting medicinal plants growing in Europe that still awaited "discovery" by the medical profession as there were in the Indies or the Americas. Marchmont Needham claimed to have collected dozens of such remedies, of "great efficacy", in conversations with "the meaner Persons and Practisers, which the Learned . . . are wont to scorn."[3] The chemist Robert Boyle felt that ". . . the Art of Physic might be improved if Physicians were a little more curious, to take notice of the observations and experiments . . . of Midwives, Barbers, Old Women, Empiricks and other Illiterate persons".[4]

But the attitude of the medical profession remained one of patronizing contempt towards many of these homegrown remedies, as it was towards those who employed them. It is hard to excuse this attitude: much less hard to account for it.

The eighteenth-century European physician was the product of long years of training. Some of this time might be spent actually studying sickness first-hand, at the bedside of the patient – the famous medical school of Leiden had led Europe in this innovation – but most was spent mastering an approach to disease which was based upon a series of elaborately formulated propositions, largely the work of Galen and Avicenna.

In recent centuries, it was true, the structure had been severely jolted. The Belgian anatomist Andreas Vesalius (1514–1564) had exposed several serious errors in Galenic anatomy; William Harvey (1578–1657) had discovered the circulation of the blood; Leuwenhook (1632–1723) in Leiden and Marcello Malpighi (1624–1694) in Bologna had studied a strange new world of nameless animalcula and minute blood-vessels through primitive microscopes.

But medicine remained a theoretical science, and early in the eighteenth century there appeared on the medical scene a new Galen: the solid, reassuring figure of Hermann Boerhaave (1668–1738), the Avicenna of eighteenth-century medicine.

Boerhaave was born in a small Dutch village near Leiden, the son of a minister, and grew up intending to enter the ministry himself. At the age of sixteen, he began his studies at Leiden University, and took his divinity degree in 1690. A glutton for learning, he studied mathematics as well as philosophy, and in turn became absorbed by medicine, avidly reading the work of every author, ancient and modern, on which he could lay hands.

Although Boerhaave appears never to have attended a single formal lecture in medicine – he was almost entirely self-taught – he presented a thesis in 1693 at the University of Harderwyk, and received his doctor's degree, by which time he was also an expert chemist.

Leiden University, which was to be his life, made the most of this prodigy: in 1709 he was appointed to the joint Chair of Medicine and Botany, in 1714 to the Chair of Clinical Medicine, and in 1718, the Chair of Chemistry. He occupied all three concurrently for some time, with brilliant distinction, as well as running the most famous consultancy practice in Europe. He died in 1738, hard at work to the end.

Only a man of immense discipline and method could have accomplished the staggering amount of work that such a career entailed, and Boerhaave was nothing if not methodical, both in his habits and in his approach to medicine. His starting-point, arrived at partly from his wide-ranging studies, and partly as a result of his anatomical observations, was the conviction that health resulted from the proper interaction of the body's solids and fluids. From this, he developed a new system of medicine which he believed took into account the most recent discoveries of the day, and brought the science of medicine up to date.

Boerhaave constantly stressed that all theory must be confirmed by observation at the sickbed, and modern medical historians paint him as the father of clinical training. But it was the beautiful completeness of his theories, not the decades of careful observation upon which they were based, which impressed the medical world of his day, and which carried utter conviction to the next four or five generation of European physicians. A student of Edinburgh University in the 1730s recalled: "I was taught to think the system of Boerhaave to be very perfect, complete and sufficient."[5]

Thus despite Paracelsus and Harvey, despite Vesalius and Leuwenhook and Malpighi, the eighteenth-century European physician almost inevitably grew up a theorist, with a confirmed belief in the importance of general principles. His proud contempt for Empiric was not merely the contempt of the professional who has received fourteen years of expensive university training for the amateur who has had none, but that of a man thoroughly conversant with the first principles of medicine for the impudent quack who was simply groping in the dark. Where doctor and quack chiefly disagreed was in the way they decided what medicine might be useful.

The professional physician prescribed for what his long training had taught him might be the underlying condition which had given rise to the patient's distressing symptoms. The blood might be too viscid – or too thin; the predominant acrimony of the humours might be "acid and austere" – or "rancid and oily". The bodily fluids might be circulating too freely – or else stagnating; there might be an obstruction of the viscera. According to his diagnosis, the physician would then prescribe medicines which might be acid or alkaline, stimulant or sedative, heating or cooling, and so on, while an evacuant of one sort or another – emetic, diaphoretic, sudorific, diuretic, purgative – was almost always considered a necessity.

To the country healer, wise-woman or "Empirick", all this learned theorizing was – quite literally – so much Greek and Latin. Instead, they prescribed directly for a particular ailment, using plants known to have a useful action in such cases. ". . . where the Practitioners of Physick are altogether illiterate, there oftentimes Specificks may best be met with, because such persons . . . for want of skill in physick . . . do almost wholly rely upon specificks. . . ."[6]

Culpeper's herbal is written largely with this class of practitioner – as well as ordinary domestic use – in mind. Instead of classifying his plants into various degrees of coolness, drying and so on, Culpeper plainly said what sicknesses they were good at making better, often quoting his own experience, as with the Celandine (*Chelidonium majus*); it can, he says, be made into an oil or ointment – "which you please, to anoint your sore eyes with: I can prove it both by my own experience and the experience of those to whom I have taught it, that most desperate sore eyes have been cured by this only medicine . . . the juice . . . rubbed often upon warts will take them away . . . the juice or decoction of the herb gargled between the teeth that ache, easeth the pain."[7]

To the professional physician, such "Specificks" were almost a rude word, since they ran counter to all this training; and one of the reasons why the European medical profession gave such a cool reception to Cinchona or Peruvian bark was precisely because it was a "Specifick" cure for malaria.

So doctors continued snobbishly to ignore many useful medicinal plants growing in their own countries. And those who were prepared to learn from "meaner Persons", or pick up useful tips from old women were, naturally, few and far between. There were exceptions like the great Thomas Sydenham (1624–1689), who claimed to have cured dropsies by garlic alone, and the philosopher-doctor John Locke, who prescribed endless reliable English country herbal remedies, by letter, for his friends the Clarke family.

The disease scurvy offers an appalling example of the tragic gulf that yawned at this time between the theoretical doctor and the humble country practitioner with his despised "Specificks".

Scurvy is a deficiency disease, caused by a lack of the Vitamin C supplied by fresh fruit and green vegetables, of which citrus fruits are a particularly rich source. In the seventeenth century it was considered a "New Disease", partly because all kinds of skin diseases were now being christened "scorbutic", but mainly because sailors on the long sea voyages which had become common were vulnerable to scurvy once supplies of fresh fruit and vegetables ran out, while poor people crowded into the rapidly proliferating slums of the big cities like London often lacked either fruit or vegetables in their diet.

While nobody knew what caused scurvy, the disease itself was grimly familiar to naval and military surgeons. James Lind quotes an accurate description of it from a Dr. Grainger, who observed nearly a hundred cases of it among the troops stationed at Fort William: "Its first appearances were, *lassitudo*, breathlessness, upon the least quickness of motion, and a taste in the mouth peculiarly disagreeable: which were soon followed by rotten, spungy, painful gums, bleeding from the slightest touch; foetid breath; pains always of their thighs, frequently of their legs . . . sometimes discoloured with purple *maculae*. Neither were much swelled, yet both were harder than usual; and so extremely painful, that the gentlest touch gave agony . . . the contagion spread, their faces grew strangely sallow, their teeth loosened, palate and fauces ulcerated, asthma increased; they fell away, slept little, old ulcers broke out again, cried out when turned a-bed, and sometimes fainted upon motion of their body. . . . what surprised me most, was, that their appetite even in these deplorable circumstances, was not greatly impaired."[8]

If nobody knew what caused scurvy, however, the remedy for it had been known in folk medicine for centuries. Throughout Northern Europe there grew a cure so well-known and so reliable that the small, creeping, round-leaved plant providing it is known, simply, as scurvy-grass (*Cochlearia officinalis*). It does in fact contain significant amounts of Vitamin C – as much as oranges – and Gerard pointed out that it is "a singular medicine against the corrupt and rotten ulcer, and stench of the mouth: it perfectly cureth the disease called. . . the Scurvie" which he then described in accurate clinical detail. Scurvy-grass, he added for good measure, was thought by many authors to have been the plant the "Caesars soldiers, when they remouved their camps beyond the Rhene found to preuaile (the Frisians had taught it them) against that plague and hurtfull disease. . . ."⁹ Scurvy-grass, according to Gerard, grew freely along the banks of the Thames, on the Essex and Kent coasts; indeed, wherever it was needed, as though specially planted by divine Providence.

Enlightened seamen knew other ways to deal with scurvy: John Hawkins wrote of the curative powers of "sowre Orange and Lemons" as early as 1593. John Woodhall, without whose *Surgion's Mate* (1617) no self-respecting ship's surgeon would have dreamt of putting to sea, wrote in it that "The use of the juice of Lemons is a precious medicine and well tried, being sound & good, let it have the chiefe place for it will deserve it."¹⁰ The Dutch, whose supremacy at sea was unchallenged till late in the seventeenth century were not often troubled by scurvy: sauerkraut was regularly served to their sailors.

The quacks of London, whose livelihood depended on a high success-rate, used scurvy-grass almost to a man, although they gave their wares impressive names like Thomas Blagrave's "Golden Spirit of Scurvy-grass", or Clark's "Compound Spirits of Scurvy-Grass", which was claimed to cure not merely scurvy but also rheums, tooth-ache, asthma, and the dreaded stone in the bladder. Since scurvy-grass could be bought from the physical herb-women for a penny a basket, the quacks who sold their Spirit of Scurvy-Grass for 6 pence a bottle, were doing quite nicely.

It may have been this very unanimity among the ignorant on the subject of cures for scurvy that made learned physicians feel that there must be more to it than met the common eye. And in 1753 the naval surgeon James Lind (1716–1794) reported on the consequences of the general theorizing spree that broke out in Europe from the mid-sixteenth century onwards. His treatise on scurvy, one of the great classics of medical literature, was written after years of experience of the disease in the British Navy, and prompted by Anson's account of a voyage round the world in which almost nine-tenths of the crew died of it.

Lind began by giving an account of the professional literature that had accumulated in two centuries on the subject of scurvy, and all the theories put forward – "galenical, chymical and mechanical, according to the whim of each author, and the philosophy then in fashion."[11] The most influential of these writers – warmly recommended to his pupils by the great Boerhaave – was Severino Eugaleno, whose work, published in 1641, was considered the standard writing on the subject for more than a century. Eugaleno thought that scurvy was a brand-new disease, sent by God as punishment for the sins of the world; that it was contagious; and that it assumed so many different forms that only careful professional examination of the pulse and urine could detect this disease lurking in so many forms.

The medical profession rose as one to this intriguing challenge, since, although Eugaleno had proposed – and declared his firm belief in – the ordinary, familiar remedies, he had not been clever enough to invent a theory that would account for their efficacy. "It was left to Dr. Willis" pursued Lind with scorching irony, "with the assistance of Dr. Lower, to clear up a subject that lay under very great obscurity, by reducing the whole into an ingenious system, which continues established and adopted even at this day".[12]

Dr. Willis, in his *Tractatus de scorbuto*, published in 1667, observed that no single description or definition of this disorder could be given, and described some of the symptoms to which it might give rise – including violent headache, dullness of the spirits, inordinate pulse, foetid breath, wasting of the flesh, and frequent and wandering pains. Its principal causes were unwholesome air, and either a "sulphureo-saline" or else a "salino-sulphureous dyscrasy of the blood", according to which repeated bleedings and a cooling regime – or, on the contrary, warmer and more volatile remedies – suggested themselves.[13]

Boerhaave's list of scurvy symptoms was even more extensive than that of Willis, divided into four distinct stages. But he was clear about the cause: it was "an extraordinary separation of the serous part of the blood from the crassamentum; the former being dissolved, thin and acrid; whilst the latter, or the grumous part, is too thick and viscid. . . ." For cure, Boerhaave recommended purges, deobstruent (opening the bowels or pores) and attenuating medicines, as well as the ordinary antiscorbutics in their elaborate apothecary preparations. But in the fourth and final stage of the disease – by which time he considered it generally incurable – he added that mercurial medicines might help.[14]

By the mid-eighteenth century the victims of all this learned theorizing could be counted in tens of thousands. There was for example, the case of the Imperial troops in Hungary during the siege of Belgrade in 1720: on miserable army rations, during the long bitter winter, thousands of them went down with scurvy. The first remedy tried was mercury, with disastrous results: "they all died in a salivation."

The army's chief physician, Kramer, then tried everything he could think of: at the end of the two years he wrote in desperation to the College of Physicians in Vienna to ask their advice. He had first administered a vomit, and followed it with "the most approved anti-scorbutic remedies": these were, however, dried, since the fresh green plants were unobtainable. Since dried plants contain no Vitamin C, nothing happened, and he had gone on to try "salts of every kind . . . hartshorn, creme of tartar, sal ammonica, tincture of bezoar, and vinegar" – because it was acid, like the lemons he could not get. There was, he said despairingly, "nothing that has been recommended by the best classical and standard authors which I have not made trial of, *except the juice of the fresh green plants*" (Lind's italics).[15]

The rations provided for the eighteenth-century British Navy, laid down by a penny-pinching Admiralty, contained virtually no source of Vitamin C: it was left to the good sense of individual officers and surgeons to see that their men were provided with fresh fruit and vegetables whenever possible. Even four years after Lind published his work, the only remedy against scurvy carried in the ships of the Royal Navy was the Elixir of Vitriol, which had been the first choice of the Royal College of Physicians when their advice was sought. The basic ingredient of this disagreeable brew is sulphuric acid: in a typical seventeenth-century recipe, quoted by Hartmann, it was brewed with spirits of wine, aloes, myrrh and English saffron. Myrrh (*Commiphora myrrha*), is both healing and astringent, for which reason herbalists usually include it in any mouth-wash, so it would have helped with the typical rotting gums of scurvy. But the sulphuric acid could only have acted as an irritant in such cases.

The result of Admiralty parsimony and College folly was that of the 185,000 men pressed into service in the navy for the Seven Years' War, 130,000 – nearly three-quarters of their number – died from disease, of whom the majority were victims of scurvy. "This alone," commented Lind angrily, "proved a more destructive enemy, and cut off more valuable lives, than the united efforts of the French and Spanish arms."[16]

Determined "to propose nothing dictated merely from theory",

Lind conducted his own clinical trial of various remedies, during a cruise in 1747, of the *Salisbury*, whose surgeon he then was. He took twelve patients, all in much the same state of scurvy, and isolated them in the same quarters on the same diet. Two were ordered a quart of cider a day; two a soothing electuary containing garlic and gum myrrh; two took the elixir of vitriol; two plenty of vinegar; two were put on a course of sea-water; and the remaining two had two oranges and a lemon each every day. "These they eat with greediness," noted Lind.

The trial continued for two weeks. The oranges and lemons ran out on the sixth day, but the two who had been eating them were on their feet at the end of the fortnight: one had already resumed his duties, the other was nursing the rest. The two on cider looked rather better. The others showed little or no improvement.[17]

Lind buttressed his case with every single example he had been able to gather from history, from correspondence with medical men, and from naval records of actual cases of scurvy and their cure. He concluded triumphantly that "Experience indeed sufficiently shows, that as greens or fresh vegetables with ripe fruits, are the best remedies for it, so they prove the most effectual preservative against it."[18]

It took another fifty years before the Admiralty finally bowed to this irrefutable evidence, and in 1795 ordered that every sailor in the British Navy should in the future have a ration of an ounce of lemon juice issued after the sixth week at sea. Within two years, scurvy in the British Navy was a thing of the past.

"Of theory in physic," remarked Lind, "the same may be perhaps said, as has been observed by some of zeal in religion, that it is indeed absolutely necessary; yet by carrying it too far, it may be doubted whether it has done more good or hurt in the world."[19]

12

The English Practice

Doctors have never been very responsive to suggestions from outside their own ranks. And the case of scurvy is another tragic instance of the price European settlers in North America paid for professional arrogance: as contempt for the "primitive" Indian became engrained in the white American mentality, the notion that he might be the possessor of useful medical secrets came to seem more and more far-fetched.

Few North American Indians suffered from scurvy. Their diet included plenty of fruit, nuts, and vegetables, and was rich in Vitamin C for most of the year. Even in the depths of winter, when snow covered the ground and most trees and bushes were stripped of greenery, the Indians knew how to cure cases of scurvy: They broke off branches from the evergreen pine or spruce trees, and drank an infusion made from them. European fur-trappers and fishermen who spent part of each year in bleak Newfoundland, northern Canada and Maine, had learned this cure from the Indians: their everyday drink was spruce beer.

This Indian remedy was noted by the indefatigable John Josselyn in 1652 for the benefit of English settlers. Yet just a hundred years later, in 1745, Dr. Cadwallader Colden of New York was reporting regretfully that scurvy "was exceedingly common in North America, & hardly anybody free of it".[1] While the "white even teeth" of the Indians were the object of general envy, the European migrants by contrast, had often lost every tooth in their heads from scurvy.[2]

Josselyn's useful hint had been forgotten, and after him few observers of native medicine in the New World were quite as well-qualified – or as sympathetic. Those few physicians who were interested to know how the Indians coped with their medical problems, or hoped to learn exciting new medicinal plants from them, were usually spare-time botanists, like Dr. Colden, Dr. Alexander Garden of Charleston, and Dr. John Mitchell of Urbana, Virginia, who swapped accounts of medicinal plants with each other and with distinguished European botanists like Carl Linnæus in Sweden, Gronovius in Holland, and Peter Collinson in England.

The most outstanding of these colonial botanist–doctors was the Scottish-born Cadwallader Colden. He was at one time Governor of New York – where in the face of local interests he tried to have sanitation and drainage measures enforced to protect the city from yellow fever – and, rare for a European, a good friend of the Iroquois. The enormous correspondence that he left is evidence of a fine and far-ranging mind, an alert scientific curiosity, and an impartial will-ingness to try any remedy, from whatever source, that might have a chance of success agains the ills that plagued North America.

Colleagues throughout the colonies sent him accounts of promising drug-plants they had come across, often with seeds and cuttings, and he tried several that later found their way into standard medicine. Pinkroot (*Spigelia marilandica*) was sent to him from Charleston by Dr. Garden who had learned of its use among the Cherokees. It was, reported Garden, excellent as a cure for worms. A century later, powdered pinkroot was a standard worming-cure for children to be found in every American druggist's shop. Poke root (*Phytolacca americana*) was another plant that excited Colden – he was convinced that poultices of its thick fleshy root would cure skin cancers. He also tried wild geranium (*Geranium maculatum*) for dynsentery cases – the roots contain astringent tannin.

When in 1758 Sir William Johnson, British government agent to the northern Indians, bought what the Indians claimed was a marvellous remedy for syphilis, Colden followed the trials of it on English troops with the keenest interest: He reported enthusiastically to Dr. Robert Whytt of Edinburgh University that syphilitic soldiers had been cured with less than an ounce of this *Lobelia syphilitica* (as it was to be known) in under a week. Whytt, who specialized in neurology, was sufficiently impressed to write back asking for some of the root to try in the Royal Infirmary.

A much earlier trial of a native medicinal plant by a European doctor had been carried out by Dr. John Tennent in Virginia. Arriving from England in 1625, he found his new patients plagued with respiratory illnesses, and ventured to test on some of his pleurisy cases a snake-bite remedy that the Seneca Indians were using. When he found that it gave good results, he published a paper on the Seneca Snakeroot, *Polygala senega*, as he called it, urged every practitioner he knew to try it, and preached the snake-root so assiduously that soon his colleagues were sick of the very sound of its name – not, perhaps, having been enthusiastic about an Indian remedy in the first place. Years after Tennent had retired to sulk in England, disenchanted by the payment of a paltry £100 for his great discovery, Dr. Garden shipped a whole bundle of the snakeroot to Dr. Colden to test.

However, by the end of the eighteenth century, after more than a century and a half of continuous white settlement in North America, few native medicinal plants had found a secure place in professional medicine, although many had made their way into common domestic use. It was not until 1772 that the first American herbal appeared. Designed as the vegetable section of a more complete materia medica, it was the work of Dr. Samuel Stearns of Massachusetts whose ambition was no less than to produce "a completer system of pharmacy, physic, and surgery . . . than ever appeared before in any part of the world."[3] Stearns perhaps saw himself as the Boerhaave of backward American medicine – "our theory stands in great need of reformation and amendment".[4] And although he claims that his herbal contained "a large number of new medical discoveries and improvements collected . . . from the Indians . . ."[5] it is plain that he had a true European scorn of these unlettered empirics, "whose want of knowledge in the liberal arts and sciences, renders it impossible for them to be regularly bred physicians. . . ."[6]

His information about Indian medicine seems to have come to him mainly at secondhand, through the "country people". Indian sources are seldom quoted directly, and Stearns was ignorant of the way they used several of the plants that they valued most highly, such as the pleurisy root (*Asclepias tuberosa*), Indian physic (*Porteranthus trifoliatus*), and maize (*Zea mays*). This was hardly surprising; while the Indian was interested in a specific cure for this or that ailment, the white physician was chiefly excited by "activity" – the more "brisk" the purgative or emetic action of a plant, the more happily confident of its powers he became.

Wake-robin (*Arisaema triphyllum*) – the transatlantic cousin of the British cuckoo-pint, *Arum maculatum* – neatly illustrated the two approaches. Its fleshy turnip-like root is violently irritant to the mouth if chewed, and if even a small amount is swallowed, it can cause violent gastro-enteritis and sometimes death. The Indian roasted or boiled it to destroy its acrimony, and then used it as both food and medicine in coughs, fevers and stomach complaints. Stearns, on the other hand, enthusiastically recommended doses of the fresh root for a wide range of ailments including jaundice and hypochondria. He notes approvingly – in the best Boerhaave style – that "it stimulates the solids, attenuates the fluids, promotes the natural secretions, and is beneficial in cold, languid, phlegmatic constitutions".[7] It was perhaps as well for his readers that he prefaced his work with that caveat that has now become standard in all medical handbooks addressed to the layman: "I . . . earnestly recommend to all persons, who are not regularly bred physicians that when they are smitten with dangerous diseases, they lean not too much upon their own understanding . . . but apply in season to some skilful physician."[8]

Finding this "skilful physician" was a problem that had vexed the colonies from the beginning. Until late in the eighteenth century, when the first regular medical school was founded at Philadelphia, a proper training meant a European training – at Leiden, Paris, or Edinburgh. But such physicians were few and far between, and many of those who did go to Europe for training failed to return, succumbing to the lure of an easy, lucrative practice in the Old Country.

In the absence of a physician, people turned to the apothecary, of whom there were soon plenty; a situation as much deplored by trained doctors in the New World as in the Old. In 1721 Dr. William Douglas wrote to Dr. Colden from Boston: "You complain of the Practice of Physic being undervalued in your parts and with reason, we are not much better in that respect . . . we have 14 Apothecary shops in Boston, all our Practitioners dispense their own medicines, myself excepted being the first who has lived here by Practice without the advantage of advance on Medicines".[9]

Since outside large cities like Boston it was difficult for a doctor to make a living without the sale of drugs to boost his income, this form of independent practice was rare. By mid-eighteenth century the typical American doctor was running his own dispensary where drugs were sold over the counter as well as by prescription – a practice that survived until well into the twentieth century.

Some doctors went even further. In the *New York Gazette* of 3 August 1752, Dr. Charles Scham Leslie advertised "a choice Assortment of Medicines" newly arrived in the *Nebuchadnezzer*, "quite fresh, and allowed to come from the most eminent Hand . . . to be sold very cheap." Dr. Leslie had clearly had his eyes recently opened to the lucrative possibilities of this line of trading: "intending to deal for the Future in that Branch of Business" continued the announcement, the good Doctor "will always take care to have fresh Assortments from London."[10]

Both doctor and apothecary were heavily reliant on a regular supply of drugs from the Old World. Until 1775 when the Continental Association forbade trade with Great Britain, newspapers in all the English colonies regularly carried advertisements of the following kind: "Imported in the *Duchess of Queensbery*, and just come to Hand, a large Assortment of Drugs with all Manner of Chymical and Galenical Medicines, faithfully prepared, also a Quantity of Almonds in the soft Shell, fresh Currans, Turkey Coffee, Prunes, Tamerind, Bateman's and Stoughton's Drops, Daffy's and Squire's Elixir, British Rock-Oil, Turlington's and universal Balsam . . . Anderson's and Lockyer's Pills . . . Cinnamon, Cloves, Mace, Nutmeg, Sugar Plumbs, Carraway Comfits, candied Eringo, Citron Allum . . . Chocolate, Bohea, Congo and Green Tea, strong and good white Tartar Emetic, with ditto dark . . . Oriental and Occidental Bezoar . . . Juice of Buckthorn, Syringes, Glyster Pipes, Nipple Glasses and Pipes etc. . . . "[11]

Earlier in the eighteenth century, apothecaries were still proclaiming their familiarity with the *London Dispensatory*, and their ability and readiness to concoct any of its elaborate compounds. But their prohibitive cost, compounded as they were of ingredients that had to be imported into Britain first, together with the near-impossibility of guaranteeing their freshness and quality, soon reduced their popularity with the colonial apothecary and his customer alike.

Their place was quickly filled by a number of the patent medicines which were having such a resounding success in England for much the same reasons. Preparations like Daffy's Elixir (a spiced tincture of senna) and James Fever Powder (an antimonial preparation), Dover's Powder – a combination of opium and ipecac – for dysentery, and Godfrey's Cordial, a sedative painkiller made of opium, were soon as familiar household words in North America as they were in England. Even the bottles were familiar – the pear-shaped bottle of Turlington's balsam or the truncated cone of Godfrey's Cordial – and by the 1750s they were imported empty to be filled by an American version of the original compound.

The complete inventory of one Virginia doctor's shop and pharmaceutical equipment has survived to tell an eloquent story of its owner's European prescribing habits and his customers in 1746. Among the most heavily-stocked items were Peruvian bark (for use against the malaria which was so common in Virginia); syrup of buckthorn – a good hearty purge; plasters of melilot (*Melilotus officinalis*), an old-fashioned but still popular country herbal remedy for abdominal aches and rheumatic pains; Elixir of Vitriol, presumably for scurvy cases; treacle water; compound bryony water (*Bryonia dioica*) (another vicious purge); and flowers of chamomile (*Anthemis nobilis*) – popular in domestic medicine for upset stomachs and children's nightmares.

There were plenty of herbal purges and cathartics – jalap, scammony, rhubarb, senna, and soccotrine or Barbados aloes (*Aloe vera*) – and alarming quantities of Blistering Plaster, or the tiny Spanish beetle called Cantharides, which produced a violent irritation of the whole urinary system. There were also daunting amounts of both mercury and antimony, in various forms.

But the only drug in the whole inventory which could have been North American in origin was sweet flag (*Acorus calamus*) or calamus, an aromatic tonic already familiar in Britain, where the roots used were usually imported from India, although Gerard had successfully grown it in his garden.

"The practice of this country" observed a French tourist in 1788 "is the English practice; that is, they are much in the use of violent remedies."[12] A Boston doctor, questioned about local medical habits in the mid-eighteenth century, put it more vividly: "the local practice" he said "was very uniform, bleeding, vomiting, blistering, purging, anodyne, etc. if the illness continued there was repetendi, and finally murderandi".[13]

It is sometimes put forward as a point in favour of American colonial medicine that the training was rigorously practical: instead of yawning on the benches of lecture-halls the young American medical student apprenticed himself to a practitioner and spent the next three years trotting behind his master as he went his rounds – getting clinical practice, instead of theory. When the practitioner was an honest and skilful doctor of long experience, no more admirable training could have been devised. But in nine cases out of ten, the student's master was an apothecary who made his living by selling drugs rather than giving sound advice, and often practised accordingly. Thus the American system translated European drugging habits to the fertile new soil of the colonies, where they flourished with the apothecary business.

On the frontiers of civilization – on remote farms, in isolated country homesteads, and in trading outposts – it was another matter. People were often obliged by circumstance to be their own doctors, to dispense with the apothecary and his patent medicines, to rely on what the country offered in the way of plant medicine, and to turn to those who could instruct them in their use – the Indians.

And far from the Eastern seaboard with its fevers and ship-borne infections, toughened by strenuous outdoor life, the white man found that he had much the same medical problems as the Indian, with whom he was often on friendly terms: the Indian suffered from the same broken limbs and wounds, frostbite and chills and rheumatism, foul sores and ulcers. Indian skill at dealing with these was, however, a revelation to many of the whites.

James Adair, an educated trader among the southern Indians, wrote of the Cherokees: ". . . they, as well as all other Indian nations, have a great knowledge of specific virtues in simples; applying herbs and plants, on the most dangerous occasions, and seldom, if ever, fail to effect a thorough cure . . . for my own part, I would prefer an old Indian before any chirurgeon whatsoever in curing green wounds by bullet, arrows &c."[14]

This low opinion of the white doctoring available was fully shared by the wealthy and agreeable planter William Byrd (1652–1704), one of the richest landowners in Virginia in the early eighteenth century. Unlike most planters, who were prepared to spend fortunes on doctors to look after themselves and their valuable and vulnerable slaves, Byrd would not allow a locally-trained doctor near his family and servants. "Here be some men indeed that are call'd Doctors: but they are generally discarded Surgeons of Ships, that know nothing above very common Remedys" he wrote in 1706 to Sir Hans Sloane. "They are not acquainted enough with Plants or the other parts of Natural History, to do any Service to the World".[15] Byrd reckoned that he could do as well as these discarded surgeons, he had the best medical library in the colony, kept up with European advances in medical science – he was proud to be a member of the famous Royal Society in London – and did his best to make the acquaintance of the neglected plants, often sending specimens to London for trial.

On a boundary survey expedition, some members of the party came down with malaria. "Our Chief Medicine" reported Byrd, "was Dogwood Bark, which we used, instead of that of Peru, with good Success."[16] Since the Peruvian bark imported into the colonies was often adulterated, dogwood bark (*Cornus florida*), became widely known as an effective native substitute, and the Pennsylvania Germans used it as a general fever remedy.

In the mid-eighteenth century, a ginseng boom which was at least comparable to the Gold Rush of a century later swept North America. As with Peruvian bark, it was a Jesuit who was responsible for its discovery: the missionary Father Jartoux, while travelling in Tartary, was given the root of wild ginseng (*Panax ginseng*), as a remedy for exhaustion. He was so astonished by its efficacy that he made enquiries, and learned that no other medicinal plant was more highly prized by the Chinese. Merchants paid huge prices for a perfect root, it was featured in numbers of prescriptions, and was considered an unrivalled tonic and panacea.

When news of this valuable plant got back to Europe the hunt was up. Soon another Jesuit, Father Martineau, who was working as a missionary among the Indians in what was then French Canada discovered what seemed to be the same plant – which was used by some Indians in much the same way. It was in fact another species of ginseng, *Panax quinquefolium*, but its action turned out to be similar to that of the Asiatic ginseng. Very soon the French were making fortunes shipping it direct to China, and the ginseng boom took off. The " 'sang-digger" became a familiar feature of the American outback, and the Indians found collecting the roots a profitable new job.

Years earlier, Byrd had discovered the virtues of ginseng, and often drank night and morning a tea that he made as the Chinese do, simmering a piece of the root in water in a silver teapot over a charcoal fire. "It gives an uncommon Warmth and Vigour to the Blood, and frisks the Spirits beyond any other Cordial. It chears the Heart even of a Man that has a bad Wife, and makes him look down with great Composure on the crosses of the World . . . In one Word, it will make a Man live a great while, and very well while he does live . . . However 'tis of little use in the Feats of Love, as a great prince once found, who hearing of its invigorating Quality, sent as far as China for some of it, though his ladys could not boast of any Advantage thereby".[17]

Among the plants Byrd sent to England, to be inspected by Sir Hans Sloane, was "a seed of the Jerusalem Oak, as we call it, which kills worms better than any wormseed I ever heard of."[18] Jerusalem oak (*Chenopodium ambrosioides*), was soon adopted on most plantations as a remedy for the intestinal parasites that plagued the slaves, particularly the children who ran around barefoot: one plantation manager directed that the slave children should have "every Spring & Fall the Jerusalem Oak seed for a week together."[19]

Another of Byrd's favourite remedies was Indian Physic (*Porteranthus trifoliatus*), which the country people were beginning to use as a home-grown substitute for ipecac – "an Excellent Vomit" according to Byrd ". . . and generally cures intermitting Fevers and Bloody Fluxes at once or twice taking."[20] Hearing of a bad local epidemic of dysentery or the Bloody Flux during one of his absences, Byrd at once wrote directions to his overseer, Mr. Booker, on how this was to be dealt with if there were any cases on his plantation: he was "to let them Blood immediately about 8 ounces; the next day to give them a Dose of Indian Physic, and to repeat the vomit again the Day following, unless the Symptoms abated. In the mean time they shou'd eat nothing but Chicken Broth, and Poacht Eggs, and drink nothing but a Quarter of a Pint of Milk boil'd with a Quart of Water, and Medicated with a little Mullein Root."[21]

This rational and successful cure may be contrasted with the treatment ordered for the Philadelphia Quaker merchant Henry Drinker, in the summer of 1807. On 2 September he began to feel "very unwell in his bowels, he voids blood in his stools", as his anxious wife Elizabeth wrote in her diary. The most celebrated physician in the city, Dr. Benjamin Rush (1745–1813), was sent for. Dr. Rush prescribed a blister, and 100 drops of "asthmatic Elexer", probably our old friend made with vitriol. Returning the following day to find no improvement in his patient, "he advised another bleeding . . . 8 ounces . . . he also advis'd rice water, and an injection at going to bed, of flaxceed tea a gill, and 40 drops liquid laudonum. . . .

"Sepr. 4 My husband has been very unwell all day, he was let blood ye 3d day successively. . . . Dr. Rush was here this morn.g and even he advis'd, if the ladunum glyster to be given at bed time did not answer ye end wish'd for, to repeat it in the night. . . .

"5 . . . Dr. Rush came he ask'd me what I thought of my husband loosing 6 ounces more blood, he was sure it was necessary . . . he ordered 6 or 8 ounces more taken. . . ." Dr. Rush also ordered a blister to be put on both Henry Drinker's wrists, two more injections or enemas, and called another doctor in for consultation the next morning. Many pills and enemas later, Henry Drinker was finally considered better, and Dr. Rush made his last visit on 3 October.[22]

It is hard to believe that Dr. Rush deserved any of the credit for his patient's recovery, though to Elizabeth Drinker, this was perfectly normal treatment. But then the human race has always believed that desperate ills require desperate remedies, and dysentery, which actually did kill many colonists, was only one of the devastating diseases that swept through whole cities bringing grief and terror to the inhabitants. The true cause of these epidemics – bacteria, flourishing in the hospitable conditions of poor sanitation and inadequate hygiene – were not even guessed at; nobody knew that yellow fever, like malaria, was communicated by the bite of a mosquito that had travelled to North America in the water-buckets of a slave-ship; there were no antibiotics.

Most heart-breaking – for doctors as well as patients – were the diseases to which small children were particularly susceptible, such as the "putrid sore throat" which raged regularly through North American cities. Writing in this century, one American doctor could recall standing at the window as a small child to watch a line of wagons going slowly down the road, each bearing an oblong box; he learned as the days went by that the boxes contained the bodies of his playmates. "Eight of the nine children in that one family died of diptheria in ten days. There remained only a baby of nine months. The mother took to carrying this child constantly even while she did the farm housework. Clutched to her mother's breast, this child seemed inordinately wide-eyed, as though affected by the silent grief which surrounded her".[23]

Faced with such cases, it takes a peculiarly brave and honest doctor to admit – even to himself – that there is nothing he can do; and the eighteenth-century doctor was prepared to try anything – the more "active" the remedy the better its chances of success, he believed. Since he was not trained to compile statistics or to make comparative trials of different therapies, the "cures" were usually credited to whatever therapy had been used.

Neither was he trained to watch for the undesirable side-effects of a drug, it was thus easy to assume, when treatment failed, that the patient would have died anyway from the disease, like Elizabeth Drinker's two-year-old son Charles: ". . . our dear little one after diligent nursing had outgrown most of his weekness and promised fair to be a fine Boy, became much oppressed with phlegm, insomuch that Docr. Redmans oppinion was that unless we could promote some evacuation he could not live, he ordered what he thought might prove a gentle vomitt, agatated him much, but did not work, and in little more than 20 minits from ye time he took it, he expired aged 2 years 7 months and one day – about a week before he was fat, fresh and hearty – he cut a tooth a day befor he dyed."[24]

When even the most certain of vomits and purges failed, what more was there for the doctor to try? And by the end of the century there were many physicians who felt the same as the esteemed Dr. Holyoke of Salem, who lived to be a hundred and died full of honour. Showing a new apprentice his shop in 1797 Dr. Holyoke remarked: "There seems to you to be a great variety of medicines here, and that it will take you long to get acquainted with them, but most of them are unimportant. There are four which are equal to all the rest, namely, Mercury, Antimony, Bark and Opium".[25]

13

The
Foxglove Saga

In the spring of 1768, a young English doctor named William Withering (1741–1799) rode out to make a professional call on Miss Helena Cooke. He was anxious to make a good impression: this was one of his first patients, in his very first practice, and from what he had learned, the young lady's illness was likely to require a long convalescence, with plenty of professional attention. The good impression was mutual; before long the doctor's calls had an interest that was decidedly unprofessional: Dr. Withering and Miss Cooke fell in love.

Like many young ladies of the time, Miss Cooke had a charming hobby: she made water-colour paintings of plants and flowers. Since she was confined to her home, she lacked fresh material, and Withering eagerly offered to be her plant–hunter. He spent much of his time on the road between patients, and flower-spotting for Miss Cooke gave an agreeable new interest to the hours on horseback. Until this time, Withering had always found botany a remarkably dull subject. At Edinburgh University, where he had studied medicine, the hours he spent with his Professor of Botany, Dr. John Hope, seemed to him the dreariest of his day. He wrote to his parents of "the disagreeable ideas I have formed of the study of botany".[1]

Under the bright gaze of Miss Cooke, however, the world of green plants took on a new charm and a new interest. Withering had plenty of leisure to devote to it, and he soon found that not only was botany fascinating in itself, but that it opened up to him a new world of professional connections and possibilities. Almost all the great botanists of the time were doctors, the hobby coming naturally to men whose professional interest already involved them with plants; and his own friend Richard Pulteney was working on a biography of the most famous of all botanists, the Swede Carl Linnæus who had at last brought order and method into the wilderness of plant classification.

In 1776, eight years after his first meeting with Miss Cooke, and four years after his marriage to her, Withering published the book that had sprung from their romance. It was called *A Botanical Arrangement of all the Vegetables Naturally Growing in Great Britain with Descriptions of the Genera and Species according to Linnæus*. The book was a great success, and deserved to be – it was the best book on the market for the amateur botanist, of whom there were growing numbers; it was written in English; it provided a complete Linnæan framework for the study of British flora; and it included useful technical details such as a sketch of the microscope Withering had devised, and notes on how to dry and preserve specimens. Best of all, in the eyes of many readers, it was unencumbered by the old Galenic lumber of the traditional herbals. Withering was brisk about these: they were so inaccurate, he stated, that a fresh start was needed. We must "take up the subject altogether new, and rejecting the fables of the ancient Herbalists, build only upon the basis of accurate and well-conceived experiment-ation."[2]

Since this was, after all, a book about botany rather than a herbal, Withering's notes on the medical virtues of his plants are brief and scattered, and many of them are a sad commentary on the degree to which Galenic medicine had sunk in contemporary practice. Yarrow (*Achillea millefolium*), is "little attended to at present";[3] betony (*Stachys betonicæfolia*), "formerly much used in medicine, but it is discarded from the modern practice";[4] the leaves of coltsfoot (*Tussilago farfara*) "were formerly much used in coughs and consumptive complaints; and perhaps not without reason" but obviously so no longer.[5]

Withering records these facts without regret, but there are other plants which he suggested deserved greater, not less, attention, and the "accurate . . . experimentation" he had proposed. One such was the foxglove (*Digitalis purpurea*), about which Withering's comment was tantalizing: "a dram of it taken inwardly excites violent vomiting. It is certainly a very active medicine, and merits more attention than modern practice bestows on it."[6]

What Withering might have added was that he himself was at that time completely preoccupied by the medical virtues of the foxglove, and had been since the previous year. He later explained why, in words that every medical student knows by heart: "In the year 1775 my opinion was asked concerning a family recipe for the cure of dropsy. I was told that it had long been kept a secret by an old woman in Shropshire who had sometimes made cures after the more regular practitioners had failed. I was informed also that the effects produced were violent vomiting and purging; for the diuretic effects seemed to have been overlooked. This medicine was composed of twenty or more different herbs; but it was not very difficult for one conversant in these subjects to perceive that the active herb could be no other than foxglove".[7]

The dropsical bloating of the body caused by fluid retention is often the result of heart disease, and eighteenth-century medicine had no effective remedy for it. Much interested, Withering determined to investigate this possible cure with the utmost thoroughness.

As a start, he combed the old herbals to see what they had to say about it, only to find that there were no more than scattered references to it, although the Bavarian Leonhart Fuchs in his *De historia stirpium* (1542) had suggested that it might be useful for dropsy and internal swellings, and digitalis had been used for some time after this on the Continent as an emetic and purgative for dropsical cases.

Enquiring further, Withering found that in the west of England it was "much used . . . by the common people" for tuberculosis;[8] but in his part of the world, and in Yorkshire, its use in domestic medicine was chiefly for dropsy, and in the form of a tea made from leaves – although the quantities used were often nearly lethal.

Standardizing the preparation, and then working out the right dosage, were the first practical problems to be solved. But unlike the average general practitioner of his time, who had never looked at a plant since his student days, Withering knew his Linnæus well enough to know where to start. The leaves, he found, were of differing degrees of activity at different times of the year – but in the case of a flowering plant this activity is likely to be at its peak just before the seeds are formed, so this was the time Withering chose. "I expected, if gathered always in one condition of the plant, viz. when it was in its flowering state, and carefully dried, that the dose might be ascertained as exactly as that of any other medicine; nor have I been disappointed in this expectation".[9]

In order to study the lethal consequences of an overdose, Withering repeated an earlier experiment, made in 1748, when one investigator had fed quantities of foxglove leaves to turkeys: the turkeys staggered about and died in fits, having voided the entire contents of their intestines: he came to the conclusion that the drug must be dangerous if it purged or vomited his patients. Over the next ten years, cautiously and patiently, he tested his infusion of foxglove leaves on dropsical cases; a move to Birmingham in 1775, which brought him hundreds of extra patients annually at a free clinic for the poor gave him plenty of scope for his clinical trials. By 1780 he was recommending foxglove to fellow practitioners, and although one of them, Erasmus Darwin, made an effort to assume the credit for its first professional use, medical history has firmly credited it to the young botanizing doctor from Shropshire.

Withering's *Account of the Foxglove*, published in 1785, is a classic of medical history, methodically recording dozens of case-histories. Most of the conclusions he came to about dosage, adverse reactions, and which cases were most suitable for treatment have been more than confirmed by subsequent research. But even with his impeccable professional credentials, and despite all his patient fieldwork, the foxglove was by no means an instant success story. Many doctors, despite all his cautions, used it as a "brisk" emetic or purge, and when their patients died from an overdose, condemned it out of hand; other practitioners, noting merely that it slowed the pulse, classed it as a sedative along with opium. In its early years of widespread use, foxglove must have claimed many victims.

In Withering's *Account of the Foxglove*, he made some pertinent comments on the future of research into other such medicinal plants – a field in which "we have hitherto made only a very small progress".[10] There were, he considered, three possible lines along which research might be pursued.

There was the possibility of experimenting on "insects and quadrupeds" – a novel approach which, as he remarked, "has not yet been much attended to".[11]

There was the Linnæan approach from "analogy, deduced from the already known powers of some of their congenera" – plants of the same family, in other words, often had similar medicinal properties. But given the limitations of contemporary botanic knowledge, Withering felt that this would be a long way round.[12]

Finally, the virtues of plants might be learned "from . . . empirical usages and experience" and this, in his view, was the most obvious and the most promising approach, since it was "within the reach of everyone who is open to information regardless of the source from which it springs".[13]

But how many doctors of Withering's time – or indeed, today –

were open to information which came from empirics and lay people? The story of Peruvian bark suggests that if foxglove had not happened to come to the attention of a botanizing doctor with a mind more open than that of most of his profession, the world's millions of heart patients might never have had digitalis therapy. The fascinating question thus presents itself: how many other country remedies – like the foxglove, unrecorded in the herbals – have never met their Withering, and have been lost forever to orthodox medicine?

Certainly the medical system that educated Withering hardly encouraged much running after empirical remedies. At Edinburgh University, which early in the century had become the most influential school of medicine in the British Isles, Withering had been taught by William Cullen, a Leiden man and himself a brilliant and scientific thinker, but with the same burning urge to reduce medicine to as coherent and logical system as his master, Boerhaave. And however original Cullen's thinking, there was nothing startlingly original about his therapeutics, in which purging, blistering and blood letting figured strongly.

Cullen was succeeded in his Chair by Dr. James Gregory, another ardent advocate of blistering and bloodletting. And the most serious challenge to Cullen's theories came from his ex-pupil, John Brown, who taught that good health was a condition of moderate excitability – the quality which distinguished the living from the dead. Too much produced what he called a sthenic condition – such as gout, malaria or typhus fever. Too little – and the patient sank into an asthenic state, which might manifest itself as measles or smallpox. Therapy was essentially simple: sthenic conditions responded to sedatives, and he thought none finer than laudanum – the alcoholic tincture of the narcotic drug opium. Asthenic conditions called for stimulants – of which the nonpareil, in Brown's view, was whisky.

All three men had enormous influence over their students – and in consequence over the British medical profession as a whole – and the respective merits of their theories were hotly debated. But whether you were a Cullenite, a Brunonian, or a follower of Dr. Gregory, the result was much the same in practice: an undue attachment to theory, and a corresponding decline in the value placed on observation, clinical experience, and the careful evaluation of drugs. More and more, doctors came to place their reliance on a mere handful of powerful drugs or techniques – a prescribing laziness grimly summed up in the contemporary skit on Dr. Lettsom:

> When patients sick to me apply
> I physicks, bleeds and sweats 'em
> Then after, if they choose to die –
> What's that to me? – I lets 'em.[14]

Dr. Lettsom had one of the most successful and fashionable practices of his day – his annual income has been estimated at £12,000 – and he could afford to quote this piece of wit with relish on his way to the bank. But as the century wore on, an increasing aversion to the often-agonizing doctoring of the day, together with a well-founded doubt of its efficacy, became evident throughout Europe in the success of a new wave of home-doctoring texts which preached much milder treatment, usually with herbs or simple kitchen remedies together with a new awareness of the importance of personal cleanliness, diet and hygiene.

One of the most popular was Dr. S. Tissot's *Avis au Peuple*, published in Lausanne in 1761, which went into one edition after another all over Europe. Its success may have inspired a Scottish physician, Dr. William Buchan, who in 1769 published his own *Domestic Medicine*. Buchan's work was hardly likely to appeal to the medical profession of which, by implication, he was strongly critical: "I think the administration of medicine always doubtful, and often dangerous," he wrote, "and would much rather teach men how to avoid the necessity of using them than how they should be used. . . ."[15] But he enjoyed a huge popular success, an up-to-date Culpeper, and in Scotland particularly, it was reckoned that almost every cottage possessed a copy of this book, with its emphasis on the importance of diet, hygiene and cleanliness, and its simple herbal remedies.

An even earlier expression of this popular movement was a slim volume called *Primitive Physic*, or *An Easy and Natural Way of Curing Most Diseases*, written by the Methodist preacher John Wesley (1703–91) and first published in 1747. Before Wesley's death, this had already gone through twenty-three editions. Wesley was the son of a rector, was educated at Oxford, and grew up destined for the Church. After experiencing a whole-hearted conversion in 1738, he determined to devote his life to preaching. But his message was too clear and uncompromising for the well-fed Hanoverian clergy, and when the churches closed their doors to him, he took to the streets and the fields, preaching to crowds of up to thirty thousand, and travelling the length and breadth of the country.

Thousands of his poorest converts could afford neither doctor nor apothecary, Wesley knew, and *Primitive Physic* was written for their benefit. In this unpretentious little book, which sold for pennies at Meeting-Houses, Wesley spelled out for his spiritual children dozens of simple and effective remedies for their ailments, together with the basic rules of what today we call preventive medicine.

The chief appeal of Wesley's Methodism was in the mushrooming industrial and mining towns and the seaports of Britain, and while these were yet to know the full horrors of the Industrial Revolution with its reeking slums, their populations were already cut off to a certain extent from the traditions of simple, effective herbal medicine rooted in rural England, and celebrated by Gerard, Markham and Culpeper.

Even the herbs themselves – the ordinary, English ones – were often hard to come by: many of those Wesley prescribed were "not to be had in Bristol" which certainly had plenty of apothecary shops.[16] These, on the other hand, had never been in short supply, and as the apothecaries themselves slowly moved up the social scale into the ranks of general practitioners, a growing army of druggists followed on their heels. By the end of the century, they were tough competition for the apothecaries, and their professional encroachment was in turn as deeply resented as the apothecaries themselves had once been by lordly physicians.

In the summer of 1794, two hundred London apothecaries gathered at the Crown and Anchor tavern in The Strand to hear complaints about this growing threat to their profession. "There was scarcely to be found a village or a hamlet, without a village or hamlet druggist. If the sale of medicines and the giving of advice was not here sufficient to support the vendor, he added to his own occupation, the sale of mops, brooms, bacon and butter." The most shocking consequences of this, to the now-proud apothecaries, was that while the cost of living had doubled in the last twenty years, the price of medicines, far from following suit, had had "a most shameful and a most fatal reduction indeed."[17]

But the proliferation of druggists had other consequences. The druggists, like the generations of the apothecaries on whom they modelled themselves, seldom bothered to stock the British herbs which their village customers could grow for themselves, and which their town customers hardly expected to pay for – as Wesley had already noted. Instead, they stocked the familiar compounds, exotics and chemicals – many of them highly toxic – which they blithely sold to all who could afford them. There was no form of control over the sale even of deadly poisons like arsenic and strychnine, other than the conscience or good sense of the purveyor.

But there was a difference, which rightly appalled the apothecaries: whereas these last had undergone a formal apprenticeship in the preparation and identification of drugs, and had the useful opportunity of seeing how they were professionally prescribed, the druggists had had no formal training of any kind. They were simply retailers, often totally ignorant of the powerful and dangerous drugs they were prescribing.

In the circumstances, Wesley's followers were often not merely wasting their money but risking their health by buying over-the-counter medicine: and Wesley's *Primitive Physic* was not calculated to enrich either druggist or apothecary. Some of his recommendations were "modern" – he had great faith in the fashionable new electric-shock therapy, and recommended it for a lengthy list of ailments, including "Blindness, Feet violently disorder'd, Gout, Head-ach, Singles and Swellings of all Sorts." A few "cures" on the other hand, were frankly magical: "Place three corals in a bag made from the skin of a cat: wear it round the neck and it will drive off a mortal fever." Some were plain common-sense: for "Costiveness" he suggests "Rise Early every Morning"; for morning sickness, "eat nothing after six in the evening." Others were old folk-remedies, like this for tuberculosis: "sleep for three nights in the cow-house, as near to a cow as possible" or goose-grease smeared on brown paper to wrap around an ailing chest.[18]

Great numbers of the remedies Wesley suggested, finally, were the simple, effective herbal remedies with which, since time immemorial, primitive and country people have healed their ailments: garlic for coughs and hoarseness, lilies or betony for a headache, valerian or peony for epilepsy, valerian for nervous disorders, turnips for scurvy (they do in fact contain Vitamin C), nettle poultices for sciatica, chamomile tea for indigestion, agrimony for kidney and bladder problems, and broom-tops for dropsy, among others.

A favourite remedy of Wesley's was tar-water, made from pine resin. Tar-water was popularized in Europe by Bishop Berkeley, the philosopher and amateur doctor, who first heard of this remedy in Rhode Island. North American Indians used pine resin in a variety of ways – among others, as a salve for wounds, boils and ulcers; in decoction for chest ailments; and as a kind of medicinal chewing-gum for upset stomachs. Bishop Berkeley adopted the remedy with enthusiasm, and came back deeply convinced of its virtues. He made his version by mixing a gallon of cold water with a quart of the sticky resin, letting it stand for three days, then pouring off the clear "Tar-Water". The Bishop recommended this remedy so whole-heartedly, and for such an astonishing variety of diseases that its therapeutic virtues were as widely and energetically debated in the 1740s as are those of acupuncture or regular jogging today.

To settle the question, Berkeley made the startingly novel proposal of a controlled clinical trial: two groups of patients in two hospitals, to be identically fed and lodged, but one group provided only with "a tub of tar-water and an old woman; the other hospital, what attendance and drugs you please".[19] Since no doctor or hospital was prepared to run the formidable risk of their treatment actually proving inferior to this empirical foolishness, nobody in the medical profession took him up on this suggestion. Wesley, however, who shared his faith, recommended tar-water as a cure for diseases as diverse as "rheumatism, pleurisy, and Inward Ulcer, the Cramp, Stoppage in the Kidney, Epilepsy, and St. Anthony's Fire."

But its chief appeal for him was probably as a healthy excuse for administering quantities of his favourite remedy, water – a therapeutic substance second to none in his eyes and efficacious in almost the entire range of human ailments, from asthma to varicose ulcers. "Cold bathing," he wrote, "is a great advantage to health: it prevents abundance of diseases. It promotes perspiration, helps the circulation of blood, and prevents the danger of catching cold."[20]

It is possible that Wesley learned to trust in both tar-water and cold bathing during the three years he spent as a young man in America, preaching in Georgia. Wesley was so impressed by the rugged good health of the North American Indians he saw there that he made a careful study of these practitioners of genuine "Primitive Physick". "Their diseases, indeed, are exceeding few; nor do they often occur, by reason of their continual exercise, and (till of late, universal) temperance".[21] He was keenly interested in the continuity of their medical practice: ". . . if any are sick, or bit by a serpent, or torn by a wild beast, the fathers immediately tell their children what remedy to apply. And it is rare that the patient suffers long; those medicines being quick, as well as generally infallible."[22]

Some fifty years later, these marvellous medicines were still largely unknown to the European physician. But two major events in world history now turned the eyes of the North American settlers towards their native flora with a new and urgent interest.

The first was the American War of Independence (1776–1783) which not only lit the flame of American nationalism: it also brought home to the Revolutionary Army medical authorities the extreme inconvenience of relying on imported drugs – a reliance which was still almost total. When Washington's armies retreated to their winter quarters at Valley Forge after the loss of Philadelphia, the military doctors drew up an emergency "Pharmacopœia of Simples & Efficacious Remedies for the use of the Military Hospital. . . . Especially adapted to our present Poverty & Straitened Circumstances."[23] Of the forty-eight vegetable drugs listed among its hundred items, only three could be said to be indigenous: the sassafras, still valued in the treatment of venereal disease; the Virginia snakeroot, used as an aromatic and bitter tonic; and the butternut (*Juglans cinerea*), a mild cathartic and aperient, which was resorted to when standard drug supplies ran out. All the rest had to be imported, most from European suppliers.

The second spur to national self-sufficiency was the Napoleonic Wars, into which Europe plunged in the closing years of the century. This time North America was not directly involved, but imports of drugs were none the less affected, some vanishing from the market altogether, others – like opium – becoming almost prohibitively expensive.

One foreigner voiced his astonishment at American disregard of the medicinal treasure in their own backyard: "It is to be wished," wrote Dr. Johann David Schöpf, "that the physicians of America . . . may also have a patriotic eye to the completer knowledge of their native materia medica. It betrays an unpardonable indifference to their fatherland to see them making use almost wholly of foreign medicines."[24]

Schöpf had served with the German troops in British service during the Revolutionary War, and stayed on afterwards to make a long plant-hunting tour of the country, after which he wrote the first *Materia Medica Americana*, in which he catalogued more than four hundred native medicinal plants. It was later suggested that he had collected his material from the Indians, but Schöpf was cagey about his sources, and not particularly complimentary about Indian medicine. There were those, he noted, who still have a very high opinion of it, and ordinary people – although not the "well-informed" – were impressed by the jealous mystery the Indians made of their doctoring. But for himself, Schöpf concluded, "I see no reason to expect anything extraordinary or important, and I am almost certain that with the passage of time nothing will be brought to light, if as is the case, outright specifics are looked for and presumably infallible remedies".[25] The Indians were simply a naturally tough race, he continued, whose physical systems threw off disease easily with the help of a few purges, perspiratives, or diuretics, administered in heavy doses.

The ethnic arrogance of Schöpf's attitude was even more forcibly embodied in one of America's most highly-respected and famous physicians, Dr. Benjamin Rush of Philadelphia. Rush had taken the trouble to enquire closely into Indian health and practices, but he did so with a mind closed by prejudice: "We have no discoveries in the materia medica to hope for from the Indians of North America," he asserted. ". . . it would be a reproach to our schools of physic if modern physicians were not more successful than the Indians even in the treatment of their own disease."[26]

14

Heroic Medicine

On Friday 13 December 1799, the sixty-seven-year-old hero of the American Revolution and former President, George Washington, woke up in the night at his home in Mount Vernon, not feeling very well. He had been soaked by rain the day before, and now he felt first chilled to the bone and then feverish, with a painfully constricted sore throat and laboured breathing. He decided that a bleeding might give him some relief and alerted his household: they at once sent for a bleeder in the neighbourhood who took twelve or fourteen ounces of blood from Washington's arm. But although the General's family was extremely anxious, he refused to allow them to trouble his doctor in the middle of the night, and the whole household returned to an uneasy sleep.

Next morning Washington was no better, and Dr. James Craik, his personal physician, arrived at 11 o'clock. It was the start of a grim medical marathon. Dr. Craik, alarmed by Washington's condition, promptly sent for two other physicians to join him in consultation. Meanwhile, he ordered two more "copious" bleedings; a blister was applied to Washington's throat; two doses of mercury were given him; and a cathartic injection was forced up his rectum – all to no avail: Washington's breathing grew more painful and laboured. The consultant physicians arrived in the afternoon, and Dr. Craik suggested yet another bleeding. In this suggestion he was seconded by Dr. Brown, but vigorously opposed by Dr. Elisha Dick, who pointed out that they had already drawn perhaps three pints of blood from a sick and ageing man. "He needs all his strength," he argued, "bleeding will diminish it." He was overruled, as the most junior doctor of the trio, and a fourth bleeding was ordered. This time, no less than thirty-two ounces of blood were drawn off – "without the smallest apparent alleviation of the disease" – the doctors later reported.[1]

A third huge dose of calomel – ten grains – was now given him, followed by several doses of tartar emetic (antimony); vapours of water and vinegar were blown around his throat; to the fiery blister on his throat was added a bran-and-vinegar poultice, and more blisters were strapped to the soles of his feet. After hours of this torture, and several vain struggles to speak, Washington at last managed to make known to his doctors his desire to be left to die in peace. Late on Saturday night – a bare twenty-four hours after he had woken with a chill and a sore throat – he breathed his last.

It has been calculated that over four pints of blood – about half his total bodily content – were removed from Washington. A blood loss of this order would today be considered a major medical emergency, necessitating immediate blood transfusions and intensive care, to avert the otherwise inevitable death from lowered blood pressure, collapse and acute shock. Even at the time, at least one of the two doctors responsible for the last murderous bleeding later had misgivings: "I have often thought", confessed Dr. Brown to Dr. Craik a few weeks later, "that if we had taken no more blood from him our good friend might have been alive now". He added, "But we were governed by the best light we had: we thought we were right, and so we are justified".[2]

The "best light" available to North American doctors of the time had already been savagely satirized – as a "Rush-light".[3] It was that of Dr. Benjamin Rush of Philadelphia, the ardent, forceful and compelling personality whose thinking dominated American medicine for nearly a century, a man of prodigious energy whose talents ranged over the entire field of human activity.

Rush was one of the signatories of the Declaration of Independence, and campaigned vigorously for national universities, temperance, the abolition of slavery, the education of women, the provision of free schools, and humane treatment for the insane. He also had one of the busiest and most successful practices in the country.

It was, however, as Professor of Medicine at Pennsylvania University for almost half a century – from 1769 to 1813 – that he exerted his most profound influence on American life – and death. Pennsylvania was only one of four North American universities training physicians, but it produced seventy-five per cent of them, and an estimated 2,300 students passed through Rush's classrooms over the years.

Rush himself, a graduate of Princeton University at the age of fifteen, had studied medicine at Edinburgh, and his students in turn carried away the theories of Brown further simplified by the powerful and dogmatic mind of Rush. To Dr. Rush, the notion of numbers of different diseases, all needing careful individual study and systematic classification, was the sheerest nonsense: there was only one disease, and that was "irregular arterial action" following on that state of "debility" which first set the stage for disease. This was true of every kind of sickness: "It is by no means necessary to know how to class epidemics in order to cure them, any more than it is to individual or solitary diseases", taught Rush.[4]

Just as it was unnecessary to study numbers of diseases, so, too, could the materia medica be simplified. He spoke scornfully of the "great and unnecessary number of medicines which are used for the cure of disease".[5] Perhaps Rush, like Withering, had found the hours spent poring over botanical specimens "disagreeable": his own students might dispense with the study. "To those physicians who believe in the unity of disease, this large and expensive stock in drugs will be unnecessary. By accommodating the doses of their medicines to the state of the system, by multiplying their forms, and by combining them properly, twenty or thirty articles, aided by the common resources of the lancet, a garden, a kitchen, fresh air, cool water, and exercise will be sufficient to cure all the diseases that are at present under the power of medicine", taught Rush.[6] All that was necessary was to prescribe for "the underlying state". And the twin pillars of the Rushian therapy were bloodletting and calomel.

There was almost no disease for which Rush did not think bloodletting helpful, from catarrh to rheumatism, from tuberculosis to earache. In pneumonia it was particularly essential ("copious bleeding – up to 140 ounces"); and Rush ridiculed the idea that perhaps bloodletting might on occasion be positively harmful to a patient: " 'Tis a very hard matter to bleed a patient to death," he reassured his classes.[7]

Since there could be no sound healthy blood unless the liver was functioning properly, medicines which acted powerfully upon this organ "are deservedly in the first rank of all articles in the materia medica," taught Rush.[8] Of these the undisputed king was mercury, the "Sampson of the materia medica," as Rush was fond of describing it. Mercurous chloride or calomel, together with antimony or tartar emetic, was by the end of the eighteenth century one of the two most popular drugs in North American medicine, and Rush's enthusiasm swept calomel into a decisive lead over all other drugs. He himself described it lyrically as "a safe and nearly an universal medicine".[9]

Calomel was considered to act in one of two ways: either by purging all diseased matter from the body, and thus disposing of the disease, or by converting an ordinary sickness into a "mercurial" fever, which, all physicians believed, got better of its own accord.

Closely allied to Rush's deep faith in "active" medicine, was his equally deep distrust of the healing power of nature. Rush had very little time for nature: ". . . I would treat it in the sick–chamber as I would a squalling cat – open the door and drive it out", he was heard to cry energetically during one of his lectures.[10]

In such practice, there could be no respite for the patient. When Nancy Drinker came down with what was almost certainly yellow fever in 1794, her mother wrote a blow-by-blow account of the non-stop barrage of "active medicines" with which her doctor assailed both disease and sufferer. After three days of calomel, rhubarb, blood-letting, castor oil and Daffy's Elixir, the patient rebelled – but to no avail. "Nancy much against taking medicine, and hard to me to urge it, but as her case was desperate, thought it best to persist – she had less reaching this morning but a constant sickness, sd. her Stomach and throat felt as if she had been eating Allum, we were much at a loss what to do, the Dr had sent sevral sorts of medicine, that if one fail'd the other was to be try'd . . . if no change took place for ye. better, to lay a blister on her Stomach . . . if ye pills did not answer she was to take powders of Jalap, if they would not stay on her stomach, Senna was to be given in an infusion. . . ."[11]

The greatest challenge to Rush's skill as a physician came in the 1790s, when four times in a decade, the city of Philadelphia was emptied by virulent epidemics of yellow fever. Philadelphia was peculiarly vulnerable to this disease, with its tropically hot and moist summers, the mosquito-breeding swamps that lay around the town's outskirts, and the constant arrival in its port of ships from Africa, and from Central and South America.

The epidemic of 1793, however, was the worst Rush had seen, and at first he was puzzled as to how to deal with it. Then he came across a note by a practitioner dealing with an earlier epidemic, in which drastic purging was urged as the only solution. Rush hesitated no longer. He began dosing his patients with ten grains of calomel combined with ten grains of jalap, the particularly vicious vegetable cathartic. (Ten grains of calomel is the equivalent of almost 650 mg: until its use was abandoned in modern medical practice because of its acute toxicity the average U.S. dose was from 120–300 mg). When his patients continued to die, he raised the dose to ten of calomel and fifteen of jalap, then to ten plus fifteen every six hours or so, followed by a bleeding.

It was related with awe that no less than three of his apprentices were busy night and day putting up powders of calomel and jalap, or rhubarb. Many of his patients died: victims it was supposed, of the yellow fever. Others, incredibly, got better: Rush assumed that calomel and bleeding had pulled them through.

Much of Rush's doctoring was in fact quite enlightened and sensible – he prescribed cold baths, fresh air, and horse-riding for some of his patients, and he often warned students against "undue attachment to great names" in medicine. But his enthusiasm for purging and bleeding, together with his conviction that "desperate diseases require desperate remedies", made a lasting impression on his classes. For generations the regular medical practice of North America relied heavily, and at times almost exclusively, on these two therapies, which were enthusiastically preached by medical textbooks up to the mid-nineteenth century.

Of bloodletting, a medical journal commented in 1837: "Among American physicians there is no one remedy of greater importance in the treatment of diseases than the lancet . . . no adequate substitute can be found for its vast remedial powers".[12] And in 1823 Eberle, whose *Treatise of the Materia Medica and Therapeutics* was required reading for every medical student, noted that "Latterly mercury has become a very common remedy in acute disorders," then added encouragingly "but even at present its powers in these affections are perhaps too little attended to by the profession in general".[13]

As the use of calomel became more common, doses grew larger: the most extreme cases on record being that of the Mississippi valley doctor who noted that he commonly prescribed four tablespoons of calomel daily to his patients. It was quite customary to give patients doses of twenty or thirty grains, and one patient of Dr. Rush survived a dose of eighty grains. A New Orleans minister, writing in 1856, vividly recalled watching a doctor, who had been called to a patient during an epidemic, at once take fifty ounces of blood from him. The patient fainted; when he came round, he was immediately forced to swallow 300 grains of calomel and gamboge.[14] (Gamboge (*Garcinia morella*), is another violent vegetable purge, of which the safe dose is calculated today to be about 6 grains at the most.)

As the frontiers of America rolled west with the pioneers, medical practice became more drastic still. Pioneer doctors were famous for their "herculean doses", Professor Cooke of Transylvania is said to have administered thirteen tablespoons of calomel to one cholera patient. "If calomel did not salivate" he cried merrily, "there is no telling what we could do in the practice of physic".[15]

The magnificient recklessness of this practice earned it at the time the name "Heroic Medicine", and in its energy and simplicity, it seemed singularly fitted for the vigorous young republic just cutting itself off from its European ties and traditions. Oliver Wendell Holmes (1809–1894), physician as well as witty writer, brooding in 1861 over the excesses of his profession, concluded that it was indeed peculiarly American. "The medical mind of the country . . . has clearly tended to extravagance in remedies and trust in remedies, as in everything else . . . how could such a people be content with any but 'heroic' practice? What wonder that . . . the American eagle screams with delight to see three drachms of calomel given at a single mouthful?"[16]

No procedure carrying such heavy risks for the patient as blood-letting, and no drug that produced such appalling side-effects as calomel would today be admitted to normal medical practice. But pathology and physiology were sciences then in their infancy. And in the case of calomel, very little, if anything, was known of the way it acted, though plenty of theorists were happy to guess. Less still was known of its long-term side-effects, but its most immediate and visible ones were a matter of record. These were, indeed, horrific: following salivation, extensive areas of the facial flesh and bone sometimes became blackened and mortified, then sloughed away, eye, cheek and all. Sometimes whole portions of the jaw rotted and fell out; occasionally the diseased jawbones fused together as if in lockjaw, dooming the victim to a silent death from starvation unless the condition was corrected by painful surgery.

The Surgical Clinic of the Medical College of Georgia saw an eight-year-old boy from South Carolina in the winter of 1849–50, with his jaws clamped rigidly together following mercurial salivation. The surgeons were compelled to make a long incision through the jawbones and remove eight or ten teeth, and their sockets. Following persevering sessions with "Mott's dilator", the surgeons were able to report some degree of success: "Patient can now open his mouth about ¾ of an inch between the incisors, the only teeth he has".[17]

He was "lucky" compared to one woman that an Irregular doctor attended. She was, he reported, "nearly destroyed by taking mercury for the then prevailing influenza. Her whole system was excessively diseased: she was almost unable to swallow; her tongue, gums, throat and jaws, swollen and sore; her breath so fetid, that it was almost impossible to stay in the room; her flesh nearly wasted away, and her countenance sunken, pale and ghastly: there was excessive debility, water running from the mouth, appetite gone, and, from the putrid state of the fluids, every appearance of speedy mortification and death".[18]

She was an extreme and an unlucky case. But individual susceptibility to calomel varied enormously, some patients being salivated by as little as a quarter of a grain, others suffering no apparent ill-effects from doses of one hundred grains. In the circumstances, it was temptingly easy for a doctor to close his eyes to the frightful visible effects of his therapy, and close his mind to any more insidious long-term damage he might be inflicting on the patient's system. As for bloodletting, the extreme debility it produced – the fainting, the weakness, the convulsions – could always be attributed to the disease for which it was prescribed. No doctor is particularly ready or willing to believe that his treatment might be disastrous for his patient, while from time immemorial, the vast majority of patients themselves have submitted to the ministrations of their doctor, however painful, with a faith as complete as it is occasionally astonishing.

15

Roots
and Herbs

Not everyone shared the prevailing faith in heroic medicine. In 1813 one visitor to Philadelphia enquired how the epidemic of yellow fever was being treated, and was appalled to learn that "the treatment prescribed by Dr. Rush was to bleed twice a day for ten days . . . am confident that the same treatment would kill half of those in health".[1] He was deeply struck by the looks of those who survived this therapy: "Those I met in the streets who had escaped the fatal effects of bleeding, mercury and other poisons, carried death in their countenance; and on conversing with them, they had never been well since they had the fever."[2]

This visitor was Samuel Thomson (1769–1843), the son of a poor and illiterate farmer from Alstead, New Hampshire. His name was soon to rouse scorn, indignation, rage, or resentment in the mind of the average North American doctor.

Thomson's childhood was bleak. His father was a harsh religious fanatic, brutally strict with his children. Samuel, the eldest, was born club-footed, and grew up knowing the miseries of being both sickly and a cripple. The heroic doctoring of the time could do nothing for him, and it was not until his father called in a local herb-doctor, the widow Benton, that his health began to improve steadily. The eight-year-old boy became fascinated by the insignificant green plants which had such marvellous healing powers and he set himself to learn all he could about them. "I . . . was constantly in the habit of tasting everything of the kind I saw; and having a retentive memory I have always recollected the taste and use of all that were ever shown me by others, and like-wise all that I discovered myself".[3]

His most exciting discovery was the peculiar property of the pale-blue-flowered lobelia *(Lobelia inflata).* He noticed with interest that simply nibbling the leaves made him vomit, and he used to give it to his workmates for the boyish fun of watching them "spit and vomit".

On one occasion the joke went too far: the man he gave it to "was in a most profuse perspiration, being as wet all over as he could be; he trembled very much, and there was no more colour in him than a corpse". He was several times violently sick, then, astonishingly, he ate a hearty dinner and worked like a Trojan all afternoon. "He afterwards told me that he had never had anything do him so much good in his life; his appetite was remarkably good, and he felt better than he had for a long time."[4] From then on Thomson had the highest opinion of this plant and its medicinal powers, which he had discovered all by himself.

There were still at this time regular doctors who prescribed roots and herbs for their patients, and Thomson was particularly impressed by a Dr. Kitteridge, whom he met in 1788, and who had a great and deserved reputation in his neighbourhood. "His system of practise was peculiarly his own, and all the medicines he used were prepared by himself, from the roots and herbs of our own country."[5]

But such doctors were already a vanishing breed, and before long Thomson could observe for himself their decline, and their replacement by the new brisk race of Rushites. One such doctor lived on the Thomson farm for a while: "During the first of his practise he used chiefly roots and herbs, and his success was very great in curing canker and old complaints; but he afterwards got into the fashionable mode of treating his patients, by giving them apothecary's drugs, which made him more popular with the faculty, but less useful to his fellow creatures".[6]

By the time Thomson was twenty-one, the calomel-and-bleeding practice was well established, and Thomson observed it with increasing mistrust and astonishment: "whenever any of the family took a cold, the doctor was sent for, who would always either bleed or give physic".[7]

Then, in his own family, the limitation of such crude and "active" doctoring were brought grimly home to him: his mother fell ill with measles, which "turned in and seated on her lungs . . . her cough was very severe and her mouth was sore, and she was greatly distressed". Several doctors were called in, but "she continued to grow worse daily, the doctors gave her over, and gave her disease the name of galloping consumption, which I thought was a very appropriate name

– for they are the riders, and their whip is mercury, opium and vitriol, and they galloped her out of the world in about nine weeks."[8]

Soon after, Thomson married a Miss Susanna Allen. When she went into labour for the birth of their first child, Thomson reluctantly sent for the doctor. The labour was a long and difficult one, and Thomson, standing helplessly by, was devastated by the "horrid scene of human butchery". It was, he wrote, "during the whole night . . . one continued struggle of forcing nature, which produced so great an injury to the nervous system, as to cause strong convulsion fits in about an hour after her delivery."[9]

Some years later, his two-year-old daughter fell ill with the "canker-rash": she went into a coma, and "the canker was to be seen in her mouth, nose, and ears, and one of her eyes was covered with it and closed; the other began to swell and turn purple." The doctor said he could do nothing for her: she was doomed. In agony, Thomson sat watching the convulsive struggles of his little girl: she was "so distressed for breath that she would spring straight up on end in struggling to breathe". Suddenly, obeying a strong instinctive command, Thomson filled a bath with steaming hot water, and sat holding her over it, while he kept a cloth wrung out in cold water over her eyes. For twenty long minutes he held her tensed little body in the steam. Then suddenly she relaxed, the struggles stopped and her breath began to come more easily.[10]

His daughter recovered, although the illness left her blind in one eye. But Thomson's faith in doctors was destroyed for good, and thereafter, when any of his family fell ill, he doctored them himself quite successfully, by steaming them, or administering his favourite emetic herb, lobelia, and infusions of other herbs.

Gradually, friends and neighbours began applying to him in sickness, and he sometimes succeeded in cases given up for lost by the doctors, though on at least one occasion, he had the painful experience of seeing his patient, a child, handed over to a regular doctor after he had already begun treating it. Thomson had steamed it and given it his herbal treatments, then left directions with the parents for continuing the treatment.

In his absence the family doctor called, poured scorn on Thomson's steaming and herbs, and persuaded the family to give him care of the child. By the time Thomson heard of the case again, the child was dead: the doctor "had filled it with mercury and run it down . . . till the child wasted away and died, in about two months . . . its parents were willing to allow that I understood the disorder best. The doctor got twenty-five dollars for killing the child by inches, and I got nothing."[11]

At this point in his life, Thomson had to make a decision. With a wife and family to support, he could continue to make a meagre but assured living from the family farm, doing a little doctoring on the side as it came his way. Or he could throw caution to the winds and set up in precarious full-time practice as a root-and-herb doctor – still a familiar breed – in competition with the Rushite regular doctors. He had wanted for years to become a doctor: only the family lack of funds had stopped him. Now he hesitated, but the call was too urgent: "[I] finally concluded to make use of that gift which I thought the God of nature had implanted in me".[12] He knew that no peaceful practice lay ahead: incidents like the case of this child had already decided him to take up arms against a medical practice that he regarded with growing aversion and horror.

As it turned out, no abler champion for natural medicine could have been found: Thomson was a fighter by nature as well as a healer, a plain-spoken, obstinate, cantankerous crusader whose pure flame of purpose now burned as brightly and steadily as that of Wesley, Culpeper, or Paracelsus, all men who in their time had hurled themselves against the entrenched battlements of the medical establishment.

Were Thomson's healing methods entirely of his own devising? When he came to write his autobiography, years later, he acknowledged only one outside source of inspiration for his revolutionary and successful practice of medicine: the widow Benton, the root-and-herb doctor of his childhood, who had spent some time pointing out to him the medicinal herbs she used, and explaining their use. She was, he always remembered, considerably more successful than the Regulars, and "the whole of her practise was with roots and herbs, applied to the patient, or given in hot drinks, to produce sweating; which always answered the purpose".[13] Her practice seems to have left a deep impression on Thomson, for in essence the basis of the therapy that he developed was the restoration of bodily heat – of which process sweating is an indication.

It was also clear from Thomson's writing that he was reading the medical literature of the day, though he always insisted that his methods were entirely of his own devising. The only master that he allowed was Hippocrates, whom he described reverently as "the father of the healing art".[14] His works are also silent on the subject of the most obvious source of inspiration: Indian medicine. Like Thomson, the Indians steamed and sweated their patients; like Thomson, they gave them massive doses of emetics; like Thomson, they used roots, barks, fruit, and leaves for almost the whole of their materia medica; like Thomson, they never used mineral poisons. And although tribes here and there resorted to moderate bleeding to relieve inflammation or pain, most Indians were as deeply opposed to the practice as Thomson, believing that to bleed was to waste the river of life itself.

It is impossible that Thomson should have known nothing of Indian medical practices: the widow Benton's knowledge of local medicinal herbs must have derived at least indirectly from them. But he never directly acknowledged any debt to them, and certainly there is no reason to doubt that he discovered the most important herb in his repertoire, lobelia, all by himself just as he described, although there are records of its use in folk-medicine before his time. He may also have felt that since antipathy and contempt for Indian medicine were deeply rooted in orthodox circles he would have been adding needless difficulties to his own practice by associating himself with it.

Instead, he elaborated a theory of his own, of the utmost simplicity: "all diseases . . . are brought about by a decrease or derangement of the vital fluids by taking cold or the loss of animal warmth . . . the name of the complaint depends upon what part of the body has become so weak as to be affected. If the lungs it is consumption, or the pleura, pleurisy; if the limbs, it is rheumatism, or the bowels, cholic or cholera morbus . . . all these different diseases may be removed by a restoration of the vital energy, and removing the obstructions which the disease has generated".[15]

To the "obstructions" he often gave the name "canker", which he visualized as a "white feverish coat" caused by cold, that attached itself to the mucous membrane of stomach and bowels, causing disease, putrefaction and death. Its formation could be halted, and the canker itself thrown to the stomach by restoring bodily heat: emetics would then remove it safely from the system.

Thus the great object of his treatment was always to raise and restore the body's vital heat: "All . . . that medicine can do in the expulsion of disorder, is to kindle up the decaying spark, and restore its energy till it glows in all its wonted vigour."[16]

Thomson's simplicity of theory – "cold . . . is the cause of all disease"[17] – earned him the contemptuous scorn of the Regulars, who dismissed him as an illiterate empiric. When one quite sympathetic doctor expressed his astonishment at Thomson's successful handling

of a case of dropsy, and asked him how he did it, Thomson replied
gravely "you know, doctor, that the heat had gone out of the body,
and the water had filled it up; and all I had to do was to build fire
enough in the body to boil away the water". The doctor burst into a
laugh, and said that it was a "system very short".[18]

There was, however, a significant difference between Thomson's
theorizing and that of the Regulars. His theory was formed only after
long observation, and he believed that it was accurate because it
constantly gave good results in practice. The Regulars, in contrast,
proceeded from theory to practice without stopping to consider
whether their theories gave good results or not when put to work.
They believed that calomel and bloodletting *ought* to cure diseases, so
they continued to prescribe them blindly – often with fatal results.

In Thomson's eyes, it was medical practice of this order that truly
deserved the name quackery: what use was all the scientific book-
learning in the world when it produced such illiterates in practice?
"Give us more practical knowledge and less theorizing; more of true
science and less speculation."[19]

The other difference between Thomson and the Regulars was
equally radical. Thomson brought back into medicine the Hippocratic
idea of the *vis medicatrix naturae*, the healing power of nature which it
was the doctor's task to assist. Following Cullen and Rush, most
Regulars believed that the enemy, disease, was to be attacked by the
weapon of strong, active medicine. Nature was simply a bystander
who often got hurt in the process, unluckily, but certainly could not be
relied on to defeat the enemy unaided.

Over the years Thomson developed, elaborated and refined his
system, till it became a regular series of Courses of Medicine, which
though not actually painful were certainly a gruelling ordeal for the
patient, and hard work for the doctor. There were various differences
from one Course to another, depending upon what disorder was being
treated, but the trio of lobelia, to make the patient vomit, cayenne
(*Capsicum minimum*), to restore bodily heat, and the vapour bath to
make him sweat were "the grand bulwark of the system".[20]

Course I – the most drastic – was Thomson's favourite. It began
for the patient with a dose of strong herb tea, after which he stood in a
hot steam bath till "a lively perspiration appears, and the veins have
become full upon the feet, hands and temples". After a lukewarm
shower and a rubdown, the patient was then put to rest in a warm bed.
The second phase began with a wineglassful of red-hot tea, made with

cayenne pepper, lobelia, and other herbs according to the sickness, sweetened with molasses, while another dose of it was given simultaneously as a rectal injection. The tea made most patients violently sick: if it failed to do so, a second and even a third glassful of the same fiery brew was administered. Between vomiting, he was given refreshing herb teas to drink. This second and very trying part of the ordeal might last up to six hours, but once his stomach was settled, the worst was over: after another steaming, a shower, and a cold rub-down, the patient usually felt completely recovered – and swallowed a glass of digestive bitters to celebrate.[21]

Besides lobelia, Thomson was eventually using about sixty-five other herbs, including cayenne, bayberry (*Myrica cerifera*) and myrrh (*Commiphora myrrha*), an antiseptic, cleansing herb of which he was particularly fond. Another favourite was sumach (*Rhus glabra*), one of the earliest borrowings from Indian medicine. He used the small red berries steeped in wine and sweetened, and thought it particularly "good for children in cases of canker, especially in long cases of sickness when other articles become disagreeable to them".[22]

Thomson had a special solicitude for his youngest patients: nasty-tasting medicines were disguised by honey, sweetmeats, or orange-juice. If the little patients detected the tell-tale taste of the emetic, Thomson advised: "let him taste some of the drinks made pleasant, just sufficient to produce a desire for more, then put in your emetic unnoticed by the patient, and let them hurry to drink it before the taste is detected".[23]

In the fevers, the colics, the quinsies, dysenteries and chest ailments which formed the largest part of any early nineteenth-century practice, the Thomson treatment was outstandingly successful – particularly in contrast with the physicking and bleeding of the Regulars. The year 1805 brought a striking chance for the inhabitants of Alstead and the neighbouring town of Walpole to compare the two, when an epidemic – probably yellow fever – swept through both towns. Thomson sweated and gave his herbal heating mixtures; the doctors, following Rush, bled copiously and gave calomel. Thomson lost "not one patient that I attended; at the same time, those who had the regular physicians, nearly one half of them died."[24]

Thomson's fame soon grew beyond his immediate circle. In the same year he made a professional visit to Richmond; in 1806 he was called to New York to treat cases of another yellow fever epidemic; after that, he began travelling extensively through the New England states. His success – accompanied as it was by blistering attacks on the calomel practice – soon ensured the hostility of many of the Regulars.

Doctors do not take kindly to being called fools and murderers, and since it was not in Thomson's nature to be either conciliating or moderate in his expression of his views, the whole regular profession soon rose against him, denouncing him as an illiterate quack. In 1808 he was accused of having sweated two children to death, and late in 1809 he was arrested and thrown into prison at the instigation of a Dr. French on a formal charge of murdering a young man called Lovel by administering lobelia.

The circumstances of the trial suggested to Thomson that he was the victim of a malicious medical plot. For nearly two months he was held in a bare unheated cell in the depths of the freezing New England winter; the presiding judge, Chief Justice Parsons was clearly biased against him, and afterwards secretly wrote a grossly distorted account of the trial which was entered in the official record, and often used later to discredit both Thomson and his medicine. The medical witness produced by the prosecution swore blandly that the herb shown in evidence was lobelia, though Thomson's own expert witness established that it was in fact marsh rosemary. Technically, Thomson was acquitted, but much of the mud slung about stuck to him, and in an effort to clear his reputation, he sued Dr. French for slander. He lost, and had to pay more than $600 in costs and damages.

This was a heavy blow, since his financial problems were already becoming acute. He had never been a rich man, had no capital, a family to support and travelling costs and other expenses to be met. While administering the Thomson treatment to a single patient could take up to half a day, his patients still only paid two or three dollars for his time.

More discouraging still was the thought that single-handed he could only treat such a tiny number of all the patients who needed him – always supposing that his enemies in the medical profession failed in their expressed object of stopping his practice. It was at this crisis in his career that Thomson revealed for the first time that genius for salesmanship and promotion which would soon come to be regarded as peculiarly American, and without which the cause of botanic medicine might have withered away in its infancy.

He needed men to spread his medical teachings throughout America, and money to pay them. There were, he reckoned, hundreds of thousands of sick people who would certainly call on him for his safe and effective treatments, if only these were widely available. The answer was to teach his system of medicine, in all its primitive simplicity, to a legion of potential patients, with a network of agents to supply his herbs. And to safeguard his own livelihood, and his control over a system of medicine which was literally his own invention, he would do what every self-respecting American inventor had been doing since the United States Patent Office first opened its doors in Philadelphia in 1796: he would take out a patent.

Thomson gave considerable thought to the exact form of the patent he was to apply for, and finally, grandly, specified a "System of Practice", as exemplified in four separate Courses of Medicine, with a detailed list of the herbs and compositions to be used in each. He then travelled to Philadelphia, and after several long sessions with the Clerk, as he wrote later, "I got it made out according to my request, and the medicine to be used in fevers, cholics, dysenteries and rheumatism; he then asked me if I wanted any additions, and I told him to add 'The first three numbers may be used in any other case to promote perspiration or as an emetic', which he did . . . completed and delivered to me on the 3d day of March 1813."[25]

Protected down to the last detail by a United States Patent, "Thomson's Improved System of Botanic Practice of Medicine" was now ready to conquer America, according to the bold and effective plan Thomson had worked out. In each city he would appoint an agent to publicize and promote the Thomson system, with the object of persuading people to pay twenty dollars for "Family Rights". Twenty dollars bought the purchaser a certificate and "the right of preparing and using, for himself and family, the medicine and System of Practice secured to Samuel Thomson by Letters Patent . . . and that he is thereby constituted a member of the Friendly Botanic Society, and is entitled to an enjoyment of all the privileges attached to membership therein".[26]

Each purchaser of a Right was given instruction in the system, and for another two dollars, he could buy the *New Guide to Health or Botanic Family Physician*, available only to Right-holders. The agents themselves took a percentage of the profits from the sale of Rights, and had the exclusivity of the Thomson herbal medicines which Thomson prepared and supplied to them wholesale from a central warehouse. They had literature for sale, and some of them ran infirmaries where patients could undergo the Thomson courses under supervision.

The Family Rights which thus formed the cornerstone of the

Thomson operation were more than a piece of super-salesmanship: they testified to Thomson's deep conviction that every man ought to hold himself intelligently responsible for his own health and that of his family, and that years of medical study were unnecessary in the treatment of sickness once you had grasped the basic principles of health in all their astonishing simplicity.

Thomson, however, was intelligent enough to perceive that while the appeal of his medicine was powerful among the labouring classes and simple country people, it was much less attractive to the educated and more sophisticated. Even those made better by his mode of treatment, who had been profusely grateful at the time, "after I had worn myself out in their service", often had second thoughts once recovered, and "began to think that it was not done in a fashionable way", while the medical profession almost to a man was violently hostile. [27] It occurred to him that if he could reach some of the leading lights in the medical world, and persuade them to give his system an honest public trial, he might make spectacular headway against such prejudice.

With his usual confidence he went straight to the top. In 1813 he wrote to the great Dr. Rush himself, asking for an interview, and explaining his purpose, and to Rush's colleague Dr. Benjamin Barton, one of the leading botanical lights of Philadelphia, and a member of the faculty of the University of Pennsylvania. Barton's grand work, *Collections for an Essay towards a Materia Medica of the United States* (1804) had recently been published, and since he was known to be sympathetic towards Indian medicine, Thomson felt that he was more likely than most of his colleagues to be at least open-minded, if not receptive, to the new Botanic practice.

As for Dr. Rush, there was nothing mean or small-minded about him for all his dogmatism: he had always advised his students to take a notebook with them on their travels in case some old woman or country-healer might be able to tell them something worth noting down, and he had told a student: "converse freely with quacks of every class and sex. . . . You cannot imagine how much a physician with a liberal mind may profit from a few casual and secret visits to these people." [28]

Thomson had a knack of impressing important people with his evident honesty and strength of purpose, and both men received him in the kindest way. Barton expressed particular interest in the herbs he was using, and promised to give his medicine a trial. Rush, as usual, was up to his eyes in work, and could spare little time for this most interesting of quacks, but Thomson later recorded that "He treated me with much politeness; and said that whatever Dr. Barton agreed to, he would give his consent".[29]

Thus for a few minutes the begetter of a medical system that in its long day slaughtered thousands, and the man whose name came to signify the most outspoken opposition to that practice, sat and conversed in friendly terms.

It is interesting to speculate what might have happened to the course of medical history if Rush had lived to keep his promise. He was nothing if not fair-minded, and if he had been impressed by Thomson's methods in action, he might single-handed have set a new, more merciful direction to the bloody course of contemporary doctoring. But within a few months, the great man was dead. With him died what faint hope Thomson may have had of winning the regular medical profession over to his way of thinking.

16

Botanic Warfare

"We have drawn blood enough to float a steamboat, and given calomel enough to freight her," remarked an Ohio physician during the great cholera epidemic of 1836.[1] Almost a quarter of a century had elapsed since Rush's death, and little had changed in the practice of regular physicians confronted with deadly infectious disease.

What had changed beyond recognition, however, was the opposition that such practice encountered, and the competition that it faced. The medical profession itself was not immune to heart-searching about the value of its heroic therapy, and these were eloquently voiced by Harvard's great botanist, Dr. James Bigelow, in a paper entitled "On Self-Limited Diseases", read in 1835, in which he called for a renewed recognition of nature's healing powers.

Bigelow was certainly no Thomsonian enthusiast. On the contrary, he had repeated, in his great *Vegetable Materia Medica of the United States*, published in 1817, all the old slanders about Thomson. But as Professor of materia medica at Harvard, he was painfully aware that the great medicinal treasures of the American flora were being largely neglected by the profession, while the Thomsonians and the practitioners whom he termed quacks were making enthusiastic use of them.

If the medical profession was beginning to have its doubts about Heroic Medicine, huge numbers of the American public were no longer in any doubt at all: they had rejected it and opted enthusiastically for botanic medicine.

Thomson's success had been as overwhelming as his timing was lucky: events in American history may be said to have conspired to bring forth Thomsoniasm.

Just as Heroic Medicine had seemed specially fitting for the ardent young Republic just breaking free of its European ties, so in the early years of the nineteenth century, Thomsonian Medicine, with its emphasis on self-reliance and energetic home-doctoring with simple herbs, seemed tailor-made for a new age of pioneering expansion. Its sheer revolutionary novelty was an additional recommendation: the weight of medical tradition counted for nothing in a land where all was thrust, expansion, innovation.

In 1803 the Louisiana Purchase had more than doubled the size of the United States by adding 827,000 square miles of territory, stretching north-west across the continent from the Appalachians to the Rockies: as America turned its back on Europe and faced west, what had once been the disregarded "back country" now became the beckoning land of the frontier – and the frontier receded westwards with the wagons of the hardy pioneers, through Ohio and Kentucky, through Iowa and Illinois, through Kansas and Nebraska.

The taxing Thomsonian courses of medicine seemed, to the cynical eyes of one mid-nineteenth-century Regular doctor, to embody the very spirit of these "restless, dauntless, active western backwoodsmen, who even judge of their 'physic' by the amount of labour it is capable of performing."[2]

The pioneer and his family, leaving behind the comforts of regular medical attention along with the Main Street drug-store, were an obvious market for home-doctoring books or systems. The ink was scarcely dry on Thomson's beautiful new patent when in 1813 Peter Smith's *The Indian Doctor's Dispensatory* came whizzing off the presses at Cincinnati, crammed with herbal remedies and aimed straight at "the Citizen of the Western Parts of the United States of America". Peter Smith boldly asserted the superiority of Indian doctoring: "the natives of our own country are in possession of cures, simples etc. that surpass what is used by our best practitioners".[3]

Hard on Smith's heels came Samuel Henry's *New and Complete American Medical Family Herbal*, published in New York in 1814. Henry had had the wit to anticipate a growing demand for "a Herbal . . . that treats upon the real Medical virtues and plants indigenous to the United States", and he cashed in on a fast-growing respect for Indian medicine among his pioneer customers: his work, he claimed, was partly founded upon his experiences as "a prisoner last war, among the Creek Tribe of Indians."[4]

In addition to these home-doctoring books, the Midwest pioneer drew on a growing fund of herbal knowledge learned in many cases almost entirely from the Indians, and passed from family to family: Madge Pickard and Carlyle Buley have indicated in *The Midwest Pioneer* numbers of native remedies in common use, including snake-root, sassafras, dogwood or willow for fevers; butternut bark for a purge; butterfly weed, also known as pleurisy-root; slippery elm or blood-root (*Sanguinaria canadensis*), for dysentery; pinkroot for worms; and pokeberry leaf tea for smallpox victims – the poke leaves were also crushed as a poultice for cuts and burns.

According to Virgil J. Vogel, for at least the first half of the nine-teenth century, "every muddy backwoods trail was trod by horse-back-riding 'Indian' doctors, toting saddlebags of herbs and root-medicines to isolated cabins and frontier communities . . . Most of these white medicine men claimed to have learned their lore from the red men; so common was this claim that, whether true or not, it suggests that Indian medicine enjoyed a high reputation among the frontiersmen."[5]

That vast additional expanse of wild unexplored America fired the imagination of the botanist as well as the pioneer – "a new country where the face of nature presents an ungathered harvest," wrote Bigelow lyrically.[6] His own costly three-volume work, published in 1817, gathered in a mere fraction of this harvest – just sixty plants – while the equally lavish *Vegetable Materia Medica of the United States*, published in the same year by William Barton, of the flourishing Philadelphia school of botanists, contained only fifty, many of which also appeared in Bigelow, so that between them the two enthusiasts actually listed only eighty American medicinal plants.

However, even these, carefully and methodically assessed, were enough to excite any Regular doctor not completely addicted to the calomel and bleeding system, for they not only confirmed the value of plants that had been used in domestic medicine for years, such as boneset and pinkroot, but added new treasures which were to be highly valued by both Regular and Botanic doctors for years to come, many of them listed in official pharmacopoeias. Among these were blue flag (*Iris versicolor*), a powerful cathartic and liver stimulant; golden rod (*Solidago odora*), useful for stomach disorders; Byrd's Indian physic (*Porteranthus trifoliatus*), soon to be widely used in dysentary cases as America's answer to ipecac, and May apple (*Podophyllum peltatum*), a violent purge. Powerful new emetics and purges, it should be added, were heavily emphasized in both works.

The works of Barton and Bigelow – fashionable coffee-table books for their day – roused interest in medical botany at a time when it had long been popular in Europe (where the equivalent volume was Woodville's elegant *Medical Botany*), and gave Thomson's system a credibility among classes who might not have considered it a few years earlier. Even Thomson's greatest liability – his distinctly common origins, his lack of education, and his republican politics – were soon miraculously transformed into a positive asset by the emergence of the self-reliant Common Man as a political force. The Common Man was Thomson's most enthusiastic follower.

In the circumstances Thomsonian medicine could hardly have failed to enjoy huge popularity among the masses, and from the year that Thomson secured his patent it swept to astonishing success, with growing numbers of agents scattered throughout the States, an efficient central organization for supplying the crude plant drugs used in the practice – many of which like cayenne were imported – and a highly efficient public relations organization, which kept it challengingly in the public eye throughout, and directed a constant savage onslaught against the excesses of Regular medicine. It had its literature: a journal, *The Thomsonian Recorder*, and Samuel Thomson's own works – his *Narrative of the Life and Medical Times of Samuel Thomson*, first published in 1822, and his *New Guide to Health*, which appeared in 1825. Both works ran through ten editions before 1835, which may be said to have been the high-water-mark of the movement.

"The manner of its circulation was like that of a patented machine", commented a Regular doctor sourly. "Agents, armed with set phrases against the use of mineral poisons, and in favour of vegetable remedies peddled the books through the country, and sold the right to their use in practice at twenty dollars per right. It spread steadily on, until it pervaded the whole country, including the Canadas. Every neighbourhood was invaded, and in every neighbourhood one or more individuals were to be met with, possessed of the requisite turn of mind necessary to constitute a Thomsonian doctor."[7]

By 1835 the Governor of Mississippi could announce that half the population of his state depended upon Thomsonian practitioners; Tennessee had twenty-nine agents, Alabama twenty-one, Indiana eleven, and New York eight, while the Regulars reluctantly conceded that one-third of the people in Ohio – one of the most densely populated of all western states – were Thomson's followers.

By 1839 Thomson claimed over 3,000,000 faithful. Even among the

Regular physicians themselves – most of whom gave as good as they got in terms of acrimonious abuse – Thomson was not without his admirers. A distinguished and unexpected convert was Dr. Benjamin Waterhouse, Professor of the Theory and Practice of Medicine at Cambridge University, Massachusetts. As the man responsible for introducing vaccination into North America – amid a storm of medical opprobrium – Waterhouse knew what it was like to incur the enmity of the profession. He had read and been deeply interested by Thomson's moving and simply-written *Narrative*, and at a time when Thomson was being howled down as a quack, Waterhouse rose courageously to his defence. ". . . this man is no Quack," he declared in a letter to the *Boston Courier*, "He narrates his medical discoveries, gives an account of his system of practice, together with his manner of curing diseases, upon a plan confessedly new; to which he adds the principles on which his new system is founded. He . . . merits attention." Waterhouse added a reproach for his own profession: "it is not beneath the dignity of any physician . . . to inquire into the truth of a series of experiments published with so much confidence, and purporting to be for the benefit of mankind".[8] Waterhouse was open-minded enough to try out lobelia and the Thomson courses himself – and to admit the fact publicly.

Writing in 1825 to a colleague in New York, Waterhouse spoke even more warmly of "Dr Thomson, who has the honour of introducing the valuable Lobelia into use, and fully proved its efficacy and safety . . . [and who] has cured and relieved many disorders which others could not, without being a regular diplomatized physician."[9]

Most Regular physicians, however, still felt that they could afford to sneer at outsiders like Thomson. It was another matter when dissent came from within their own ranks. And in New York that same year, as it happened, two "regular diplomatized physicians" opened their first practice "upon a plan confessedly new". One was Dr. Hans B. Gram, the first homoeopathic doctor in the New World; the other was Dr. Wooster Beach (1794–1868) who was to found the medical sect known as Eclecticism, for so many years to come a festering thorn in the side of Regular American medicine.

Homoeopathy was the discovery of a German physician, Samuel Hahnemann (1755–1843). A precociously brilliant man, he had mastered eight languages and turned himself into an outstanding experimental chemist by the time he obtained his medical degree in 1799. He had followed the orthodox training of the day, with its insistence on powerful drugging, bleeding and blistering, but he soon grew first disillusioned, then appalled by the failure of these methods in practice. Far from curing his patients, he felt, he was becoming "a murderer or a malefactor" a thought so terrible to him that he gave up practice and concentrated on his chemical work and his writings.[10]

In 1790 he produced a translation of the Scot Dr. Cullen's materia medica, adding notes and comments of his own. One of these notes – on cinchona, the specific cure for malaria – ascribed cinchona's effectiveness to its tonic action on the stomach. Hahnemann demolished this suggestion in a few lines, and invited his readers to consider this fact: he had dosed himself with cinchona regularly for several days – and brought on in himself all the symptoms of intermittent fever – which subsided when he stopped taking the drug.

In his wide reading, Hahnemann had previously come across the medical theory that like cures like: it is common in German folk-medicine – from which Paracelsus probably borrowed it – and is also found in Greek medical writings. The case of cinchona seemed to Hahnemann to confirm it. He had always been deeply interested in the action of drugs upon the human body, and after endless experiment he arrived at the conclusion that cinchona worked because it created an artificial illness in the body similar to malaria, which stimulated the body's own defence mechanism – the *vis medicatrix naturae* central to Hippocratic medicine. Other drugs, he reasoned, might be used in the same way, once their action in a healthy person had been determined; and to establish this "drug-picture", Hahnemann – by this time a professor at Leipzig University – instituted a series of "provings" with a chosen band of pupils. Over a period of time, they dosed themselves with a particular drug and made elaborately detailed notes of their reactions – physical, emotional, mental. To define this old-new therapy, Hahnemann coined the tag *Similis similibus curentur* – let like be cured by like.

Cautiously, he began testing his theory on patients. It succeeded, and, in the process, he made yet another discovery, again almost by accident: the smaller the dose, the more effective. He began diluting his drugs more and more, until he was in effect administering a medicine in which not a molecule of the original substance remained.

The science of immunology has today established beyond all doubt that the human body has marvellous and elaborate defence mechanisms which are activated by an alien substance – be it germ or drug. Vaccination is an orthodox application of Hahnemann's discovery, as is desensitization therapy in allergy; you and I apply it hopefully when we take a hair of the dog that bit us. Even homoeopathy's great stumbling-block – that a medicine without a single molecule of the original drug could still have its effect – is being accounted for in molecular chemistry.

From his provings, Hahnemann gradually built up a collection of about ninety-nine remedies. Some were taken from minerals such as arsenic and sulphur; some from animals – the most famous of which is Lachesis, taken from the venom of a particularly deadly tropical snake; and the majority from plants, such as yellow jasmine (*Gelsemium sempervirens*), the poison nut (*Strychnos nux-vomica*), and poison ivy (*Rhus toxicodendron*). He found that however poisonous in normal doses the action of a drug, it was therapeutic in his minute doses*; he also discovered that at a certain degree of dilution, the characteristic healing effect of a plant disappeared, to be replaced by a totally different action. Thus a homoeopathic dose of opium might be given to arouse a near-comatose patient, and whereas a herbalist uses yarrow mainly for severe feverish colds, the homoeopath uses it for haemorrhages of all kinds.

As might be imagined, the orthodox medical profession of early nineteenth-century Saxony found Hahnemann the most odious of medical heretics for a number of reasons. He was an eloquent critic of the bleeding and purging medicine they relied on; he attacked their most cherished theories; and he was a dangerous rival, attracting numbers of patients away from the Regulars. These alone would have drawn down on him the united fire of the profession, while his most un-heroic doses of medicine guaranteed the deadly enmity of the apothecaries, but to make matters worse, Hahnemann had unfortunate personality defects – he could be vain, pompous, irritable – which made him an easy target for snipers. The apparent absurdity of his theories, finally, alienated many who might have been interested, particularly when Hahnemann blandly insisted that his "natural law of cure" should be judged only in practice: "it matters little what may be the scientific explanation of *how it takes place.*"[11]

Evidently, his treatment did work – which fact the Regulars found

*He thus anticipated by nearly a century the Arndt-Schulz biological fundamental law formulated by two German scientists, Rudolf Arndt, a physiologist, and Hugo Schultz, a pharmacologist. After repeated experiments, the two established the law that for all poisonous substances large doses kill, moderate doses paralyse, and small doses stimulate.

the most enraging of all. By 1813 homoeopathy had become a force to be reckoned with in Germany – homoeopaths were highly successful at treating the typhoid fever that Napoleon's tattered remnant of an army brought back with them from Moscow.. And slowly, news of Hahnemann's theories spread throughout Europe, attracting many doctors who were dissatisfied, as he had been, with the medical practice of the day.

Among these was a young Danish medical student, Hans B. Gram, son of a Danish immigrant to the United States. Gram had returned to Copenhagen for a European medical education, learned of Hahnemann's teachings, and soon became convinced of their truth. He crossed the Atlantic again to open North America's first homoeopathic practice in New York in 1825. Three years later, one of his students, John F. Grey, opened a second. Quietly, inexorably, Hahnemann's natural law of cure established itself in the New World.

The young American Wooster Beach had probably never heard of Hahnemann, but he shared with him and with Samuel Thomson a horrified aversion to Regular medical practice, and a strong religious conviction that he had a personal mission to change the face of medicine. A tall, heavy-boned swarthy-complexioned man, Beach came of respectable New England middle-class stock, his family being related to the Woosters of Connecticut, one of whom – General David Wooster – had died while serving with distinction in the Revolutionary War. Beach seems to have been a precocious youth, eager for learning and plunging into medical studies which had a deep fascination for him. He was soon questioning the validity of the Heroic system: ". . . my soul was filled with indignation at these instruments of cruelty and misery, administered under the specious pretext of removing disease."[12]

He burned with reforming zeal, but he had no idea what possible alternative there might be to the heroic method. Then he heard from a relative of an old German herbal doctor, Jacob Tidd, whose practice at Amwell, New Jersey was said to be getting remarkable results using only the local medicinal plants.

The more Beach learned about Tidd, the more eager he became to know more about this superior, kindly practice, and he finally called on the old man, and begged Tidd to take him on as a pupil. Tidd refused: he was always turning away such applications, he told Beach. Studying the well-tailored young man before him, he added sardonically, "Doctors wish to be gentlemen, but if I take any one to learn, I want another hog like myself to root around the mountains in search of medicines; they wish to be gentlemen, but they ought to be the servants of all men".[13] He sent Beach away – not once, but twice – and the young man first took up teaching, and then went into business. But for the next seven years, he was continually haunted by this vision of a new medicine, and at intervals he pestered the German doctor to change his mind.

Providence, he always believed, led him to make a last call on Dr. Tidd, just at the time the old man's grandson had emigrated westward, leaving him with no assistant. Tidd may have been touched as well as impressed by Beach's persistence: at any rate, he finally took him on as an apprentice, and over the next years, Beach worked alongside him, absorbing a long lifetime's experience in the treatment of sickness with medicinal herbs.

After Tidd's death, Beach moved to New York, where he enrolled as a medical student at the Barclay Street Medical University. "I concluded this was best," he wrote later, "were it only to detect the errors of the modern practice".[14] There were, of course, other excellent reasons, among them the fact that Beach had no special desire to find himself a legal outcast. The activities of Samuel Thomson had brought about a flurry of restrictive legislation in many states, under pressure from State or local Medical Societies, and in New York it was illegal to practise medicine without a diploma. Any undiplomatized practitioner who made a charge for his services was liable to a fine of twenty-five dollars, and he was permanently at the mercy of discontented patients or jealous rivals.

Beach's burning ambition was to reform medical practice generally – not to alienate the entire profession by savage attacks from without – and he was convinced that he would be in a stronger position to do so if he were himself a diplomatized doctor. The faculty occasionally listened to criticism from within their own number: against the onslaughts of "illiterate quacks" like Samuel Thomson, they simply closed ranks in complacent hostility.

Thus in Beach's eyes, Thomson's very success, founded as it was upon "a total subversion of all medical science . . . and the ignorance, prejudices, and dogmas of a single individual",[15] had been actively prejudicial to the cause of medical reform.

Having studied the Thomsonians in action, Beach was determined to avoid what he judged to be their major error: the forthright rejection of any kind of intellectual activity. Samuel Thomson was an instinctive healer, and his near-pathological mistrust of the theorizing that had produced Heroic Medicine had taken him far in the opposite direction. He insisted that his followers should study patients, not books; that his system of medicine was now complete and in need of neither change or improvement. He would have agreed enthusiastically with Wesley's view that doctors made "a needless mystery" out of a knowledge that ought to be available to every man. "The moment," urged Thomson, "you blend the simplicity of my discoveries with . . . abtruse sciences such as chemistry . . . that have nothing to do with medicine, that moment the benefit of my discoveries will be taken from the people generally."[16]

To Beach, this was astonishing arrogance: how could the most gifted, the most brilliant of natural teachers ever put away his books with the curt statement that all medical knowledge stopped here? Beach had not yet been to Europe, but he had read widely and avidly in his subject, and he was aware that new worlds were opening to research in the fields of pathology, physiology, and anatomy, while even in Thomson's own special field – that of medicinal plants – Linnæus had laid the foundations for a new scientific appraisal which to Beach held out glorious possibilities. If chemistry offered tools to unlock the medicinal secrets of plants, how could any Botanic doctor afford to dismiss chemistry as having "nothing to do with medicine."?

A "gentleman" to his finger-tips, too – as Jacob Tidd has perceived – Beach was probably anxious to dissociate himself as completely as possible from the low-class, ill-bred "steamers" who made up the majority of Thomson's followers, and whose doctoring was done in so very "unfashionable" a way. They themselves were well aware of this liability: as one of their journals complained: "The fashionable calomel gentry drive up to the door, are conducted with etiquette to the bedside of the patient, and upon the point of a beautiful silver-steel penknife deal out divers little powders, and then mount their 'go-cart' and leave, and when they get home mark down $2 or $3. But this will never do for the Thomsonian physician, he must take off coat, go the work, and see that the patient's relatives are sometimes violently opposed to having a 'steamer' called in, and would about as lief see the poor sufferer die, as cured by means of 'roots and herbs' ".[17]

From the patient's point of view, there was little to choose in sheer unpleasantness between bleeding and blistering on the one hand, and the Thomsonian's scalding drinks, his devastating emetics, and his exhausting "courses" on the other. Admittedly the Heroic practice could kill you, while the other often made you better . . . but distant ills often seem worth risking for the sake of present comfort.

One way or another, Wooster Beach's determination to put as great a distance as possible between his own and Thomson's methods is completely understandable.

The Censors who examined Beach for his diploma recommended him warmly to the New York Medical Society: ". . . he has studied the practice of Physic and Surgery the term required by law, . . . he possesses a good moral character, and . . . he has sustained an examination before us which does him honor."[18] He was now enrolled as a member of the New York Medical Society; armed with his diploma, he began to practise.

At first, he hoped to bring his fellow-members around to his own point of view: truth must prevail, once it was sufficiently publicized, he felt, and he devoted his enormous restless energies – and much of what must have been a considerable family fortune – to publishing the truth in a variety of newspapers, periodicals and tracts. To his disappointment, all he succeeded in doing as far as his Regular medical colleagues were concerned was to arouse their intense hostility, and to find himself branded one of the odious Botanic outcasts.

It was a bitter blow, and he found himself forced back onto familiar Thomsonian ground: if you can't convince the profession – appeal to the patients. But he was still determined to take on the doctors on their own turf, and to conduct his campaign along respectable, scientific lines. If the truth could not be preached successfully, perhaps it might be demonstrated. Accordingly, he had constructed a charming two-storey building on a plot of ground in what was then "a central and pleasant part of the city", between Broome and Grand, which he proudly named "The United States Infirmary".[19]

Its opening in 1827 was defiantly announced in his religious newspaper *The Telescope*. "Various attempts have been made from time to time by different individuals to rescue medicine from its present degraded, and lamentable state; from various causes, however, their efforts have not been fully crowned with success. But we are now happy to . . . introduce a better System of *Medical and Surgical practice*." The new institution "has been founded (from the most disinterested motives) for the *treatment of diseases generally, by a new and improved method*. The remedial sources are chiefly to be derived from the vegetable kingdom."

There was to be a Surgical department, where operations would be performed "by improved methods, by which the suffering and danger consequent upon fashionable surgery, will be obviated"; the Infirmary would be open day and night; and the poor would be treated and prescribed for at no charge.[20]

Beach had a new name for his practice: while explaining to a friend his notions of combining what was useful in the old practice with what was best in the new, the friend exclaimed "You are an eclectic!" to which, according to legend, Beach replied, "You have given me the term which I have wanted: I *am* an Eclectic!"[21]

He had already gathered round him a little band of young and enthusiastic doctors who shared his ideals, among them Dr. Thomas Vaughan Morrow, a young Kentuckian, and Dr. John Steele from Pennsylvania, and in 1829 he felt sufficiently confident to erect another building alongside his little Infirmary, this time a large and handsome three-storeyed structure, which he first christened the "Reformed Medical Academy," later changing it to the "Reformed Medical College of the City of New York."

New York State, however, no doubt under pressure from the New York Medical Society, who were by this time violently anti-Beach, refused to charter the new college, so that Beach was compelled to send out his students armed only with a certificate of membership in "The Reformed Medical Society of the United States." The last thing he desired to do was turn out troops of Botanic Irregulars, to be easily confused with the despised Thomsonians, and Beach began to examine other possibilities.

Ohio, the Thomsonian stronghold, at once suggested itself, since the state laws in this pioneer country were much more liberal and the regular profession less deeply entrenched. After enquiries, Beach heard of a moribund academy in the small town of Worthington, Ohio, already chartered as Worthington College and empowered to grant degrees. Discussions followed, the building was offered to Beach, and he opened a full-scale medical college, which under the direction of Morrow was soon thriving, with people coming from miles around for treatment. In 1835 the *Western Medical Reformer* was launched to publicize Eclectic ideas, and in 1837 an infirmary was added to the College, where in-patients could be treated, and students given proper clinical instruction.

Eclecticism made headway fast. In 1836 Professor Morrow could claim happily: "There are now, in different sections of the United States, about 200 regularly educated scientific medical reformers, who have gone forth from the New York and Worthington Schools; besides, a considerable number of old school physicians, who have come out and openly declared themselves decidedly in favour of the improved or botanical system of medical and surgical practice."[22]

Up to the mid-1830s Samuel Thomson, now a venerable patriarch in his sixties, could afford to ignore the new competition of the Eclectics and the familiar attacks of the Regulars: he could point to the growing thousands of his believers, and the hundreds of thousands saved from a physic-and-bleeding fate as his system's best vindication. But even among the faithful, not all was peace and union. Like many men of deep and stubborn convictions, Thomson was never inclined to be tolerant of those whose views differed from his own. And this jealous intolerance increased with age, so that bitter feuds between Thomson and his supporters – even his own sons – were soon delighting Eclectics and Regulars alike. His books were pirated, and many of his agents cheated him, while the Annual Conventions – a typically American device, invented by Thomson, for rallying the faithful and boosting their personal loyalty to him – soon became a forum for dissension.

The first convention had been held in Columbus, Ohio, just before Christmas 1832, designed by Thomson to publicize the great success his followers had had in treating the cholera epidemic of that summer. Among others relating their triumps, a young practitioner from Richmond, Alva Curtis, related how he had lost only one out of 200 patients, many of them suffering from the advanced or collapse stage of the disease. Curtis, an able and charming man, was promptly enlisted by Thomson to edit the *Thomsonian Recorder* for him.

The convention was a triumphant success, so impressive were the assembled numbers of Thomsonians and their well-documented claims to therapeutic triumphs that one state after another now repealed those very Practice Acts originally designed to save the Regulars from Thomsonian encroachment. By 1835 New York was one of the few states where such laws were still in force.

But Curtis' appointment turned out to be a major mistake from Thomson's point of view: Curtis had ambitious plans of his own for the movement, and used his new position to advance them. In 1835 he gave the utmost prominence in the *Recorder* to a resolution in favour of a medical school passed by that year's convention. The very idea was anathema to the old man: he rushed into print to crush the scheme, and Curtis resigned. But the younger man had accurately gauged the mood of the movement – the clamour for a medical school became widespread. Greatly encouraged, Curtis set up a "Botanico-Medical School and Infirmary" in Columbus, Ohio, and he was swiftly followed by another "Curtis-ite" down in Georgia, where the Southern Botanico-Medical College was chartered the same year. This split in the ranks of the faithful was made final at the 1838 convention, when Curtis and his followers formally broke away to set up the "Independent Thomsonian Botanic Society". An angry and bewildered old Thomson dissolved the ungrateful convention for ever, his dreams crumbling around him.

The last years of his life were clouded by animosity and feuding. One of the worst of these quarrels was with a former follower, Morris Mattson, who in 1841 published *The American Vegetable Practice* full of slighting remarks about Thomson. The old man's son John published an immense 834-page tome called the *Thomsonian Materia Medica*, by way of riposte, and dedicated it to one of the warmest and most respectable of Thomson's former champions, Dr. Benjamin Waterhouse. But the book's pseudo-scientific pretensions drew down upon it the delighted scorn of the Regulars, the Eclectics and the neo-Thomsonians alike.

Tired and disappointed, Thomson survived this last blow by little more than a year. For some time he had been subject to attacks of diarrhœa, which he had always managed to control "by his own medicines, and always by his own directions," but by the beginning of August 1843, there was no controlling it any longer. Week followed week, and all his medicines did him no good. On 23 September he announced that he needed one of his own courses and dutifully embarked on it the next morning: it seemed to do him good, but when asked how he felt on Sunday morning, he replied dully that "he felt as much refreshed as a boy who had been whipped". By Monday morning he had a high fever, and the nurse reminded him brightly of his own verse:

> See, when the patient's taken sick,
>   Coldness has gained the day;
> And fever comes as nature's friend,
>   To drive the cold away.

Thomson managed a weak smile, but his condition was deteriorating fast, and though he continually ordered fresh treatments for himself it was with no enthusiasm. He did not wish to live, he said, and on the morning of 4 October he slipped quietly away, "like going to sleep".[23]

In 1836 Thomson had once more applied to Waterhouse for a reference, when he sought to renew his patent. Waterhouse had generously complied – in much more restrained terms than earlier – but he had added a gentle reproof of the acrimonious botanic warfare now raging: "I wish the regular physician had a better opinion of the Thomsonian discoveries in the vegetable kingdom, and that the empiric practitioners had a better opinion of the regular or scientific physicians. The conduct of Hippocrates is a bright example for both. Experience must be enlightened by reason and theory built upon close and accurate observation."[24]

It was a counsel of perfection not much attended to in the American medical world of his day.

17

The
Age of Calomel

In 1800 a country physician, Dr. John Chambers, of East Dereham in Norfolk, published a *Pocket Herbal Containing the Medicinal Virtues and Uses of the Most Esteemed Native Plants*. He intended it for the home-doctoring market — no less than forty-seven clergymen appear on his list of subscribers — and he dedicated it to those ever-busy "Ladies, who . . . seem to place their chief happiness in promoting that of others, and to employ both their time and their talents in the relief of the distressed."[1] At first glance his book seems a modest contribution to that long and honourable line of English herbals whose ancestors are Gerard, Markham, and Culpeper.

Chambers, indeed, writes warmly of this tradition of gentle medi-cation with plants, suggesting to his readers that the plants here recommended might be ". . . a more safe and pleasant instrument in the pursuit of their humane exertions, than . . . in Mineral Drugs, by which it is to be lamented that the use of Herbs has been almost entirely superseded".[2] And the first 240 pages of the book are a delightful evocation of an England largely rural, on the very eve of the Industrial Revolution, where plants were still the medicine of the poor, "*Common Cowslip* . . . Grows in pastures and flowers in May . . . The country people boil this in ale, and give it in Giddiness of the Head, with success . . . *Jack by the Hedge* . . . it grows under hedges and flowers in May. This plant is eaten by our country people with their bread and butter, and is very wholesome."[3]

But there is a joker: tucked away at the back of the book are "A few Remedies, Not of the Vegetable Kingdom," presumably for those advanced readers, whose trust in wholesome herbs was no longer as complete as it once was.

Many of these remedies were far from being either safe or pleasant. His *Universal Alterative Drops*, for "bad habits of Body" contain ten grains of corrosive sublimate, that most vicious of mercurial preparations. For "Obstructed Menses", he offers remedies which he might have learned from any unscrupulous back-street abortionist, combining calomel with tincture of a certain plant abortifacient so venomously poisonous that it was certainly responsible for many deaths. And for a purge, Dr. Chambers suggests a combination of three of the most strongly active substances ever used in medicine: scammony, antimony and calomel. Three grains of this, he lightly suggests, "will safely clear an infant just born of its meconium, which . . . by retaining it lays a foundation for future diseases."[4]

Prescribed by doctors, the minute amounts carefully weighed out by experienced apothecaries, such prescriptions were, to put it mildly, hazardous to a patient. Yet calomel, opium and many other poisonous drugs – vegetable as well as mineral – were on free and open sale to anyone with a few pennies in hand, and the time to call on their local apothecary or druggist – where they were dispensed as freely as aspirin or cough mixture is today.

The "Ladies" to whom the reckless Dr. Chambers entrusted his potentially lethal prescriptions were certainly prescribing for their neighbours as enthusiastically as ever, like the Rector's wife in George Eliot's *Middlemarch* "much too well-born not to be an amateur in medicine".[5] But they no longer relied chiefly on their physic garden, and in most well-to-do households, the still, the pestle and mortar and the hanging bunches of dried herbs had been supplanted by the home medicine-chest which turned the housewife into her own apothecary.

Made of beautifully polished wood, lavishly fitted with brass, velvet and cut glass, hundreds of these medicine-chests have survived to testify to their enormous popularity. Some of them were supplied by leading chemists, like Savory & Moore or John Bell (which survive in London to this day), while others bore the label of the Apothecaries' Hall. They came supplied with little booklets of instructions for their use, and supplying refills for these chests was a service advertised by many druggists.

Among the more popular were The Family Dispensatory Chests which bore the seal of approval of Dr. Richard Reece, whose *Medical Guide* – first published in 1802 and already through fourteen editions by 1824 – was written for use with the chests. The Family Dispensatory Chests contained "those drugs &c with which one person, at least, in every village ought to be provided," together with graduated measures, scales and weights, a "Lavement Bag, with Pipe",[6] and other useful odds and ends. Its contents indicate the growing popularity of those "Mineral Drugs" which were slowly pushing herbs out of domestic as well as professional medicine. Of the sixty items, only twenty-four are plant-derived preparations, including the familiar purging quartet of rhubarb, senna, castor oil and jalap; essences of cinnamon and peppermint, tinctures of ginger and camomile, powdered Peruvian bark, and the highly costly Lenitive Electuary. And of these twenty-four, only one – the Compound Spirit of Lavender – may be said to be homegrown, English doctors by this time having learnt thoroughly to despise any herb that did not have an exotic origin, and hence a high price in the apothecary's stocklist.

Very few of the mineral preparations would be available today other than on prescription: they included, naturally, laudanum, or the tincture of opium, and calomel, or mercurous chloride, which by the beginning of the nineteenth century were the two most frequently prescribed drugs in England.

There is some excuse for the reckless abandon with which opium was prescribed, since it was a splendid painkiller, while its fatally addictive nature was still not widely realized. But the growing reliance of English and American doctors on calomel for every human ailment from syphilis to an upset stomach makes one of the blackest chapters in all of medical history. It may be explained by the earnest belief of doctors at this time that "activity" was everything in a drug, and the more you meddled with nature, the better. But it cannot be excused on the grounds of ignorance of mercury's deadly side-effects. On the contrary, in a horrifying exhibition of doublethink, some of the very doctors who pointed out its perils, and condemned its abuse most sternly, were themselves guilty of spreading the calomel gospel with enthusiasm.

Among these, unluckily, was one of the most popular compilers of home-medicine books, designed for housewives and other "amateurs in medicine". Dr. Thomas Graham's *Modern Domestic Medicine* first appeared early in the century and in his preface he preaches the "soothing plan of treating diseases". Those drugs which most powerfully allay irritation, he states, "are the most speedy and effectual in the cure of diseases", and he concludes severely that "it is this fact chiefly which has urged me to oppose, to the best of my ability . . . the frequent and excessive use of mercury, a practice far more general and destructive than is commonly appreciated".[7] The key word here, however, is "excessive": it turns out that in Dr. Graham's view no other drug could soothe and tranquillize the disordered system quite as successfully as mercury; he recommended its use in no less than forty-six different ailments, as various as asthma, gout, cancer, jaundice, madness and smallpox, and many of them perfectly trivial, such as headache, indigestion or a stitch in the side. The medical profession had come a long way since the days when Paracelsus doubted whether "so desperate a remedy" should ever be used for syphilis.

Unlike Dr. Graham, Dr. Reece appears to have had almost no reservations at all about the calomel which featured so importantly in his Family Dispensatory Chests. "Of all the mineral productions used in the practice of medicine", he wrote warmly, "mercury is by far the most valuable".[8] His favourite remedy was the Antibilious pill, containing three grains of calomel, to be taken three at a time, and he thought the drug likely to be particularly useful in childish rickets or convulsions "which frequently arise from an accumulation of slime in the intestines".[9]

Ah, the intestines! No other part of the human body held so deep a fascination for the nineteenth-century doctor – probably because the "activity" of his drugs had so obvious an effect in this area. Apart from diarrhœa and constipation, many other diseases were traced to a malfunction of this important length of tubing, to be goaded back into normal activity by a barrage of powerful drugs. Dr. Reece devoted an entire book to the subject: his *Practical Dissertation on Costiveness*, published in 1826, alerted thousands of readers to the perils of ignoring this health-threatening state from the very moment of birth. "Costiveness is . . . so common among newly-born infants, that it is a practice with accoucheurs to send an aperient mixture for the infant with the medicines for the mother," he wrote approvingly.[10] And he stated as a fact that "there is no complaint more general, especially among females . . . than costiveness".[11]

This universal costiveness – except, presumably, in the new-born – was fairly certainly the result of the lifelong battering with strong purges and aperients that nineteenth-century bowels underwent: an iatrogenic – doctor-induced – disease if ever there was one. And a great contributory cause is likely to have been the enormous popularity of laudanum, which produced constipation as a side-effect; "judiciously administered . . . this is certainly the most valuable drug we possess," wrote Reece, ". . . more or less employed in almost every disease incident to the human frame".[12]

These two drugs, together with antimony, bleeding and blistering, constituted the general therapy of the day, and most people accepted it without complaint, assuming with the usual blind trust of patients since the beginning of time, that the doctor knew best. Indeed, many patients had actually come to prefer meddling medicine to any other kind, as is shown in George Eliot's *Middlemarch*, which neatly sections the different layers of medical practice in one English town in the early part of the century. ". . . Since professional practice chiefly consisted in giving a great many drugs, the public inferred that it might be better off with more drugs still if only they could be got more cheaply, and hence swallowed large cubic measures of physic prescribed by unscrupulous ignorance which had taken no degree".[13] The apothecaries of Middlemarch included Mr. Toller, "a well-bred, quietly facetious man . . . given to the heroic treatment, bleeding and blistering and starving his patients, who commonly observed that Mr. Toller had lazy manners, but his treatment was as active as you could desire . . . he was a little slow in coming, but when he came he *did* something."[14]

With most of the medical profession leading them, and the most up-to-date home-doctoring books egging them on, it is hardly surprising that the "Ladies" who had once so confidently consulted their Gerard and Markham now left them to gather dust on the shelf while they tried their hand at a rather more potent medicine.

In educated circles, the simple herbal medicine was beginning to seem distinctly old-fashioned now – as it had for decades among doctors – and the early years of the nineteenth century saw the passing of an age. There were still herbal practitioners to be found in some cities. But all over England, traditions of native plant use that had been handed down in countless families, over countless generations, were dying out: they survived for the most part only in isolated villages, in cottage circles and women's talk, or else were preserved in a popular name – marsh woundwort, staunchweed, self-heal, eyebright, boneset. Only the poorest of the poor – England's labourers and drudges – still turned to the fields and hedgerows for relief of their ailments, and most of them would have gone to the apothecary if they could.

Herbal medicine is as old and as universal as man himself. In Western Europe it was now entering upon the last stages of that decline in importance that had begun in the age of Paracelsus. Increasingly, it would strike the average doctor as, at best, quaintly old-fashioned; at worst, as a perverse and dangerous form of quackery threatening to lure people away from effective modern medicine with its laboratory wonders.

There were still plant-derived drugs on which doctors everywhere relied: opium for pain relief, Peruvian bark for malaria, and a handful of useful purges – like senna, castor oil and rhubarb. Foxglove was slowly securing its place in the pharmacopœia; and a quartet of poisonous plants, all of them powerfully narcotic, continued to command both the respect and the interest of the profession on account of their high degree of "activity": aconite (*Aconitum napellus*), deadly nightshade (*Atropa belladonna*), hemlock (*Conium maculatum*), and henbane (*Hyoscyamus niger*). But enormous numbers of herbs which had been known and valued in medicine for centuries, were now steadily being relegated to history, while their place was taken by one of the growing number of chemical preparations.

It is impossible today not to feel both astonishment and indignation at the short-sighted and cavalier manner in which the medical profession of Britain – like that of half Europe – at this time turned its back on the enormous therapeutic resources of the plant world. Even at the time, isolated voices were raised in protest.

Sir John Hill, the most lovable and clever of the eighteenth-century herbal quacks, was one of the most eloquent. He was particularly indignant that the botanic study of plants was becoming a fashionable drawing-room hobby while the vital properties of the plants were neglected, and he said so in the Preface to his *Useful Family Herbal* published in 1789: ". . . It grieves a man of public spirit and humanity, to see those things which are the means alone of the advantages of mankind studied, while the end . . . is forgot. And in this view he will regard a Culpeper as a more respectable person than a Linnæus."[15]

Hill was perfectly aware that Culpeper and many other herbals were hopelessly unscientific – "there is not the most trifling herb which they do not make a remedy for almost all diseases" – [16] but this seemed to him an urgent argument for much more research into medicinal plants, rather than for ignoring their potential altogether, at a time "when physic is becoming entirely chymical, and . . . lives are thrown away daily . . . which might be saved by a better practice".[17]

The same thought was echoed more forcibly some thirty years later, when John Waller published his *New British Domestic Herbal* in 1822: "Although we cannot deny that, in skilful hands, very considerable advantages have accrued to Medicine from chemical preparations, it is, nevertheless, a melancholy truth, that the healths of thousands, and the lives of not a few . . . are yearly sacrificed to the rage for preparations of mercury, arsenic . . . and almost every deleterious mineral under Heaven . . . so far has this rage for poisonous drugs gained ground, that scarcely any article from the *vegetable* kingdom is thought worthy to enter into the prescription of a Modern Physician, that is not recognized for a dangerous and active poison: hence the daily use of aconite, hemlock, henbane . . . &c."[18]

The science of pharmaceutical chemistry made vast strides in the early years of the nineteenth century, but it was much the same handful of potent plants that fascinated the pharmacists, and when they learned how to break plants down chemically, and isolate their active constituents, it was to such plants that they turned their attention first, in the hope of producing even more powerful drugs in standardized form.

Careful clinical work with plants, on the other hand, such as had given digitalis to medicine, had come virtually to a standstill, a fact noted with grief by Dr. William Woodville, whose lavish and beautiful five-volume *Medical Botany*, published in 1832, may have been the last herbal, properly so-called, to be written by an English regular physician for a century and a half. "It is a lamentable truth", he wrote, "that our experimental knowledge of many of the herbaceous simples is extremely defective; for as writers on the materia medica have usually done little more than copy the accounts given by their predecessors, the virtues now ascribed to several plants are wholly referrible to the authority of Dioscorides."[19]

If the chemical practice could have been shown to be dazzlingly superior to the "herbaceous", there might have been some justification for the strong preference of most English doctors for the former. But to dispassionate observers, such as Woodville, it was blindingly obvious that this was not the case: ". . . it would . . . be difficult to show that this preference is supported by any conclusive reasoning, drawn from a comparative superiority of chemicals over Galenicals."[20]

Other critics were much more outspoken. Dr. James Hamilton, the distinguished Edinburgh physician, attacked the use of calomel for trivial ailments in his *Observations on the Use and Abuse of Mercurial Medicines* published in 1819. In this work, one of the earliest scientific studies of drug side-effects, Hamilton warned doctors that although some of the more immediate and dramatic results of calomel therapy – such as bloody diarrhœa, emaciation, salivation and debility – were mercifully rare, its long-term action on any patient's constitution might be much more insidious, and quite as deadly, particularly in children.

He also suggested that a great many of the major health problems of the day, as well as much general ill-health and debility, were due to constant dosing with calomel. He was frightened by the alarming rise in the incidence of convulsions – "all those fatal conversions to the head, which of late years have so frequently taken place in the fevers of children"[21] – and by "the daily increasing ravages of hereditary scrofulous disorders"[22], that tuberculous infection of the lymph nodes in the neck which produced the huge disfiguring ulcers known as The King's Evil. Hamilton became more and more convinced that both could be laid at the door of calomel, and he strongly suspected that this drug might also be a factor in the upsurge in numbers of deaths from ordinary tuberculosis.

Hamilton was that rarity, an orthodox physician clear-sighted enough to see that there were failings in his own profession, brave enough to say so, and generous enough to admit that practitioners outside the pale of orthodoxy might actually be doing better. And one of his closest and most interesting friends was a lively, unconventional Scotsman named Charles Whitlaw who spent most of his grown life in the blackest books of the medical profession.

Whitlaw was trained in boyhood for a career in horticulture and landscape gardening, and to complete his training he crossed the Atlantic to study the splendid botanic gardens of Philadelphia. He arrived in the great heyday of the Philadelphia botanizing physicians, fell under their spell, and soon found gardening much less interesting than this new passion. Linnæus became "my great master" as he always called him; but it was the medical aspect of the Swede's writings that interested him, in particular Linnæus' many observations on how the toxic or therapeutic effects of a plant varied from one species to another.

To a man of Whitlaw's country upbringing and agricultural bent, this was a fascinating new field to explore, and equally exciting were the numbers of new medicinal plants, unknown to Linnæus, whose properties were at last being learned from the Indians and widely discussed in American botanical circles. With characteristic energy and curiosity, Whitlaw went straight to the source, and in the intervals of a successful American career as a landscape gardener, he devoted all his spare time to researching these potent plants and learning about their use from the Indians themselves.

He was much struck by the vapour baths which the Indians resorted to "in the various species of inflammation", and made notes of how they set about it: "A few heated stones, in the first instance, are heaped together, round which something similar to a soldier's tent is erected. The person or persons to receive the bath are seated round the stones, upon which are thrown herbs, and water sprinkled with the hand". He tried it himself and found it "suffocating in the extreme," but he could see that it worked. It seemed to him probable that the "principal virtue of the Indian vapour-bath consisted in the herbs when thrown upon the heated stones, being converted into gas".[23] He thought it obvious that drugs taken by mouth must do more harm than good, if the stomach was disordered and the patient constipated.

Filled with these new ideas, he began experimenting with different combinations of herbs and vapour baths. He does not say who his first patients were, but by 1820 he was established in London, with a Committee running his Vapour Bath Institution, and patients flocking to try this novel cure.* By 1830 he could claim that over 60,000 patients had come under his care, and every disease in every stage of its progress had been treated by him, while his agents had set up similar Vapour Bath Institutions in towns throughout Britain – Devizes, Manchester, Salisbury, Weymouth, Poole, Hastings, Romsey, and Edinburgh among them. These patients were treated with herbs whose use Whitlaw had learned from Linnæus, as well as many of the herbs being used by the Thomsonians in America: among them was lobelia, although Whitlaw never mentioned Thomson in his own writings. Like Hahnemann, Whitlaw tried his herbs on healthy people first, not the sick.

It may have been at Edinburgh that Whitlaw and Dr. Hamilton first met. Dr. Hamilton was by this time President of the Hunterian Society, and a highly distinguished figure in the ranks of the medical profession. But he was much interested by reports of Whitlaw's success with scrofula cases, which had always puzzled and disturbed him. He took the trouble to go to London and inspect Whitlaw's

---

*The Medicated Vapour Bath has survived as therapy in Germany, where it is still practised with beautifully designed modern equipment. In the mid 1970s a British homoeopathic doctor, Dr. Lambert Mount, introduced the idea into his practice, opening a clinic at Tunbridge Wells. It did not, however, prosper, and to the best of my knowledge nobody else in Britain has attempted to practise this particular treatment since.

Bayswater clinic himself, and when the Baths Committee asked him
for his impressions, he sent a generous reference: ". . . I can state, that I
have seen several persons with numerous scars of ulcers, who had been
cured by his means. I have likewise known others labouring under that
dreadful malady whilst under his care, and have marked in them a
progressive amendment."[24]

Hamilton did more than write complimentary letters: he sent
several of his own patients to Whitlaw for treatment, and always spoke
in the highest terms of the Vapour Baths – a fact that did not endear
him to the Royal College of Physicians who had struck off their
register another admirer of Whitlaw, the highly respected botanizing
physician Dr. Thornton, "because of his association with an itinerant
quack or vendor of American herbs in London".[25]

Whitlaw was indifferent to the opinion of the Royal College, but on
arrival in New York in November 1824, with the object of reorgan-
izing his American supplies of herbs, he was astonished to find that
their animus had pursued him across the Atlantic. In a violent denunciation of "all species of quackery" at his inaugural address, Dr. David
Hossack, President of the New York Medical Society, singled Whitlaw out for special mention, congratulating the College on its tough
action: "Dr. Thornton's conduct, in aiding the Whitlaw imposition on
public credulity, richly deserved this mark of disapprobation", thundered Dr. Hossack, who had his address printed and widely circulated.[26]

Challenged by Whitlaw to "divide . . . a hundred patients, and try
who could cure them soonest", Dr. Hossack responded with a dignified silence, and Whitlaw went to Washington where, taking a leaf
from Thomson's book, he patented his system.[27] He then set up a local
Committee, who bought from him the right to run the first Medicated
Vapour Bath in America, and was soon numbering Senators and
Congressmen among his patients.

There are so many points of resemblance between the Whitlaw and
Thomsonian systems – the steaming, the herbs, the patent, and the
agents busily spreading the good news – that it is hard to believe that
Whitlaw knew nothing of Thomsonian methods. But there were two
major differences of approach. While Thomson poured huge draughts
of medicine down the throats of the sick, Whitlaw medicated his
patients purely by way of steam that had been impregnated, by a
special device of his own invention, with the volatile oil of specific
medicinal herbs. And whereas the semi-literate New Hampshire

farmer appealed mainly to the working-classes, Whitlaw was a widely-read and highly articulate man, with excellent social connections. He appealed first and foremost to the educated, made converts in the highest places – dukes, as well as regular doctors – and picked the most prosperous country towns and respectable watering-places of Britain for the establishment of his Vapour Baths.

For all that, his fame died with him some time around the 1840s. Most of the Vapour Baths appear to have closed down soon after his death – lacking the impetus of his driving personality to keep them going – and within the decade, the British medical profession had identified an entirely new species of herbal quackery. Much to their delight, its ringleader was called Albert Isaiah Coffin.

18

"Coffinism"

The Victorian Age and Dr. Coffin arrived in London almost simultaneously. In June 1838 the short, slightly plump nineteen-year-old Victoria was crowned Queen amid scenes of extravagant enthusiasm. After the succession of eccentric, crotchety elderly gentlemen who had occupied the throne for so long, her subjects looked forward with vivid hope to a bright new future, presided over by this earnest girl.

It was a highly interesting moment in British history, as every foreign visitor allowed, among them Dr. Albert Isaiah Coffin, a tall, rather delicate-looking forty-eight-year-old American.[1] In appearance and manner he was quite ordinary – "There was very little refinement or cultivation in him at that time", it was later remarked – and when he tried to gather an educated London audience, and lecture it on the beauties of the Thomsonian system of botanic medicine, of which he was a practitioner, the attempt was a flop: London remained unmoved.[2]

Never one to be easily discouraged, Coffin at once changed tactics, left London, and went to "the thickly populated districts of the north", where in England's new urban slums he tried again, deliberately addressing himself, this time, to an audience of working-men and their families.[3]

Many of those who listened to Coffin had grown up in the countryside, and could remember a mother or a village wise-woman who doctored them with herbs. On fine Sundays, when everyone flocked to the green meadows and woods outside the towns, there were those who could still put a name to and vaguely recall the use of plants that Gerard had written about. And on city market-days, the herb-vendor with his stall piled with bunches of dried medicinal herbs was still a familiar sight.

Such audiences took the jaunty American botanic doctor to their hearts. Hull was the scene of his first triumph; at Sheffield the welcome was warmer still (he always afterwards had a special affection for Sheffield); and Coffin finally settled in Leeds, with a fast-growing network of agents to sell his herbs, and thousands flocking to hear his lectures.[4]

Throughout his life, Coffin remained curiously reticent about his youth and his years in America. But from time to time, with a flourish, he would produce a fragment of autobiography, from which a highly-coloured and no doubt skilfully-edited early history of this remarkable person can be pieced together.

Born in America in 1790 or 1791, Albert Isaiah Coffin was the son of a Jewish couple "engaged in agricultural and farming occupations", and he was brought up to a life on the land. Like Thomson, he found it uncongenial: "I certainly disliked the employment and anxiously longed for emancipation for such thraldom". One of his father's friends was a Dr. E——, a neighbour who used to drop in some evenings for a chat. The doctor was a kindly man, and he soon realized that when he mentioned medical matters, the restless teenager – who was clearly bored with farmwork – sat up and listened. When questioned, he admitted that he should love to be a doctor himself. The doctor secretly gave him a great pile of medical textbooks – Bell, Thacher, Ainsworth – and night after night, the boy sat up studying. He filled many sheets of foolscap paper with questions that puzzled him, leaving spaces for the doctor's answers, and after a year of this novel form of tuition, his chance to show how much he had learned came.

His sister fell ill, the doctor was summoned, and at once turned to the young Coffin and asked what he made of the case. " 'There seems,' said I, 'to be an inflammatory action in the hepatic region, or inflammation of the liver, and the epigastric region sympathizes.' – 'What would you give?' said he. 'I should give,' I replied, 'expectorants and diaphoretics.' 'Well, go, my lad to my medicine-bags . . . and put them up.' I did so accordingly." Coffin's parents watched in amazement while Coffin unwrapped, weighed, measured and mixed medicines, before throwing in a touch of his own – he applied hot bricks to his sister's feet. His very first case got better – the whole story of his nocturnal cramming came out, and the doctor acquired a hard-working, enthusiastic apprentice.

But days and nights of sitting over his textbooks undermined the young Coffin's health. He caught cold after cold, and then a steady, chronic cough and catarrh, which was finally pronounced to be tuberculosis. "I was at this time . . . reduced to 60 lbs. weight, and as to my fingers I could see daylight through them," Coffin used to say impressively at this point in his reminiscences . . . "I expectorated three pints of matter a day, and sometimes a pint of blood . . . all said I must die and I believed it."

Destiny now stepped in. "There was a portion of the tribe of Seneca Indians that obtained their livelihood by basket and broom making . . . on one occasion an old gipsy-looking woman of this tribe, came to our house and requested a draught of cider . . . while the Indian was drinking, she espied me and said to my mother, 'Is that your son?' She answered it was, and permission being granted, she came in and felt my hand, saying 'White man no cure you'. I myself felt assured of it, however I begged my mother to take the woman away."

Outside the boy's room, the Indian woman cross-questioned Coffin's mother on his illness, then offered to cure him for a gallon of cider. More to please his mother than with any real hope, Coffin agreed that she should try, and the woman disappeared into the woods, returning later with an apronful of herbs, including branches from the prickly ash (*Zanthoxylum americanum*). With these, she made a strong decoction, and gave Coffin a wine-glassful to drink. Soon "a comfortable glow [was] diffusing itself over my whole frame . . . a pleasant moisture bedewed my hands and I felt as one reprieved from a sentence of death. I exclaimed with joy, 'the medicine will cure me' ".

He recovered – to find, like Thomson, that his faith in regular medicine was dead, and in its place was a new conviction: there was a natural way of healing, drawing on a green materia medica, which was vastly superior to anything written in the books, and the Indians seemed to know all about it – the illiterate old Seneca woman had succeeded where the book-learned physicians had failed. He wanted to know more.

"I immediately formed my resolution, threw in my lot amongst those roving tribes . . . imbibed their tastes and habits, and diligently gleaned from them all the information I could regarding the various herbs, barks &c., with which they were acquainted".

To his surprise, he learned that he was not the first white man in this field: he heard about Samuel Thomson – then almost ready to apply for his patent – and rushed to meet "that truly great and clever man".[5]

Presumably, though he never actually said so, he became a Thomsonian agent and practitioner, eventually settling in the small town of Troy in New York State. If he learnt nothing else from the great man, he certainly learned to value publicity: in 1832 he wrote to the newly-launched *Thomsonian Recorder* to boast that in 200 obstetric cases, he had lost neither mother nor child.[6] And when cholera reached Troy in the summer of that year, he had an inspiration: he published each day a racy account of his numbers of successful cures in a *Bulletin of Health*, in striking contrast to the town doctors who could only publish their failures in a daily bulletin of mortality.[7] There came a day when his own name might have featured on this last: he caught the cholera himself, and was soon "reduced to a mere skeleton . . . blue to my elbows". In this crisis, however, no old Seneca woman was now needed, and he cured himself with the sound Thomsonian remedies of lobelia, composition powder, stomach bitters, and plenty of good cayenne pepper.[8]

But Coffin was born for a wider stage than this small-town practice could offer him, and at an age when most of his contemporaries were settling into retirement, he launched himself energetically on a new career. In 1837 he sailed for France, his bags crammed with Thomsonian remedies, to bring the new medicine to the Old World.

Post-Napoleonic France, however, had strict medical ordinances, and his packets of Composition Powder were confiscated as unlicensed compound medicine by the Customs men at Le Havre. He stayed, undeterred, and opened a shop for the sale of the rest of his stock, spending his spare time learning about European herbs from the local shepherds. At the age of forty-seven, he also went courting – and married an American woman named Sarah. But a burglary in which he lost £300 in cash – a huge sum in those days – was a final blow: he abandoned France, and sailed for "dark, physic-laden, pill-swallowing England".[9]

Had Coffin lived today, he might perhaps have been a successful television personality. Racy, vivid, cosy, down-to-earth, switching from comedy to high seriousness in an instant, he appealed to his working-class audiences as one of them – he used to take off his jacket and roll up his sleeves to underline a point. Coffin's lectures must have been first-class entertainment, as is obvious from the surviving accounts of them.

Lecturing to a Sheffield audience in the summer of 1847, he spoke of a recent serious illness: "those who attended me expected I should

close my disease with death. But cayenne pepper fetched me out.
(Loud applause.) I did not send for Dr. Bickersteth, or Dr. Lewis,
although they lived very near – and indeed there are twenty-six
doctors living in my street. (Laughter.) I did not send for any of them;
but my wife – for so many years the partner of my toils – rolled up
her sleeves, and turned doctor, and here I am. (Applause.) I feel very
weak; but begin to feel stronger, and believe I shall have to pull my
coat off. (Laughter and applause) (Dr. Harle: Don't pull it off.) Our
friend Dr. Harle says, don't pull it off. (A voice from the gallery: I
think you had better put your hat on.) I will have them all off. (Here
Dr. Coffin took off his coat amid laughter and applause.)"

Having won over an audience, Coffin would become serious and
speak of his determination to fight medical monopoly: "My object
was to benefit the working classes, and I believe that I have done them
more good than they could derive from the old practice of medicine.
(Applause.) I believe the working classes are the only classes who
deserve to have any good done to them. (Renewed cheering.) (The
Chairman: You'll catch it now.) The chairman says I shall catch it now;
but I can say that there is not any man works harder than Dr. Coffin.
(Loud applause.)"[10]

Coffin exploited his genius for popular journalism too: he launched
a monthly (later a fortnightly) called *Coffin's Botanical Journal*, in which
his message was rammed home in the same vivid, colourful style – the
above account, in fact, is reprinted from an early issue. By way
of entertainment, both lectures and the *Journal* were crammed with
horror stories with a happy ending, in which, after some luckless
patient had been brought to death's door by the blistering, bleeding
and physic of "regular" medicine, he was restored to health by a
simple Coffinite using wholesome herbs.

Coffin modelled his British career closely on the example of Thomson: soon after his arrival, he set up a herbal depot in High Holborn,
run by one of his earliest converts, Mr. W. B. Ford, under his personal
supervision. He wrote and published a *Botanic Guide to Health*, again
closely modelled on Thomson both in theory and remedies, but
featuring common European herbs such as agrimony, clivers (*Galium
aparine*) and *Parietaria officinalis*, or pellitory-of-the-wall, as well as the
American ones he imported in huge quantities, usually from the
Shaker settlements in the United States.

In every town where his magnetic personality and his growing fame
brought eager audiences, he appointed agents and set up local "Friend-

ly Botanico-Medical" societies, who bought his *Guide* and his herbs, practised medicine accordingly, and held regular meetings.

Some of his converts were themselves medical men, like Thomas Harle, a Manchester surgeon who had been nineteen years in practice when he heard of Coffin, went to jeer, and stayed to become Coffin's right-hand man, and an enthusiastic witness to the cause. "Previously he found he was not able to cure disease, and he was sorry to confess it, but now he could cure disease . . . properly cure it, and without leaving any ill effects upon the system such as always result from calomel, opium and other poisons."[11]

Many of Coffin's agents – simple, working men – developed into first-class and dedicated herbal practitioners, like William Fox of Sheffield whose two sons were still well known practising herbalists in Sheffield early this century. Much of the strength of Coffinism came from its appeal to the wives as well as the men: Coffin was a teetotaller himself, urging temperance on all his followers, and his meetings were family affairs, with the ladies dispensing tea and light refreshments, and often themselves being recruited as practitioners.

The movement spread like a prairie fire. By 1850 there were branches in every major city in the industrial North – the Coffin heartland – as well as in London, where he now had a handsome house at 24 Montague Place; the *Guide* had gone through twenty printings, and the now-fortnightly *Journal* claimed 10,000 readers.

All the eloquence and organizational ability in the world, however, could not for long have recommended a system of medicine which failed to work in practice. "Coffinism" demonstrably did, as time after time ordinary working people came forward to testify, not only in the pages of the *Journal*, or at public meetings, but while giving evidence in the court cases which soon began to be the "regular" answer to Coffin's success.

At first the medical establishment refused to take this transatlantic pretender seriously. "Coffinism", as they inevitably nicknamed it, was only one of a number of medical "heresies" rampant at the time, such as Mesmerism, Hydropathy and Chronothermalism, and certainly less of a threat than homoeopathy, which had arrived in London from Europe in 1832 in the engaging person of Dr. Hervey Quin, who was attracting a growing and – what was worse – fashionable following.

But the wretched Coffin constantly obtruded himself on their notice: indeed, it was part of his plan to do so. (A friend once warned him, "Doctor, the medical men are saying nasty things about you", to which Coffin replied happily, "I don't care a d— what they say about me – so long as they say something").[12] Eventually, he could no longer be ignored; something had to be done to put the ignorant quack in his place. The big guns of the *Lancet* were wheeled round and trained on Coffin; the statute books were hurriedly searched for legal weapons.

Irregular practitioners at this time were still protected by the old Henry VIII statute – the "Quacks' Charter" unless it could be shown that a patient had died as a direct result of their treatment. But after digging around for a while, the establishment came up with an opening for legal action: under an act passed in the reign of George III, a person could be charged for practising as an apothecary unless duly licenced by Apothecaries' Hall. Soon, cases were being brought on this charge, and at first the regular practitioners, who almost invariably instigated them, imagined that they only had to put any of these common bricklayers and foundrymen turned herbalists into the dock to expose both their ignorance and the awful peril to the public that they represented.

Their tactics backfired badly. As often as not, it was the medical witnesses who were shown up as ignorant: Coffin ran rings round the "expert" evidence brought in to testify that lobelia was a poison; juries sometimes refused to convict Coffinites out of sheer sympathy even when the evidence told against them, while the courtrooms were often packed with an audience intensely hostile to the medical profession.

In one such case in the autumn of 1853, in an inquest on a three-year-old boy, it was alleged by the Faculty that his death had been caused by the improper treatment given him by a Mrs. Ann Mansfield, particularly her administration of lobelia.

It emerged in the evidence that the little boy, whose "legs were paralyzed by taking cold while in Victoria Park", had been under regular treatment for months, first as an in-patient at the London Hospital, and then as an out-patient at the Orthopædic Hospital. He was next treated by a Mile End Row surgeon who saw him three or four times, but, according to the father, "did not benefit the child"; the "expense being too heavy, he discontinued taking him." Mrs. Mansfield by contrast had taken the boy into her own home, given him the best treatment in her power, stayed with him night and day till his death, according to the child's own mother, and made no charge at all, but left it to the parents' generosity. Dr. Letheby, an eminent professor of Chemistry and Toxicology, and an old foe of Coffin, was brought forward to pronounce that lobelia was a powerful poison and ought not to be administered except with great caution and in very small doses; he had no hesitation in attributing the child's death to lobelia.

The Coroner – on this occasion, sympathetic to the Coffinites – announced that he had had a child himself with the same disease, who had died despite the best professional care; a juror added that he had lost three children who were under the care of the medical faculty, while another "wished they could hold inquests on the bodies of those who had died whilst under the care of medical men". Other jurors declared one after another that they had taken far greater quantities of lobelia, with no ill-effects whatsoever; and the foreman of the jury stated that Mrs. Mansfield was a very respectable woman who had cured a great number of people. A verdict of death from natural causes was returned, and Professor Letheby retired discomfited.[13]

There was nothing new in this resentment by the poorer classes of a medical establishment whose fees put trained professional care far out of their reach, leaving them to the care of a few conscientious but overworked medical officers, or else to those quacks whom the *Lancet* had denounced in ringing terms as responsible for the slaying of "thousands and tens of thousands among the poor and ignorant".[14] To whom else should they turn? And their resentment was skilfully exploited by Coffin, who used any weapon that came to hand in his bold onslaught on what he saw as a vicious and uncaring monopoly.

But it was not only resentment that Coffin appealed to when he addressed his working-class faithful: he appealed to their dignity, to their generosity, to their intelligence, to noble instincts that were too often ignored. He set out not merely to convert them, but to educate them. And when it spoke on matters of health and hygiene, his *Journal* was far ahead of its time.

Among contemporary abuses strongly criticized by Coffin, both in his lectures and in the *Journal*, were the adulteration of food with noxious chemicals; the social evils arising from the employment for long hours in the cotton mills of women with babies and small children; the low standards of industrial safety; the industrial diseases produced by jobs like knife-grinding and lint-making ("a threat to the lungs"); and the folly of tight lacing (at one of his lectures, Coffin produced a female skeleton with its ribs squeezed together by years of this fashionable absurdity).

The *Journal* also campaigned vigorously for improvements in general sanitation, and particularly in the cleaning and water supply of industrial cities; it applauded the action of the enterprising Dr. Snow who, merely by removing the handle of the Broad Street pump and thus cutting off contaminated water supply, was able not only to halt a local cholera outbreak but to demonstrate its origin. The *Journal* campaigned vigorously *against* vaccination – which seems reactionary until it is recalled that this was at the time a particularly hazardous procedure with many casualties, performed by transferring infected matter straight from the open sore of a smallpox victim into the arm of a healthy child.

But it is in his views on the care and health of children that Coffin – in common with all nineteenth-century medical botanists, whatever their label – found himself most dramatically at odds with received medical opinion, and criticized them most forcefully. He deplored the habit of forcing castor oil and calomel down the throats of new-born babies, or of purging children at all; while the profession ritually lanced baby gums to "ease" teething, Coffin maintained that it was a natural process and required no meddling; while the profession prescribed calomel for worms, Coffin advocated a moderate diet and no sweets; while the Regulars treated costiveness with endless purging, Coffin suggested rye bread; while the profession prescribed corseting and drugging for rickets, Coffin warmly recommended fresh country air, and plenty of it. He insisted that all children should be encouraged to take regular exercise, run about and shout, and he thought it absolute folly for infants to be fed on anything but breast-milk.[15]

Unlike England's legislators and many members of the Royal College of Physicians, the Coffinites had constant first-hand experience of the slums of the big manufacturing cities, from which they drew most of their patients. And the scandal to which they drew their readers' attention, over and over again, was the appalling rate of child mortality in Britain. It was bad enough in London, where only sixty per cent of children survived to their fifth birthday. In Manchester, this figure dropped to under fifty per cent; and in "cotton" towns like Ashton-under-Lyne, the survival rate was as low as forty-three per cent.[16] The cause of these depressing figures was plain: desperate poverty, and working mothers, who relied on child-minders during their long hours at the cotton mills. "The practice of mothers labouring in the mills" it was reported, "is all but universal"; pregnant women worked up to the last moment, and went back as soon as possible after their babies were born. Occasionally three or four women clubbed together for a wet-nurse – an observer saw one of these so exhausted "as to be unable to walk across the room" – so that thousands of babies died of malnutrition. More often, the babysitter was a young girl, or else old women who were paid around 2 shillings weekly for the half-dozen or so children they regularly minded.[17]

Mothers and child-minders alike relied on one comforter for the restless, fractious babies: Godfrey's Cordial, containing laudanum in a base of water, aniseed and treacle. "Godfrey" was a familiar household word in Manchester; druggists, grocers, even pubs sold it as "children's draughts, a penny each"; bottles of "Mother's Quietness", "Infant's Preservative", or "Soothing Syrups" – the names as anodyne as their contents – sometimes contained even stronger doses, and half-emptied bottles were often brought back to have a little more laudanum added.[18] The *Journal* drew its readers' attention to the lethal effects of this constant doping, quoting cases of babies so susceptible to opium that they died of narcotic poisoning after doses containing no more than two drops of laudanum. Many small children became helpless addicts, stupefied and slowly wasting away: there was a general tendency to ascribe these deaths to "natural causes".[19]

The medical botanists as a matter of principle never used or supplied narcotic vegetable poisons although, as they pointed out bitterly, such potentially lethal substances as laudanum and prussic accid were on cheap open sale, while regular doctors used a whole arsenal of poisons, vegetable killers such as hemlock, belladonna – deadly nightshade – as well as minerals like arsenic, antimony and mercury.[20]

There was indeed a certain black humour in a situation where the Coffinites were watched like hawks for a single death that might be laid at their door, while, as the *Journal* pointed out, a doctor might "bleed, and blister, and administer poison in twenty different forms, and he may lose his patient at the last, and yet no coroner's inquest will be held in *his* case; no inquiry will be made: the victim of diplomatized ignorance may be laid in a premature grave, but the parchment license will secure entire immunity. . . ."[21]

The injustice of such a state of affairs was never felt more keenly by the Coffinites than at the time of the Cholera Report in 1853. After the second major Asiatic cholera epidemic in 1848–49, which killed more than 55,000, a committee was set up by the Royal College of Physicians, under Dr. William Gull of Guy's Hospital, to report on the various methods of treatment adopted in this and the earlier epidemic, and their success – if any. Their report finally appeared in the wake of another almost equally disastrous epidemic, and two years later it was published as a White Paper.

It was a dismal record of failure, from which the physicians who drafted it had been able to extract only one crumb of comfort – it served to show which therapies had *not* been successful, for future reference. But while all the regular therapies of calomel, bleeding, opium or alcoholic stimulation had proved a good deal worse than useless, and the report admitted as much, it was completely silent on the two therapies which *had* been strikingly successful – those of the medical botanists, and the homoeopathic treatment with minute doses of camphor. [22]

The first pandemic of the deadly Asiatic cholera reached Europe, and then the United States, from the Far East in 1829. Caused by the microscopic comma-shaped *vibrio choleræ*, which is transmitted in contaminated food or drinking-water, the disease struck with frightful speed: the victim might be perfectly fit one evening and dead before breakfast the next day. The first symptoms were agonizing cramps in the stomach, a deathly chill, and an incessant purging diarrhœa so violent that eventually only "rice-water" – water with dissolved salts and flakes of mucous membrane in it – was being voided. The cholera victim dies from dehydration, from loss of alkali, or from loss of potassium – usually from all three combined.

The Botanic doctors – like many of the Regulars – were ignorant of these scientific explanations, but their methods cured most cholera cases, as the Regular's calomel, brandy and opium never could. Dr. Coffin and his followers wrapped the patient up warmly with a hot brick at his feet; plied him with hot herbal drinks and rectal injections of oak bark, tormentil, cayenne, bayberry, raspberry leaves, ginger, myrrh; if these produced no improvement, they gave lobelia emetics; and when the crisis was over, prescribed for their prostrated patient strengthening drinks of arrowroot or slippery elm. [23]

Dehydration was countered by the repeated drinks ("a wineglassful every half hour") and injections; potassium and alkaline losses were made up by the herbs specified, rich in both; most of the herbs were also highly astringent; and ginger and capsicum would equalize the circulation and prevent a fatal collapse. [24]

It might be imagined that any conscientious Regular doctor at this time, faced as he sometimes must have been with the contrast between his own high failure rate and the impressive success of the Botanics, might have been only too happy to learn how the Irregular did it, and follow suit. Medical history suggests, unfortunately, that Regular doctors are seldom willing to learn such lessons. On the contrary: if a successful new remedy or treatment in a particularly dreadful disease is offered by an outsider – an "irregular" – his claims will be ignored by most of the profession and, if possible, concealed from the general public with indignant cries of "flagrant quackery". If he persists, he will be actively persecuted, the Inquisition at its most zealous having nothing to teach any medical establishment faced with "heresy", and patients' interests counting for nothing in the balance with professional *amour propre*. It has happened over and again in this century with unorthodox treatments for cancer, and it happened in Victorian England during two epidemics of cholera. One instance should be cited.

In October 1853 the *Association of Medicine Journal* ran a long story under the heading "Coroners' Inquest: Improper Treatment of Cholera by an Agent of Coffin, the Herbalist." Readers learned that one George Burt, of 13 Dunk Street in Whitechapel, had died of an attack of cholera after treatment by a greengrocer named John Stephens, an agent of Coffin. Burt had been drinking hard for a fortnight, and was seized in the evening with severe pains in the stomach. Mary-Anne Stephenson, who lived with him, got him two-pennyworth of ginger brandy, "after which he went to sleep for a short time. He continued in severe pain till two o'clock in the morning, and during that time his bowels were repeatedly open. She then went for Stephens, who attended. He gave deceased some powders, which he said he was to take every quarter of an hour, he also prescribed a mixture. He left and called again between ten and eleven o'clock on Saturday morning. When he came, he looked at the deceased. He remarked that he could do no more for him, and went away. As he was going down the stairs, she observed deceased to be dying. She called to Stephens, who returned. When he saw that the deceased was dead, he took the mixture away."

Called in evidence, according to the report, the indefatigable Dr. Letheby testified that the lobelia had certainly hastened his death: it had already been responsible for twenty-two deaths in Britain. The Coroner remarked severely that "some steps ought to be taken to prevent ignorant persons practising in the medical profession"; and although the verdict was one of natural death, it was added that this may have been accelerated by "improper medicine".[25]

The story was picked up by the respectable *Morning Advertiser*, and distributed widely to English breakfast tables. "So much for the intelligence of the poor classes" was its comment. "Coffin and his agents drive a flourishing trade. . . What state of law can that be which suffers so bare-faced and false a pretension to go unpunished?"[26]

John Stephens was one of the ablest and most intelligent of Coffin's followers, and he wrote an indignant reply. Far from Coffin driving a "flourishing trade", he pointed out, Stephens had actually distributed, before cholera even arrived in Dunk Street, 339 packets of cholera powder free to the local poor, supplied by a benefit society specially set up by Coffin. The facts of the case itself, he reported, were as follows:

"On Saturday morning, just after the clock struck six (and not at two as reported), I was called to visit a patient who, I was informed . . . had been suffering all night from a severe attack of cholera, attended with violent cramps. When I arrived at half-past six, I was greeted by his wife with the exclamation, 'Oh Sir, I am afraid it is too late to do any good; oh my poor "Bill" '. I found him violently cramped, cold, clammy, death-like, tongue thickly coated, dark yellow. Four persons were in attendance; they had given him ginger brandy in the night. I did my utmost to save him, but without any hope of success. He died before eleven the same morning, and I received the thanks of all present for my services. The medical officer and the registrar, I believe, instigated the inquest. During the week I attended twenty cases of actual cholera, several of which were very malignant; and so great was my success that for four days from Thursday, the 27th, to Monday the 31st, the medical officer of the district had not a patient in or near Dunk Street. At least one hundred persons were cured of diarrhœa by the powders I distributed."[27]

Neither the medical *Journal* not the *Morning Advertiser* included in the account of the inquest an exchange between the surgeon, M' Champneys, who had performed the autopsy, and a gentleman in court. In reply to a question, M'Champneys admitted that *he had lost eight or nine cases: and that Mr. Stephens . . . had lost only two or three.* He was then asked whether it was true that the people residing in Dunk Street refused to take his medicines and took Botanic remedies in preference. His reply was in the affirmative.[28]

But Coffinism laid itself wide open to unfair discrimination of this kind. Although Coffin often urged his agents to keep proper notes of case histories and send them to the *Journal*, few bothered to do so, and there was no Coffin Hospital which could produce figures, statistics, and detailed observations of Botanic treatment. The movement had produced no literature – Coffin's agents still pored over his *Botanic*

Guide to Health as if it were the last word in medical discovery. Thus although by the 1850s there were hundreds of enthusiastic practitioners of Botanic Medicine in England who owed no allegiance to the American, and were indeed strongly critical of his methods, he always behaved and spoke as if there were no truth outside Coffinism.

The sad fact was admitted, even by some of his most loyal followers: a quarter of a century after he had triumphantly launched the cause of Botanic Medicine in England, Coffin was now one of the greatest obstacles to its progress.

19

Dr. Coffin
versus Dr. Skelton

"Our unparalleled success has brought into the field a host of adventurers, each of whom has presumed or pretended to give *something new*", wrote Coffin irritably in the *Journal* of 27 March 1852. "Books or 'Guides to Health' have been published, and each has hoped, by some vast improvement, to arrive at the same height of fame that we have done, forgetting that, if our system was true . . . any deviation from it must be error".[1]

Thus Coffin the infallible in full cry, in unmistakable echo of the embittered patriarch Thomson; and the parallels were tragically close. Like Thomson, Coffin quarrelled with and alienated some of his ablest lieutenants; he clung tenaciously to his earliest ideas, and was jealously unwilling to admit that any improvement or development might be possible; he lived to see others assume his pre-eminence; and, finally, he was to die lonely and neglected by the great movement he had originated.

Among the cleverest and most dedicated of Coffin's early recruits had been John Stevens and Richard Johnson. Stevens joined him in the early months in London, and then accompanied him to Leeds, where he worked tirelessly in the great cause. But a few years later, the two men parted company, Stevens moving to Bath and the West Country – Whitlaw territory – where he set up his own import business in American herbs, and drove himself to an early death by his exertions. Richard Johnson worked as Coffin's printer for three years in Manchester but disagreeing with the great man, moved to Glasgow and started his own business there: he was soon joined by another Manchester "defector", Luke Seddon.[2]

Coffin could ill afford to lose men like these: Stevens in particular was a young man of remarkable talents, much admired by his colleagues, who published several books before his early death, including the *Reformed Practice of Medicine*. But Coffin appears to have resented such talent as a threat to his own position, and this narrow-minded jealousy soon brought about exactly what he most feared: the rise of a rival candidate for the leadership of British Botanic Medicine, in the person of John Skelton.

Neither jealousy nor petty-mindedness entered into the make-up of John Skelton, a practising herbalist from the West Country. Born in 1806 in the small village of Holberton in Devon, Skelton was the son of well-to-do parents – his grandfather was gardener to the wealthy Bultell family at nearby Fleet – and, like Thomson, Skelton had learned plant medicine at the side of an old village doctoress and midwife – in this case, his grandmother. Hand in hand with his grandfather, the small boy went hunting in the fields, meadows and woods for the herbs his grandmother needed: "I was almost instinctively trained to know their various medicinal properties", he wrote later. "Even now, though forty years and more have passed since I first commenced this delightful labour, still I should know in what spots to find the very same herbs which I gathered in those early days".[3]

When Skelton was ten, his parents moved to Plymouth, perhaps so that their obviously gifted and exceptional son could be given a better education than the village school offered: his later writings suggest a classical education as well as access to a good library. In his teens only one occupation interested him – that of medical herbalism – and by the late 1830s, he was one of a dwindling number of practising herbalists, probably running his own small shop and working to support a wife and family.

Skelton knew of Whitlaw, and may even have worked with him; with his interests, he must have heard of Thomson. When he learned that an American Botanic practitioner had arrived in London to set up a completely modern system of plant medicine based on Thomson's teachings, he went to hear what it was all about. He was not much impressed by Coffin at first, but the American's boundless energy and optimism were infectious, and for all his failings Coffin never lacked a certain charisma: the younger man succumbed to his spell, even bringing his wife as a patient, and the two men became friends and allies in the great cause, although Skelton – who by this time had a considerable reputation and a flourishing practice of his own – preferred to remain independent.[4]

Coffin's stamina was always astonishing. After a full day in the consulting room, he must have spent endless hours at his desk dealing with business matters, working on his books, writing for the *Journal*, he would prepare for yet another of the exhausting lecture tours with which he spread the gospel, gathered recruits and cheered the faithful. But even his seemingly inexhaustible energies finally succumbed – he was already in his mid-fifties at this time – and in the winter of 1847–48 he returned to London badly in need of a long rest, and searching for a replacement who could carry on in his absence. Skelton was his choice.[5]

Skelton had followed the dazzling progress of medical botany in the North with rising excitement, and whatever reservations he may have had about Coffin's methods, he was as anxious as the American that the great work should not be suspended. After some discussion, he agreed to take over for a term of two years, and moved to Manchester for a close study of the Coffin system. For the next two years, he travelled around the big industrial centres of the North and the Midlands, among them Sheffield, Rotherham, Blackburn, Bacup, Oldham, Wakefield, Stockport, Leeds, Birmingham, Manchester and Leicester.[6]

He was brilliantly successful, and tributes to his leadership and professional skill poured in. At the end of a three-month stay in Bradford, he was presented with a handsome gold watch, and a public eulogy in which Coffin was not even mentioned. In his reply, Skelton loyally rectified this omission, saying of Coffin: ". . . it is to his great moral courage and determined perseverance that we are indebted for our success . . . may our great founder's name be venerated by us all; and our children be taught to lisp it when their grandsires and sires shall sleep in the silent dust".[7]

But Skelton was becoming aware that behind its jovial and triumphing facade, all was not sweetness and light in the Coffin movement. In Manchester, both Stevens and Johnson probably discussed with him their resentment of Coffin's high-handed ways and his rigid anti-intellectual stance. They had pulled out by the time that Skelton, his two-year agreement at an end, left Manchester and moved to Edinburgh to establish an independent business in 1850. There he soon had first-hand experience of Coffin's small-minded jealousy.

The great man had returned to England late in 1849 much restored by his travels. He found the movement flourishing, but three of his key men had deserted, and Skelton was the name on everybody's lips.

Coffin was not pleased, and he was less pleased to learn that Skelton had now struck out on his own, a formidable rival. Hurrying North, he summoned Skelton back from Edinburgh, and requested that he go to work for him in Wales. Still hoping that they could work together in harmony, Skelton agreed and went – only to realize that Coffin had simply wanted him out of the limelight: when after six weeks his funds ran out – he was not a rich man – an appeal to the Doctor produced only silence.[8]

Hurt, surprised and disappointed, Skelton returned to the North of England, to a delighted welcome from his many friends. After a twelve-month stay in Blackburn, he returned to Leeds in the summer of 1851, taking up residence at 11 East Parade. By the spring of 1852 he had established a successful herbal import business, had almost as many agents as Coffin, and in a monthly magazine, *Dr. Skelton's Botanic Record and Family Herbal* (it was also a cumulative part-work herbal designed to be collected and bound together), was eloquently expounding his own, far more constructive ideas on the work that needed to be done to secure the future of medical botany.

These were dark days for Coffin, made no brighter by the arrival in London of a much more brutal critic than Skelton – Dr. Wooster Beach, preaching Medical Reform and Eclecticism. Beach had visited London earlier, in the course of his grand tour of inspection of European medicine. Now he was back for a long stay, to promote Eclectic medicine and his own massive works simultaneously in Britain; and several English Medical Botanists were already adding M.D. after their names, secure in the possession of a piece of parchment issued by his Reformed Medical College.

Flush with gold medals from a score of European princelings, and elated by the warm welcome he had received in orthodox medical establishments in London, Beach had confidently looked forward to a dazzling triumph when he returned in person to England to preach the new mild medicine. Much to his indignation, he found that medical botany had now become irrevocably associated, in the mind of the Royal College as much as that of the great British public, with the odious name of Coffin. Beach had devoted considerable energy to lambasting the illiterate Thomsonians in America: here, it seemed, it was all to do again. With a series of blistering pamphlets, he waded in. It was ridiculous for Coffin to claim, Beach pontificated, that he had introduced medical botany to the country of Culpeper and Gerard; every old countrywoman practised it, and Coffin was doing more harm that good by resurrecting that Thomsonianism which had been so thoroughly exposed in America.

In 1852 Beach launched a monthly journal, the *Medical Reformer*, in which he returned to the attack, and these withering comments were repeated later in his *British and American Reformed Practice of Medicine*, published a few years later. "Everything done by Coffin and his illiterate agents has tended to deceive the public, and bring the cause of medical reform into disrepute among the intelligent portion of the community. In consequence of the quackery practised by this man, it has been found more difficult to introduce the Reformed Practice than if he had never appeared."[9]

With much of this, no doubt, Skelton warmly agreed, and when he called on Beach on his arrival in 1851, he had been agreeably impressed by the man: ". . . most affable and kind . . . a generosity and humility that stamped him to our mind as a man of great natural goodness".[10] Skelton had been deeply impressed, too, by Beach's accounts of the high standing that Eclecticism had achieved in America, the number of distinguished converts it had made in the ranks of the regular medical profession, its confident numbers of Medical Colleges and Hospitals, and its stated objective of progress through scientific research. If medical botany was to succeed in Britain, rather than merely to survive as a minority sect, this surely was the path, and these were the goals to aim at.

From this time on, Skelton and his followers began to call themselves Eclectics, and to look across the Atlantic for leadership, for inspiration, and for the practical benefits of fellowship with a recognized and successful group of practitioners.[11]

But Beach's vicious attack on Coffin struck Skelton as both small-minded and unfair. Medical Botany in England had enemies enough as it was, and although Skelton himself was engaged in a gentle public row with Coffin at the time, he found the transatlantic polemical style intensely distasteful, and said so: ". . . they snarl at each other, call names, attack motives, destroy each other's influence, forgetful that in so doing they are only . . . retarding the progress of the cause. It is not too late now for this to be done, if the spirit could be created; but we have little hope in either of the men. . . ."[12]

Annoyed, Beach turned on Skelton. In a review of his just-published *Family Medical Adviser*, Beach condemned it as mere potted Thomsonianism, "which has been entirely rejected by all the enlightened Botanic physicians in America". What a pity it was, he added acidly, that a man of Skelton's talent *"should be so misled* and deceived by ignorant and inexperienced leaders. . . ".[13]

Coffin, meanwhile, seemed bent on displaying just those limitations of which Beach had accused him. The Bradford Botanic Society had invited him to address a meeting on Easter Monday 1852, and Coffin was at first delighted to accept – till he saw a handbill on which, to his jealous fury, the name of Dr. Skelton figured almost as prominently as his own. Since it was Skelton who had brought Coffinism to Bradford, and he was enormously popular there, this was hardly surprising, but Coffin wrote crossly declining to have anything to do with "new-fangled ideas" – a dig at Skelton's new-found Eclecticism. The Society replied with a copy of their rules to prove that they were still true-blue Coffinites, and loyal students of the approved *Guide*, but to no avail.

As the day fixed for their meeting approached, the peaceful Medical Botanists of Bradford were amazed to find the street plastered with posters blazing out Coffin's refusal to be involved with those who practised contrary to his own system. The Society hit back with an angry poster of its own, and Coffin, after brooding for a while, made a very foolish mistake. In an effort to shore up his crumbling authority, and rally the faithful round him, he announced an entirely new organisation, to be known as Drs. Coffin and Harle's Accredited Agents' Medico-Botanic Society. He circulated its rules – a copy of which was at once brought to Skelton – and announced that the first meeting on 19 August, would be held in Bradford.

A glance through the Rules confirmed Skelton's belief that in Coffin's hands, Medical Botany had sunk to the level of an attempted trading monopoly. The preamble was a lengthy attack on those who introduced "deleterious or adulterated articles . . . pernicious compounds . . . into the practice [simply for gain]". Rule 1 limited members to the use of "only those remedies . . . procured from the establishments of Drs. Coffin and Harle"; and Rule 4 – which provoked angry laughter in Skelton – said that no agent was to attend a person "whose system is so far reduced or exhausted by disease as to prevent the possibility of recovery". (This was presumably intended to discourage some of the more incompetent Coffin practitioners from tackling cases beyond their ability, and inviting yet another Coroner's inquest.)

Skelton was normally both tolerant and courteous. On this occasion he was too angry to be either. Publishing the rules, accompanied by his sardonic comments in the *Record*, he added his own set of "rules" for those who wished to succeed in the Coffin organization:

1st.   Purchase all your goods of Drs. Coffin and Harle.

2nd.   Read no books on Medical Botany but Dr. Coffin's *Guide to Health, Treatise on Midwifery, Lectures,* and *widely-circulated Journal.*

3rd.   Abuse Drs. Beach, Skelton, Stevens and Noble*; call Richard Johnson a vagabond and Skelton a knave, and be sure to give Dr. Coffin the credit of introducing the Lobelia Inflata and Medico-Botanic system into England. Do this, and your passport to the "accredited" is safe.

Skelton went on to hint that the Coffin hierarchy was a Jewish clique, and that Coffin had surrounded himself with insignificant men, while alienating those of real talent. He summed up, with regret, "Drs. Coffin and Harle, and their agents, have narrowed instead of widened the sphere of their own usefulness, not only to the injury of the cause, but doubly so to themselves . . . I know that in thus speaking I shall not be regarded over-favourably; time, however, will determine who is in the right."[14]

With regal disregard for these criticisms, Coffin went ahead with his plans.

August 17 and 18 were evenings that lived long in the memories of Bradford Medical Botanists. Dr. Coffin, on the other hand, no doubt did his utmost to forget them. On the seventeenth, his "Accredited Agents" assembled to hear him lecture, with their new President, Mr. William Brown, in the chair. But the Mechanics' Hall was packed with Skeltonites spoiling for a fight, and the meeting was hardly opened when one of them leapt up and proposed that Dr. Skelton should take the chair. Instantly confusion broke out, and the meeting was only calmed when Skelton himself climbed onto the platform to point out that since the audience had paid their twopences and fourpences for admission, they had a right to their opinion. The chair was reluctantly given to him, and during a lull in the continuing uproar, Skelton challenged Coffin to a meeting the following night to discuss his conduct. Coffin was compelled to agree, and next day the town was once more plastered with posters, this time announcing "Dr. Coffin, versus Dr. Skelton and the Medico–Botanic Society of Bradford".

---

*Luke Noble, of Brighouse, was another "defector", and a warm supporter of Skelton.

Half Bradford crowded into the Mechanics' Hall that evening to see the notorious Dr. Coffin trounced by one of his own fellows – and their expectations were fully realized. Dr. Coffin may have hoped to win this audience as he had won so many tough, sceptical North Country workingmen in his time. He began with a touching appeal to their good nature. "There is no doubt but that I may have done wrong", he admitted with manly candour; "if I have you must condemn me, that is all, and I cannot help it; there is no doubt also but that I am a little foolish in some things, as well as other men, for I have been so long petted and caressed by the public, that I dare say I may think a little too much of myself. . . ." Had he not devoted his life to the good of the working man? How could it be said of him that he had attempted to crush them? Why, here was a sovereign given him by a lady towards an infirmary in this town, so that the poor might have their medicines at a cheaper rate, etc.

This was simply not good enough: Skelton sternly recalled him to the point at issue, and for the next hour the audience watched half in pity, half in contempt, while Coffin floundered, hesitated, fumed, ranted and rambled. "We could have freely wept over his failings", was Skelton's comment. Finally, "the doctor's years, grey hairs, venerable appearance and mortification produced what nothing else could have done, viz. a smooth exit from the scene of contention".[15]

The Bradford debâcle was a fatal blow to Coffin's position: after August 1852 it was to Skelton that the best men in the movement looked for moral leadership, and they could have chosen no finer man.

The most outstanding personality to emerge from the Medico-Botanic scene in England or the United States, Skelton brought to the cause a keen grasp of the wider issues at stake, as well as strong religious convictions, and an innate nobility of mind that raised him above petty in-fighting or personal vanity. Time and again over the next two decades, when the movement was in danger of fragmentation, Skelton pulled it together by the sheer force of his persuasive and moderating personality. He reminded its members not only that there could be unity in diversity, as long as basic principles were adhered to, but that diversity itself was a necessary consequence of that freedom they were demanding for themselves: "Union of action must arise . . . from freedom of the will; men must deal with whom they will; read what books they will; and bring experience and mind in fair competition with others if they would gather strength and promote the progress of the cause. If we set up a monopoly we cannot progress."[16]

This monopoly was in itself a major obstacle to all progress in medicine, of whatever system: "What right have we to assume that all knowledge is ours, or that what we think or teach is perfect? Whoever assumes such gives evidence of his unfitness; every day that comes brings with it something for us to learn, and the wise man will often blush at his own ignorance."[17]

The narrow intolerance that had medical herbalists squabbling among themselves as with hydropaths, homoeopaths and allopaths alike was deeply alien to Skelton, who struggled to make them understand that a party locked into attitudes of resentful opposition and hostility could never make headway, but merely evoke the same hostile stance in reply. Skelton noted approvingly from Sheffield, during one of his visits, that there was now a homoeopathic Dr. Holland – "a gentleman of most excellent talent" – with a highly successful practice in the city. "This is a good sign in progress," he commented. "Division of opinion is the best guarantee for freedom of action".[18]

Above all, Skelton grasped the vital need for Botanic Medicine to enlarge its intellectual horizons, and keep pace with advances in medicine: "At present the Coffinism of England, like the Thomsonianism of America, is reduced to a very narrow circle, whilst the principles of medical science, based upon the botanic or vegetable practice, are enlarging every way".[19]

In their own chosen territory – that of medicinal plants – almost all the exciting investigative advances were being made by orthodox pharmacists in North America and on the Continent, where the dreams of Paracelsus and the "chymists" were being unlocked with a chemical key – to reveal a microcosm of fascinating chemical complexity. The "chymists" had been right: each healing plant had an "active principle" – a single constituent, or a small clutch of them – which could, in the laboratory, be separated from the rest of the plant matter by chemical techniques, and used in what was assumed to be a purer, more concentrated, and therefore more effective form.

In 1803, a twenty-year-old German apprentice pharmacist, Friedrich Wilhelm Serturner, experimenting with crude opium, extracted white alkaloid crystals that successfully put animals to sleep. He called it morphine, and went on to extract another alkaloid – he called this "the specific narcotic element of opium" – to which he gave the name narcotine.

Morphine and narcotine, it turned out, were only two of the more than forty that have now been identified. Morphine is a powerful pain-killer; codeine is a much milder pain-killer and, like narcotine, a useful cough sedative. Papaverine is an anti-spasmodic and others are still being investigated. It is morphine which is totally addictive if misused.

Using Serturner's technique, other alkaloids – as they were christened in 1818 – were soon isolated from medicinal plants that particularly interested physicians: aconitine from aconite, emetine from ipecacuanha, strychnine from the poison nut, atropine from deadly nightshade, conine from the hemlock, and quinine from Peruvian bark.

Salicin from the willow (*Salix alba*) – used worldwide in folk medicine for the relief of aches, fevers and rheumatic pains – had been isolated earlier in the century, from which in turn salicylic acid was prepared. In a pharmacological breakthrough, these white crystals were produced synthetically in 1852 – and pharmacists all over the Western world began consciously to look forward to the day when the laboratory would replace the physic garden as the source of all the principal materia medica. Both salicin and salicylic acid, it turned out, had an unpleasant tendency to irritate the stomach, and the taste of both had a bitterness that no amount of treacle or sugar could disguise, but physicians who would never have considered using extracts of willow bark now began to use these new test-tube derivatives of the graceful weeping willow, and found them highly effective. By the time acetylsalicylic acid – a much less irritant version of salicylic acid – was produced in 1899 by the German company Bayer, and given the name of aspirin, there was already a steady demand for this popular drug.

Much of this work was done in Paris by two outstanding French pharmacists, Joseph Pelletier and Joseph Caventou. And another Frenchman, François Magendie, not only brilliantly advanced physiology – the study of the way living organisms and their various parts function – but also virtually invented modern pharmacology – the study of the action of drugs in the human body.

Magendie and his colleagues were enthusiastic about the potent new plant medicines emerging from their laboratories, and stimulated by such discoveries, a completely new branch of pharmacy was developing which was devoted to the chemical exploration and elucidation of medicinal plants.

In regular medical practice, one of the great drawbacks to the use of plant drugs has always been the difficulty of producing anything like a standard dose. The old herbalists, it turned out, had been absolutely right when they insisted that a particular plant had to be gathered not only at a certain time of year, but even at a certain time of day or night: modern pharmacognosy has demonstrated striking variations in the potency of a drug plant even within a twenty-four-hour period.

In his prolonged study of the foxglove Withering had shown that by selecting plants with care, and picking them at a particular season, it was possible to achieve a reasonably standardized dose. But Withering belonged to what was already beginning to seem a remote rural age, when doctors as well as apothecaries might be familiar with and even themselves harvest the native drug-plants they used.

The physician and the apothecary who worked in the bursting cities of the mid-nineteenth century could no longer feel as confident of their sources of plant drugs, and when the drug in question was one as powerful – and as potentially lethal – as digitalis, the question of standardization assumed a crucial importance. Synthesis in the laboratory, and the production of a pure substitute for the variable original had been the impossible dream of the "chymists": it now struck the medical profession as the exciting modern answer to this age-old problem. At a time when medical science was making explosive advances on every front, it was an answer that no longer seemed out of the question.

Thus the new science of pharmacognosy – far from ushering in at last the great age of plant medicine – simply tended to confirm the alienation of the nineteenth-century medical mind from drugs that did not come neatly packaged in liquid or powder form, and in perfectly standardized dosage.

Although the discoveries of this new science were crucial to the future of Botanic Medicine, and the Eclectics of America were already taking advantage of them, the Medical Botanists of Britain were hardly in a position even to grasp their significance, let alone make a contribution of their own. This want of intellectual thrust was, in the eyes of Skelton, even more inexcusable in Coffin than it had been in Thomson, since it left them powerless to give their movement scientific credibility, or to justify their opposition to mineral medicine. A great opportunity was slipping from their grasp.

In Skelton's view, Thomson could have established "a great first principle for medical science", if he had sufficient grounding in pharmacy to prove by experiment "that substances contained in the mineral kingdom were also contained in the vegetable and animal kingdoms, and that in order to build up and sustain the animal body, nature had established it as an infallible law that all its nutritive force should be derived from organized life, and that all violations of this law tend to disorganize and destroy the living structure."[20]

Intellectual activity of this kind was far beyond the reach of Dr. Coffin, who was happy to proclaim his ignorance: "So far is it true that pathology is the foundation of medicine", he remarked complacently, "that we are in the daily habit of curing diseases of whose pathology we know nothing at all, probably never will know anything".[21]

Yet it was advances in these very sciences that he affected to despise – pathology and physiology in particular – quite as much as the constant sniping of the Irregulars, that finally brought home to the Regular medical profession the dangerous futility of such therapies as bloodletting and blistering.

And Skelton was driven to a dismal conclusion: "Coffinism has never possessed a power to raise itself above the prejudices and opposition of the ignorant and interested, hence its continuous condition of antagonism. . . . In its own sphere it is well enough, i.e. in breaking down monopoly, and pointing out the errors of the old practice; but in *building up*, reforming, improving medical science, winning medical liberty, and enlarging the sphere of England's medical mind, it is of no use whatever".[22]

Skelton was intensely reluctant to take on Coffin, not merely because he was desperately anxious that the movement should not tear itself apart by internal dissension, but because he was a man who was proud to acknowledge a debt, and England owed a debt to Coffin, just as America owed a debt to Thomson. "Every man in the movement must respect him for his indefatigable exertions", wrote Skelton in all sincerity.[23] To the last he hoped that Coffin might find himself capable of rising to his great mission. But these hopes were defeated by Coffin himself, and nobody mourned his inadequacy more sincerely than the man who supplanted him.

Even after the movement had shaken off its allegiance to Coffin – apart from a few staunch followers – Skelton was reluctant to step into his shoes, and far from at once taking on the formal leadership –as everybody was anxious for him to do – he was at pains to avoid it, contenting himself with giving general guidance from his *Record*, and nudging the movement gently in the right direction. Moreover, he did his best to keep open lines of communication to the Coffinites, and in this he was delighted to find an ally in the intelligent and resourceful John Stephens – "our very excellent fellow-labourer" – the hero of Dunk Street, who, although deeply loyal to Coffin was as anxious as Skelton to build bridges.[24]

The great need for a united front was shown in 1854, when Mr. Brady's Medical Reform Bill was presented to Parliament. The avowed object of this Bill was to stamp out quackery by making it illegal to practise medicine unless you were registered – in other words, the product of a regular medical school – and since it was calculated in 1851 that there were approximately 6,000 unlicensed practitioners in the country – as opposed to only 5,000 regular doctors, apothecaries and surgeons – there was clearly a need for some kind of regulation.[25] But it was equally clear to Skelton, Coffin and their followers, that in their own case the move arose from the vindictive jealousy of the medical establishment – so often demonstrated by malicious and needless coroners' inquests and court cases, as well as by the running abuse in the official medical journals.

Apart from the Coffinites there already existed at this time two Botanic organizations: the Friendly Medico-Botanic Sick and Burial Society, founded in 1853 as an early form of medical insurance scheme for working-class members, to which most North of England supporters of Botanic Medicine belonged; and the National Medical Reform League, largely London-based, founded in November 1853 with the object of demonstrating to the nation at large that "the treatment of disease by means of simple herbs, roots and barks, though applied in a crude state, by parties making no pretensions to professional skill, has proved far more safe and effective than the mineral and depletive practice."[26] Two ex-Coffinites, Richard Johnson and Luke Noble, were on the executive of the National Medical Reform League, and both groups would have liked to have Skelton play a leading role in their affairs, but he resisted offers from both, contenting himself with simple membership of the Sick and Burial Society. It was this organization – no doubt at his goading – that in March 1854 orchestrated a deluge of petitions to Parliament from all over the country, protesting against the attempted monopoly of medicine. Many M.P.s were sympathetic to the cause, more were no doubt influenced by this astonishing display of popular support, and Lord Palmerston himself had no particular sympathy for Establishment arrogance: the Bill was defeated.

But schemes for a new bill were immediately set in motion, and the fight was clearly far from over. The Cholera Report, published as a White Paper the following year, and written as though neither Botanic Medicine nor homoeopathy existed, was a further blow. The homoeopaths had friends in high places, and a hospital which could produce detailed clinical records: Lord Duncombe rose angrily in the House of Lords to know why its vastly more successful records had not been included in the returns. But no such appeal was made for the equally effective Medical Botanists, and it was poor consolation at this moment to know that their name was blessed and their system honoured by all Dunk Street, and thousands more nameless survivors of this dreadful disease.

Such events brought home even to Coffin the desirability of raising the status and educational level of the movement. In 1855 he began to speak of a School and a Faculty, by 1858 he was talking of "an hospital and a medical board of scientific men",[27] and in 1860 his *Journal* carried its first detailed chemical analysis of a herbal remedy – wintergreen (*Gaultheria procumbens*), the little shrubby American plant, of which the oil soothes rheumatic pains so powerfully.[28]

For all Coffin's jaunty and optimistic talk, the future was not in his hands and he knew it. His faithful failed to respond to his calls for money to build the great Coffin hospital. It was all happening elsewhere, and when in 1864, the British Medical Reform Association was founded, with steady Mr. Ford of Derby at its first President, the name of Coffin appeared nowhere on its list of executives or members.

In his heyday, Dr. Coffin had cut a splendid figure in London.[29] He enjoyed being famous, he enjoyed his crowded, hectic, useful life, he loved to entertain in his big impressive house. And the wit, the flashes of eloquence and the gusto of the irrepressible Dr. Coffin brought him a wide circle of friends. Years later, a practising herbalist recalled a glimpse of this Victorian celebrity: ". . . a fine-looking old gentleman, well dressed, a long heavy fur-lined coat, open at the chest, displaying a large kind of brooch in plenty of shirt front, a big well-lighted cigar in his mouth, and a bundle of letters carried in one hand well in front of him made him a conspicuous figure as he walked slowly along."[30]

But as fame, wealth and importance fell away from him, his life must have been increasingly lonely. There were no children to cement what does not seem to have been a particularly happy marriage. And by the time the British Medical Reform Association had made it clear to him that he was no longer wanted, he was an old man, who may have known that he was under sentence of death from the stomach cancer that finally carried him off two years later, in August 1866.[31]

Outside the circles of Medical Botany, he was already a forgotten man. Inside the movement, few people still had a good word to say about him. It was left to Skelton to publish his most generous epitaph. In the October issue of Skelton's *Eclectic Journal* there appeared a black-bordered announcement: "It is incumbent upon us to notice the death of one whose name will ever be remembered wheresoever Medical Botany is known. . . . Dr. Coffin . . . his exertions in the early part of his career were very great, and many have derived much benefit through his instrumentality; and although he might have had some failings, it is the duty of everyone to draw the veil of charity over them, and remember him for the good he had done. May he rest in peace."[32]

20

Fruitless Medication

On 7 May 1847, some 250 American doctors filed into the long galleried hall of the Academy of Natural Sciences in Philadelphia, and sat down to consider four proposals. They had been summoned from twenty-four different states at the urgent suggestion of a New York physician, Dr. Nathan Smith Davis (1817–1904), and they represented some forty medical societies and twenty-eight colleges. Before the end of the day – their gaze occasionally flickering up to the skeleton of the gigantic curly-tusked mastodon towering over the Chair – they had voted the American Medical Association into being. They then moved on to consider the second and third proposals: the desirability of high and uniform standards for all medical schools, and the need for stiffer entrance requirements.[1]

The Regular medical profession – now represented in this infant Association – had every reason for concern. Under pressure from the Thomsonians, most States in the 1830s had repealed legislation that restricted medical practice to those officially licensed. This freedom had spawned a host of dubious medical colleges. Between 1830 and 1845 their number had doubled, many of them low-grade commercial concerns, furiously competing for students by attractively short curricula, easy entrance requirements, and degrees handed out almost automatically at the end of the first – and only – term. The result was a glut of graduates, all perfectly entitled to write M.D. after their names, many of whom knew next to nothing about medicine. The glut was worrying at a time when even the best doctors were finding it hard to make a decent living – in the United States there were five times as many doctors proportionately to the population as in France. Equally disturbing was the fact that many of these brand-new doctors were Irregulars – neo-Thomsonians, Eclectics or whatever – who spent much of their time hurling abuse at the Regular doctor and his methods. The deepest cause for concern to the 250 doctors in Philadelphia that spring day, however, could be summed up in a word that appeared nowhere in the four proposals they were considering: homoeopathy. Only in the last was it even hinted at: the Code of Ethics which they voted to accept included a clause forbidding professional intercourse with physicians "whose practice is based on an exclusive dogma, to the rejection of the accumulated experience of the profession".[2]

In the decade since its arrival in New York in 1828 with the Danish Hans Burch Gram, and in Philadelphia five years later with Constantine Hering, homoeopathy had known a dazzling success. By 1844 the homoeopaths had united to found, in New York, the American Institute of Homoeopathy, and in Philadelphia itself the Hahnemann Medical College was turning out numbers of graduates educated to the very highest standards. Unlike most of the Irregulars, who drew their support mainly from the labouring classes, homoeopathy, with its elegant, educated physicians – many of them converts from the ranks of the Regulars – appealed to the highest in the land, "the refined, the learned and the wealthy".

The homoeopaths offered their patients not merely the charm of a novel medical theory, but almost the only painless therapy available. The Regulars at this time were still addicted to bleeding, blistering and drastic purging, the Thomsonians and neo-Thomsonians insisted on their notorious courses, their emetics, and their endless fiery draughts of filthy-tasting medicine. Even the Eclectics, who were fierce about the perils of mineral medicine, often turned out to be every bit as merciless as the Regulars. Althought their blisters and purges were made from vegetable ingredients, they "corded" their patients' limbs until they fainted instead of bleeding them, and when they salivated, it was with extract of blue flag, rather than calomel.[3]

The homoeopaths could not even be accused of poor training, since their Institute made it a condition of membership that the candidate should have passed through a full course of Regular medical study first. Thus whatever success the American Medical Association might have in raising the standards of education would simply result in better-trained homoeopaths, *pari passu*. By the time the 250 doctors had assembled in Philadelphia – the choice of this homoeopathic heartland as venue was in itself a declaration of intent – the followers of Gram and Hering were already sweeping all before them, and even talked of converting the entire medical profession to their views.

The most striking success of homoeopathy – and the best publicized – had been its treatment of Asiatic cholera, epidemics of which had devastated the States in 1831 and 1832 successively. Hahnemann in Europe had had carefully-detailed first-hand accounts of the cholera sent him by his followers in Russia before it reached Western Europe, and on the basis of their observations he had prescribed camphor as the homoeopathic remedy, to be taken in one-drop doses every five minutes in the initial stages of collapse and diarrhœa. This remedy was used with impressive success by homoeopaths both in Europe and America, and although at first the Regulars greeted the idea of camphor as a cholera cure with merry laughter, they soon began surreptitiously using it themselves – although some of them hedged their bets by giving their patients calomel in camphor-water. By 1851, a physician from Cincinnati admitted to the Convention of the American Medical Association that all his colleagues agreed with him – camphor had been one of their most valuable remedies in the cholera epidemics of 1848 and 1849.[4]

A higher cure-rate, and the painless therapy of tiny doses of medicine were not the only reasons for the success of Hahnemann's followers in America. Homoeopaths – then as now – had an attractive habit of listening to everything their patients told them, and making careful notes of even the slightest symptom. When they prescribed, it was from an impressively large repertoire of drugs, mineral as well as vegetable, to which they had already begun to add some of the native medicinal plants: fever root (*Triosteum perfoliatum*), may apple (*Podophyllum peltatum*), bloodroot (*Sanguinaria canadensis*), and the Thomsonian *Lobelia inflata* were among the earliest provings recorded in the first volume of the new Institute.

As nothing else could have done, this adoption by the hated foreign rivals of their own American flora at last galvanized the Regular profession into taking an active and intelligent interest in it themselves. At the very first meeting of the American Medical Association – or A.M.A. as it is known now – Dr. Nathan Davis put forward a resolution that committees should be set up to record the indigenous medical botany of their country.[5] So wholeheartedly was it adopted that in the A.M.A. records only two years later, reports on native medicinal plants took up hundreds of pages. And for the rest of the century, as Harris Coulter has shown in his vivid historic study of

American homoeopathy, there was a steady flow into regular practice of plant drugs which had been first used by the homoeopaths or the Eclectics.

It was not only the Regulars who were conscious of the homoeopaths breathing down their necks: the Thomsonians, too, soon found their patients clamouring for gentler treatment. Before Thomson died in 1841, the movement had already split, and after the loss of his towering and forceful personality, the "true" Thomsonians, the "steamers" and "pukers", dwindled rapidly in number and in influence. It was left to the neo-Thomsonians, led by Alva Curtis, whom Thomson had both disliked and distrusted to carry on the great work, along lines that Thomson himself heartily disapproved.

Not content with success, Curtis aspired to gentility for Thomsonianism, and was determined to see the movement endowed with the respectable trappings of schools, hospitals, dispensaries and a literature, so that it might compete on equal terms with rival systems of medicine. In 1835 he began instructing students in his own home, in 1838 he formally severed his connection with the venerable patriarch, and in 1839 he founded the Literary and Botanical Institute of Ohio. In 1840 a branch was opened in Columbus as the College of Physicians, and in 1841 the whole Institute moved to Cincinnati, where it was soon reorganized under a totally new banner as the Physio-Medical Institute. By this time the very name of Thomson had been quietly hauled down from the masthead, and the engaging colours of Medical Reform run up instead.

But Alva Curtis was not the person to breathe life and heart into a struggling group of dissidents, however sincere his desire to promote the medical creed in which he believed. Quick-witted, arrogant and small-minded, his talents were better suited to gutter-press journalism, and in his hands the *Columbus Thomsonian Recorder* – from the moment that he took it on in 1832 – became exactly that. Year after year the *Recorder* lambasted every rival in sight – ex-fellow Thomsonians, struggling Eclectics, homoeopaths and Regulars were all assailed with fine impartiality. The tone of the movement became shrill, bitter, contentious, and its followers, adopting it, laid themselves wide open to ridicule.

"The Lobelia Practice," disdainfully noted Dr. Dickson Smith of Macon, in 1859, "had nothing to recommend it to the good sense and favor of the people save the noisy clamourings of its self-constituted founder; and . . . so notorious . . . is the habit with Thomsonians, of boasting, and abusing other people, that almost every page of their books and journals are full of it."[6] Dr. Dickson Smith – as he explained in a spirited pamphlet – had referred to the Lobelia Practice in an article contributed to the *Savannah Medical Journal*, but "passingly . . . with no disposition to attack that system, or call in question the truth or absurdity of its doctrine"; and his remarks had been accompanied "with complimentary credit to modern Thomsonians for having abandoned such 'heroic routine' ". These and other remarks – mild by Curtis standards – had provoked columns of abuse in the local press from one M. S. Thomson, M.D., of the Reform Medical College of Macon, Georgia. After the fourth such attack, Dr. Dickson Smith published a contemptuous riposte, in which, after listing the rise and almost immediate decline of several Curtis colleges – he exposed the pretensions of a vast thousand-page tome, the *Reform Medical Practice*, published two years earlier by the Reform Medical College. Hundreds of pages, he showed, had been lifted wholesale from such standard Regular authors as Eberle, Watson, Dunglison and Wood. It was a demolition job, done with thoroughness. "The Lobelia Practice", concluded Dr. Dickson Smith triumphantly, "possessing no inherent, intrinsic worth is waning into insignificance, amid the blazing sun-light of noon-day Science!"[7]

The Eclectics, at this time, were not much better off. As the history of Botanic Medicine shows over and over again, small fervent groups of believers can be torn apart by dissensions which would be painlessly digested by larger, established organizations. In 1859 the Eclectics of America were engaged in a passionate wrangle about the drugs they prescribed.

Since their earliest days, the Eclectics had made a point of developing a materia medica based on indigenous plants, and even regular pharmacists paid tribute to their work. Their journals, such as the *Western Medical Reformer*, published by the Eclectic Medical Institute at Cincinnati, were full of monographs on plants that were being tested and approved by Eclectic practitioners. But like the Thomsonians, they now found to their dismay that the public appetite for herbal remedies in "enormous and too often nauseating doses" was waning.[8]

The earlier Eclectic doctors had made up their own remedies from plants they gathered themselves or ordered from wholesale suppliers like the Shakers, and other specialists in botanic drugs, but by the 1840s most of them relied on ready-prepared drugs from manufacturers like Law and Boyd of New York. As Eclecticism spread, many drug firms sprang up catering specifically to this market. They, too, were well aware of customer-resistance to huge doses, and when in 1835 a young Eclectic physician named John King (1813–1893) accidentally discovered what seemed like the ideal means of obtaining a plant's full range of therapeutic action in handy powdered form, the drug houses were instantly interested.

The discovery gave Dr. King no pleasure to recall. One autumn day he and some colleagues were attempting to prepare a hydro-alcoholic extract from a huge mass of may apple or *podophyllum* root. The process was only half completed when dusk fell, and they decided to leave it till the next morning. When they looked at their cold mixture again by daylight, fragments of dark, rather brittle stuff were found floating in it, and they all speculated idly on what possible medicinal value, if any, these might have. At this moment a seventeen-year-old girl, who happened to be present, announced that she was feeling unwell.

Since podophyllum was particularly prized by the Eclectics as a remedy for biliousness and other liver complaints, the twenty-two-year-old King – probably jokingly – suggested that they try it out on her, gave her a sizeable dose of the dark crumbly stuff, and thought no more about it. An hour later he looked at his "patient" – and was appalled to find her doubled up in agony, vomiting, chilled, with excruciating stomach cramps and a feeble pulse: she was obviously dying.

"To say that I was greatly alarmed would but feebly describe my mental condition", wrote King, years later. He ran to fetch help, found all his medical colleagues out of their offices, and returned desperate but slightly calmer to his patient, having worked out meanwhile a plan of action. By repeated doses of salt water and potash, hot poultices to her wrists and ankles, and a hot fomentation of bitter herbs applied to her stomach, the girl was eventually brought around, sweated profusely, and weakly declared that she felt a little better. A week later, after much anxious nursing, she was almost completely recovered, although she suffered from the after-effects for years.[9]

It was eighteen months before King had the nerve to try his potent resin of podophyllum again – "in much smaller quantity – but this time it gave most excellent results".[10]

The plant alkaloid quinine, derived from cinchona, morphine, and a vigorous resin of jalap were by this time loudly acclaimed by the Regulars. Might not the Eclectics have the honour and glory of launching a class of American "ultimates" to replace their enormous and unappealing doses? Dr. King set to work, and in 1846 he was able to write in quiet triumph to the *Western Medical Reformer*: ". . . our medicines are as capable of being prepared in diminished quantities as any other, and when thus reduced, are much more effectual in their results". As an example he cited the blue flag, whose root contains "resin and mucilage; in the former reside its purgative and alternative properties, in the latter its diuretic. Then why administer the crude root in powder, in which these properties are combined with woody fiber and other inert substances, when a few grains of the proper constituents will answer?"[11]

King was more optimistic than his own experience warranted. In fact the two resins he mentioned, together with that of may apple, *podophyllum*, and of the black Cohosh root, *cimicifugin*, were almost his only successes in this particular line; two other attempts to produce resinous concentrates – with the black root (*Leptandra virginica*), and Goldenseal (*Hydrastis canadensis*) – produced more or less inert substances.

King's initial enthusiasm for what he called "Concentrated Principles" opened the floodgates, however. The Eclectic drug houses leapt into action, and by the early 1850s the market was awash with alkaloids, resinoids, resins and concentrated medicines. Marvellous claims were made for them, although many of them were inert, others worse than useless, and the name of King, the leading Eclectic pharmacologist, was invoked to justify their existence. The neo-Thomsonians – or Physio-Medicals, as they now called themselves – were carried away by the general enthusiasm and followed suit.

Even Regular drug houses now sat up and took notice, and the American Chemical Institute of New York entered the field: for the next decade, every physician throughout the States was deluged with promotional literature. In the language of today's pharmaceutical companies it was a bonanza. But even though King himself publicly denounced these excesses, the damage was done. Too late, he found that the Eclectics were reaping a whirlwind. Furious debate broke out in their ranks, and the resinoid issue undermined their public credibility and threatened to shipwreck the whole movement. By the mid 1850s, student enrolment at the Cincinnati Eclectic Institute was dropping disastrously.

Among those most strongly critical of the "new" medicine was Dr. John Scudder (1829–1894), who had graduated from the Institute in

1856. He later wrote of his conviction that at this time "much of Eclectic Medicine was an unmitigated humbug. It was the day of so-called *concentrated medicines* and anything ending with the suffix "in" was lauded to the skies. It was claimed that these resinoids were the active principles of the plants, and as they would replace the old *drugging* with crude remedies and teas, they must prove a great boon. But they did not give success, and finally, after trying them for a while, the practitioner would go back to the crude articles and old syrups and teas with success."[12] Scudder spoke from his own experience. In desperation he had begun making his own alcoholic tinctures from fresh plant material.

Among those who warmly agreed with his conclusions was Dr. Cleaveland, the Institute's Professor of materia medica; among those most enthusiastic for the new concentrates was Dr. Robert Newton, its Professor of Surgery, who with his personal wealth had underwritten Eclectic fortunes for the past decade. Newton was bitterly opposed to the idea of the modern, forward-looking Eclectics going back to dreary old-fashioned tinctures and compounds: Cleaveland was equally adamant that this must be done, and in 1856 the two sides literally came to blows, and Cleaveland and his followers decamped to set up a rival college.

Wooster Beach, the founding father who had been elected President of the new National Eclectic Medical Association in 1855, might have been able to heal the breach. But he had withdrawn from active involvement in Eclectic affairs: his favourite son – the one he counted on to carry forward the great work of Reform after his death – had been drowned in the East River, and Beach never got over his early death.

The two sides were eventually reconciled, but the Institute's prospects were now grim. As Scudder wrote: ". . . We reached the lowest ebb about 1861 . . . classes had dwindled down until the receipts would hardly pay the expenses. The *Eclectic Medical Journal* had run down from 1,800 to 500 subscribers, and suspended for six months in 1861."[13] It was Scudder himself who finally stepped into the breach, and helped point the way ahead again. A warm and attractive person who was adored by all his students, and a man of passionate integrity, he had been King's shrewd choice for the key role of Professor of materia medica.

It was clear to both Scudder and King that the whole Eclectic materia medica had to be drastically rethought, and when King first proposed his theory of "Specific Medication", Scudder adopted it with enthusiasm. All the old compounds and conglomerates were to go: in their place, Scudder proposed that physicians should study and learn to rely on "the direct action of single drugs", uncombined with others. Such an approach required very careful diagnosis, as well as a knowledge of the specific action of each remedy upon the body.[14]

There were to be no more "heroic" shocks to the system, no more violent cathartics, emetics and blisters. Instead, medicine was to be gentle and kindly. "I look back on the old methods of drugging, with the same feelings of disgust and horror that I look back upon the thumb-screw, the cat, the rack," wrote Scudder.[15]

A mild and kindly practice; specific medication with small doses of single drugs; ultra-careful diagnosis; to many observers the shade of distinction between this and downright homoeopathy seemed fine indeed, and Scudder was bitterly attacked for betraying Eclectic ideals. But he stuck to his guns, and after ten years intensive work, he and King decided the time was ripe: specific medicines were now ready to be marketed for the use of all Eclectic physicians. This time, however – the resinoid scandal still painfully fresh in their minds – they resolved to keep the manufacture firmly under their control, with the medicines protected by a copyright label.

King had for some years been using plant medicines specially formulated for him by a brilliant young pharmaceutical chemist, John Uri Lloyd, who worked for one of the Regular houses. In 1870, King and Scudder approached Lloyd with a proposition: would he care to join the Eclectic drug house of H. M. Merrell & Co. to work out for them "the best plant medicines possible"? They warned him candidly that this move might well be his ruin professionally, with Regular friends cold-shouldering this associate of quacks and charlatans.[16]

But Lloyd immediately accepted what he considered an unprecedented research opportunity, and Scudder and King explained what they wanted. After a careful study of the specific attributes of each medicinal plant, they wanted "exact" representatives of their desirable parts, "free from inert constituents": in other words, tailored chemically to produce an elegant balance of the active principles and the most important constituents, although this tailoring was to be minimal.[17] Lloyd was always careful to distinguish this balancing from the allopathic method of extracting a single potent principle. They had learned, he wrote, "by bitter experience, that a poisonous fragment or ultimate, broken out of or created from a plant by chemistry, did not represent the therapeutic qualities of the structure from which it was derived".[18]

In their new devotion to "kindly" medicine, the Eclectics caught the feeling of the time. Homoeopathy had been making heavy inroads on the Regulars' confidence in their heroic techniques. Confronted with their successes, using what he and other physicians regarded as completely inert medicine, Dr. James Bigelow had as early as 1835 coined the theory of "Self-Limited Disease" to account for them: in other words, most diseases eventually go away of their own accord, whether treated or not. (Interestingly enough, the theory of diseases as self-limiting is now once more in respected vogue among the medical profession – and apparently for much the same reasons. In the first place, to account for the profession's discreet abandonment, little by little, of the extensive drugging it has been practising for the last twenty-five years; in the second, to account for the success of rival therapies such as herbal medicine.)

By mid-century, moreover, the deadly futility of bloodletting had been demonstrated both by pathology and by statistical studies. As the Regular medical profession everywhere began to put away the lancets they had plied so zealously, for so long, an ingenious face-saving formula was devised to justify this apparent volte-face. In recent times, the public was told, the types of fevers had themselves undergone a change; from an excitable inflammatory nature – in which bloodletting could only do good – they had mutated to a typhoid kind in which it would be disastrous.

"There are," said the highly-esteemed Regular authority, Dr. Watson, dusting his copy of Cullen, "waves of time through which the asthenic and adynamic characters of disease prevail in succession, and we are, at present, living amid one of its adynamic phases."[19] Dr. Dickson Smith put it into American for his readers: "There is an evident tendency in diseases of late years to assume a low typhoid character – a tendency to prostration of the powers of life . . . [which] enjoins the necessity of husbanding the strength of the patient, frequently from the very commencement".[20]

This apparently preposterous theory was soon seen to contain an alarming truth: by mid-century the state of health of the average American was disgracefully poor. Coulter quotes the results of the War Department's examination of recruits for the Mexican War in 1856: there were nearly twice as many rejections of Americans as European recruits for being "too slender and not sufficiently robust", or for "malformed and contracted chests".[21] Oliver Wendell Holmes thought that the most important question facing physicians in 1867 was "why our young men and women so often break down", and he admitted with distress that in his native Boston "every other resident adult you meet in these streets is or will be more or less tuberculous".[22]

Fifty years earlier, the Scottish doctor Hamilton had endorsed Whitlaw's suggestion that constant dosing with mercury made people fatally susceptible to tuberculosis. In both America and England, the general population who consulted Regular doctors were all likely to be frequently dosed with calomel from earliest infancy. It is certain that women consumed the lion's share, since it was freely prescribed in all menstrual problems from puberty onwards, together with bloodletting. According to another American doctor, bloodletting was also "the established remedy for various complaints and inconveniences" in pregnancy.[23]

So it comes as no surprise to learn that after generations of Heroic Medicine, the women of both England and America tended to be a sickly lot. "A truly healthy lady is now . . . uncommon, especially in cities . . ." remarked one doctor in 1866.[24] Florence Nightingale – admittedly an exacting critic – spoke of the common sight of "a great grandmother who was a tower of physical vigor, descending into a grandmother perhaps a little less vigorous but still sound as a bell, and healthy to the core, into a mother languid and confined to her carriage and house, and lastly into a daughter sickly and confined to her bed".[25] And Coulter quotes the American Thomas Wentworth Higgins, writing in 1861: "In this country it is scarcely an exaggeration to say that every man grows to manhood surrounded by a circle of invalid relatives, that he later finds himself the husband of an invalid wife and the parent of invalid daughters, and that he comes at last to regard invalidism as the normal condition of that sex – as if Almighty God did not know how to create a woman".[26]

A horrid doubt seized the American medical profession. Was this what their drugging and bleeding and blistering had done to the once-vigorous young nation?

In a much-publicized, prize-winning "Essay on Rational Therapeutics," Dr. Worthington Hooker of New Haven, Connecticut, ventured to suggest, in the most polished and elegant language, that much of Heroic Medicine had been a ghastly mistake, and that the modern doctor, simply by doing less, achieved more for his patients: "The deliverance from the suffering that formerly came from fruitless medication is of itself no small gain. The amount of life saved would be seen to be very great if we could obtain correct statistics."[27] And of calomel – still regarded by thousands of Regular doctors as their "sheet-anchor", he wrote: "Some of the more valuable acquisitions which the profession has made in therapeutics during the present century are the discriminating limitations that it has been able to put upon the use of this remedy."[28]

Oliver Wendell Holmes, addressing the Massachusetts Medical Society in 1860, was even more outspoken: apart from opium and a small number of specific drugs, ". . . I firmly believe that if the whole materia medica, as now used, could be sunk to the bottom of the sea, it would be all the better for mankind – and all the worse for the fishes."[29]

His words produced such a storm of abuse and protest that he was obliged to qualify them slightly. But the Regular profession at this time was certainly becoming a great deal less confident in its attitude to drugs generally, and by 1870, as Coulter points out, the *Buffalo Medical and Surgical Journal* was stating as a fact that "Men of high reputation in the profession . . . rely mostly on nature and hygiene".[30]

Prescribing habits contracted, and many doctors learned – like Gui Patin two centuries earlier – to rely on a small but trusted range of drugs – *pauca sed probata* – such as quinine, opium, iron, iodide of potassium, digitalis and mercury, though this last was often now prescribed in near-homoeopathic doses.

In the last decades of the century, there was an increasing Regular use of such homoeopathic and Eclectic drugs as aconite, gelsemium and hydrastis, many of which received an honourable place in the standard textbooks of materia medica.* Hardly surprisingly, the general American public made fewer and fewer distinctions between one school of medicine and another, and by the end of the century, the Irregular minority was formidably strong, with demand for both Eclectic and homoeopathic physicians rising steadily. John Uri Lloyd wrote in 1905 that "when it comes time for graduation exercises at the Eclectic Medical Institute, we cannot furnish one man where we have calls for twenty-five".[31]

Moreover, while the 15,000 Irregular doctors prospered and often

---

*In Louisa M. Alcott's *Little Women*, first published in 1868, the Hummels' doctor advises Beth to "go home and take belladonna right away" when he realizes she has been nursing the baby who died of scarlet fever. Belladonna was the homoeopathic near-specific for scarlet fever.

had huge waiting-lists, the 60,000 Regular doctors often found it a hard struggle simply to stay alive, with their average income running at under $1,000. To members of the American Medical Association it was depressingly clear that in the first half-century of their existence they had achieved almost nothing. Too many schools were still turning out a glut of ill-trained graduates, while the standing of their profession had never seemed lower. To them, more and more, the Hahnemann doctor came to seem the archenemy – maddeningly successful, rich and respected. An incident in the 1890s exactly illustrated the situation.

It began when the A.M.A. decided that it would be a suitable gesture to raise a monument to the great Dr. Rush in Washington. A committee established to find the money suggested a target of $45,000, but raised only a miserable $392 the first year, and did little better the following with $498. Ten years later, the Rush movement fund was still many thousands of dollars short of its target.

The American Homoeopathic Institute then decided that they too would raise a monument – to their beloved Hahnemann. Almost effortlessly the money rolled in, by 1896 they had collected $75,000, and the monument was going up in Washington for all to see. Gritting their teeth, the A.M.A. redoubled their efforts, the total crept up slowly to $15,000 – and Rush, too, rose in stone, some years later. Between the Regular and the Homoeopath there was little doubt who, in terms of wealth and status, was the poor relation.

21

Regulars and Rivals

"If Allopathy, as taught and practised at the present day, with all the advantages of support and patronage in high places, together with . . . colleges, hospitals and dispensaries . . . to give it a position, is unable to withstand the force of illegal practitioners of 'quackery' . . . it is full time it was swept away. . . ."[1] So ran a confident letter to the *New Era of Eclecticism* published in 1870, about yet another memorial presented by the medical profession to the Government about the workings of the 1858 Medical Act. When this Act was drafted, the Regulars had made strenuous efforts to have written into it provisions to make unlicensed practice a legal offence. They had not succeeded, and among the most enthusiastic of the "unlicensed quacks" who continued to practise were the members of the British Reform Medical Association.

This body entered the 1870s with high hopes, prepared to battle valiantly for the great cause of Medical Freedom, and secure in the knowledge that most of its members could write M.D. after their names, thanks to a useful arrangement concluded with the Eclectic Medical College of Pennsylvania. Created as a University in 1867, the College was by all accounts impressive, with a strong faculty, capacity for 300 students, its own hospital, and a clinic for out-patients. It boasted the largest and most magnificent Museum of Normal and Morbid Anatomy in America, and a well-ventilated dissecting room with "an abundant supply of material". Its directors, Professors Joseph Sites, Henry Hollembaek and John Buchanan, kept up the most cordial relations with the Association in Britain, and would have welcomed any of its members who could have raised the money to pay their fare across the Atlantic and the expenses of two terms plus board and graduation fees. (If the student were rich enough, he could also have paid $200 dollars to attend a very special course, and learn "a new scientific and radical mode of treatment for the cure of Malignant Diseases, especially Cancer . . . so definite that it succeeds in 99 cases in 100".)[2]

One of these English "Pennsylvania Doctors", it was true, had been obliged to reveal in a Court case at Leicester that although he possessed a beautiful diploma, carrying the College seal and the signatures of six of its professors, and certifying that he had attended two full courses of lectures and been examined accordingly, he had not actually engaged in any such exertion. He had answered some questions sent to him from Leeds, gone there once to be examined in person, and paid over some money – he could not exactly recollect how much.[3] But the Association would no doubt have contended that all of its members were most conscientiously trained at home anyway, and that it was the malice of the medical establishment that forced them to such underhand shifts.

They were in any case proud of the Eclectic connection. One of their founder members, John Blunt of Northampton, had himself gone over to America and brought back a supply of the New Concentrated Organic Compounds for his patients, while Dennis Turnbull, their President in 1870, published in the second issue of their magazine, the *New Era*, a ringing statement of the Eclectic aims of the Association. They were quite free, he declared, "to select, at will, from one and every system of medical practice, that remedy, or those remedies, which seems to them best adapted to cure the malady."[4] Their first President, W. B. Ford of Derby, presided over the Eclectic, Botanic, Medical and Phrenological Institute at 46 Saddler Gate, Derby; and many of their adherents belonged to the Midland Botanic and Eclectic Association, of which another member, a certain Mr. Jesse Boot, of 38 Goose-gate, Nottingham, was President.

Surging with life and energy, the Association even determined to bring about a union of all the Irregulars to protest against medical monopoly, and old John Skelton, now in his sixties but as alert and vigorous as ever, chaired a two-day conference at Birmingham of a new Medical Freedom League, which resolved to send a memorandum of its views to both Houses of Parliament.

The first decade of the Association's existence had seemed, indeed, like the hopeful dawn of a new era of medical freedom and progress. By 1880, however, the prospect contemplated by the Association looked much more like a sunset. The *New Era* itself had closed down, lamenting in its very last issue that the College that they had made ambitious plans for, and which was so necessary to their great hopes had never materialized: "A goodly number of men gave their names at the first as willing to help us, but these one after another, either from lack of zeal or from the pressure of business, ceased to take interest in the affair."[5]

No more was heard of Pennsylvania degrees, or of Eclecticism itself. The new "Specific Medication" announced by King and Scudder in 1870 was probably responsible for this split. Few of the English Eclectics could have afforded to import and prescribe the quite high-priced and copyrighted Eclectic preparations of H. M. Merrell & Co., even if they wished to do so. Acceptance of the new teachings of King and Scudder would also have meant throwing out half their materia medica – the familiar compounds and mixtures and composition essences which they had been happily and successfully prescribing for years.

Thus the Concentrated Remedies were quietly dropped, and even those British herbalists (still at heart the children of Thomson and Coffin), who had once styled themselves Eclectics, now quietly reverted to the old familiar mixtures of whole-plant tinctures and infusions. In so doing, they found that their natural transatlantic allies were, after all, the Physio-Medicals who had never used anything else.

But the Association no longer had either funds or energy to reach out across the Atlantic. For most of its ninety plus members, the struggle to stay afloat financially was certainly their chief preoccupation. This decline was due to a number of factors.

The Industrial Revolution was at last bringing a measure of prosperity to the working classes who had once been the city herbalists' most loyal customers. Now in the 1870s and 1880s, with money to spend, they began switching their allegiance to the glamorously packaged and enticingly advertised new patent medicines. Long-overdue legislation on public health and sanitation was responsible for a steady decline in those highly infectious killer-diseases which had once raged through slums, and in treating which the herbalist had been so strikingly effective – there were no more cholera visitations. Thirty years earlier, Coffin and Skelton had been able to fill page after page of their journals with lurid accounts of medical murder by calomelization and bleeding. While there was still much to criticize in Regular medicine, its defects were no longer as startling as they had once been: as in

America, the abandonment of the old heroic methods cut much of the ground from beneath Irregular feet. Even to his most loyal customers in this glorious new scientific age, the herbalist with his horrid dark-brown mixtures was beginning to look a little old-fashioned, and ambitious young Jesse Boot of Nottingham felt that it was time to move on to better things. "I had an idea," he wrote later, "that the herbalist and chemist at that time was very much out of date . . . I thought the public would welcome new chemists' shops in which a greater and better variety of pharmaceutical articles could be obtained at cheaper prices".[6]

Even rural England felt the effects of the Industrial Revolution in the slow decay of centuries-old patterns of living. Flora Thompson's *Lark Rise* lovingly describes the way village life was changing in one small Oxfordshire hamlet in the 1880s. The village women still kept a medicinal herb corner in their cottage gardens, stocked with horehound, peppermint, and pennyroyal, tansy, balm and rue, they drank cowslip and camomile tea and brewed up yarrow beer. But it was only the older women who still used wild herbs for medicine, and gathered them at the right season for drying – "the knowledge and use of these was dying out."[7]

To the regular medical profession, of course, the botanic medicine still practised by Boot's former colleagues – they had now restyled themselves, simply, the National Association of Medical Herbalists – looked ludicrously out of date, the quaint therapy of a byegone age. In an article in *The Practitioner* in 1870, Dr. W. Boyd Mushet treated his readers to an amused glance through "Obsolete Materia Medica", full of "quaint and absurd medicaments". Among the "many trivial medicines", now "obsolete among physicians", he listed horehound, agrimony, elecampane, garlic, marsh mallow, comfrey and coltsfoot; and he noted with evident disapproval that "these remained, and remain, to some extent established in the opinion of the public, and are still vended by Coffinists and herbalists". He conceded that some of them "doubtless possessed active qualities, and exerted an effect upon the system", but pointed out that of these, "if ordered at all at the present day, the essence is retained by the employment of their leading principle, the offensive article in substance being rejected".[8]

By the end of the century, "vegetable" was virtually a rude word in medicine, with synthetic laboratory medicine slowly edging out the original plant. In a textbook on pharmacology published in 1893, Professor Lauder Brunton noted, at the beginning of the section on

organic materia medica, that it contained "organic compounds artificially prepared, *and not merely extracted* from Vegetable Substances
containing them. Although it is small, it contains some of the most
important remedies we possess, and in the future will probably replace
to a great extent, and *perhaps entirely*, the Vegetable Materia Medica."
(my italics)[9] And although Lauder Brunton conceded that for the time
being medicine would have to continue to rely "at least to a certain
extent. . . [on] new remedies of plant origin", he looked forward to a
future when "we may be able to make artificially drugs which will be
able to produce on the organism any effect which we desire".[10]

But the quaint old-fashioned medicine refused to go away. The
medical herbalists of Britain still commanded the loyal support of
thousands and thousands of the British populace, and although they
were a weak impecunious body lacking political muscle, it was astonishing how they contrived to get under the skin of the medical profession. Throughout its existence, the records of the Association –
today the National Institute of Medical Herbalists – show a continuous record of harassment, vexation and attempted legal suppression
by the medical establishment, and in the last years of the nineteenth
century and the first decades of this, finding the resources to fight back
took all its energies.

In 1881 a Royal Commission on the Medical Acts was set up, and
the Association, alert against another attempt against their existence,
sent a moving and dignified appeal to the Commission's Chairman,
Lord Camperdown; ". . . your Memorialists . . . wish to draw your
attention to a section of Medical Practitioners in Great Britain who
practise the Herbal System of Medicine . . . [They] wish to point out
to you that they are not merely sellers of herbs but . . . by their
education and study into the nature of plants and by the knowledge of
their beneficial and curative effects have adopted the Herbal System of
Medicine". They drew attention to their strict rules that recognized
"no Practitioner who has not passed a successful examination
in Herbal Medicine, Materia Medica, Therapeutics, Anatomy and
Physiology etc. and who are of good moral character". And they
pointed out that although "in large manufacturing districts there are
vast numbers of people who have only Herbal practitioners for their
Medical Attendants, and that Club and Benefit Societies have passed
Byelaws to enable their members to employ Herbal Practitioners and
do receive certificates from them," they were still debarred, under the
1858 Act, from giving medical evidence in courts of law, holding

medical appointments, giving sickness notes or death certificates, or legally claiming unpaid fees.

Lord Camperdown was sympathetic: he asked for a fuller statement of their grievances, and finally agreed to receive one witness to give evidence. Francis Crick, one of their most distinguished and, they hoped, impressive members, was chosen, and the Royal Commission, who questioned the sixty-one-year-old gentleman for over two hours, gave him "a most cordial and liberal reception".[11] Heartened by this success the Association found itself a tame M.P., Mr. Burt, to watch over its interests in the House of Commons, and when in 1886 an Amendment came up which would have made it actionable to practise medicine unless professionally qualified, they were able to make such successful representations that the bill was withdrawn. They were equally successful in saving their favourite lobelia from being put on a new Poisons Schedule in 1886.

But the Charter they battled for in the 1890s, which would have given their members the status of registered practitioners, was bitterly opposed by the medical establishment, and for all their lobbying and petitions, they were obliged to settle instead for simple registration as a limited company in 1895, in which year they had to counter another attempt in Parliament at legal suppression.

A further blow was the passing in 1911 of Lloyd George's National Insurance Act. Lloyd George refused even to receive a deputation, or hear their views, and although there was nothing in the Act which technically forbade Approved Societies from paying benefit on a Herbalist's Certificate, one local Insurance company after another began refusing contracts to herbalists.

By 1913, only one Local Insurance Committee – that of Worcester – was still allowing its members to patronize the local herbalist, who happened to be the Association's Secretary, Charles Burden. In no time at all Burden was reporting to the Committee that the local doctors were threatening to prosecute him under the 1911 Act for accepting insured persons. Legal counsel no doubt pointed out that they did not have a leg to stand on, whereupon they brought proceedings instead under the old 1815 Apothecaries' Act – originally designed simply to protect the apothecaries against their semi-rivals the druggists and chemists, and so often unsuccessfully invoked against the Coffinites. This time the apothecaries won, and when Burden appealed, they won their Appeal as well, facing the members of the Association with the very real threat of being legally picked off, one by one, following this test case.

They wrote anxiously to the Prime Minister Mr. Asquith to protest: ". . . the recent decision will deprive thousands of His Majesty's subjects from being treated by the system of medicine they desire . . . and give a monopoly to one system of Medicine, which never seems to have been intended by recent medical legislation." They tried to arrange for a public meeting of protest, but this was October 1914, and it could not be done – "all the Halls in Worcester being occupied by the military".[12] The Government had more urgent matters than the future of herbal medicine to preoccupy them, and when no further prosecutions followed, the Association began to relax again. But World War I also underlined their lack of standing: when European imports of important medicinal herbs were cut off by wartime conditions, they were not even consulted by the Government about the list of herbs the Government was officially recommending should be grown at home, although this represented, as they pointed out "only a very small proportion of those in actual use in medicine, and in constant public requirement."[13]

One of their most acute problems, at all times, was poverty. There are no glittering prizes in the profession of herbal medicine, and the men and women it attracts – then as now – are seldom ambitious, politically motivated, or wealthy. Subscriptions had always to be kept to a minimum, and even then there were members who could not raise the two or three guineas. They could not afford the dignity of registered offices or full-time clerical staff, for long periods of time they could not afford any kind of official journal, and simply finding the train fares to London and the price of a hotel for the frequent delegations was often an appalling strain on the Association's resources.

For the same reason, the long-cherished dream of a College was wrecked time after time by financial problems. When at last, under the goading of the enterprising William Webb, a school was finally opened in Southport in 1911, it was in one room of a house that Mr. Webb himself owned. The rent of ten shillings a year was kindly waived by him, and the Association nervously declined to lay out £150 – as he urged – on a bargain lot of laboratory equipment. The school was nonetheless opened with a flourish – Sir Jesse and Lady Boot (as they had now become) were among those who sent regrets that they could not be present – but only a year later, it was already in financial difficulties over equipment that its principal had rashly spent some £50 on, and in 1915 it closed. The Association filled the gap with the postal tuition courses it ran, did its best to keep its educational standards high, and examined its candidates rigorously at the annual conferences. But the lack of a permanent, well-endowed school was keenly felt as a brake on advancement.

For the British herbalist, early in this century, life must often have seemed like one long rallying-call to action for yet another crisis. But this bred an extraordinarily strong sense of unity and family spirit in the Association, while the repeated attempts of the medical profession to drive herbalists out of practice, were frustrated by Parliament. Time and again its members – perhaps demonstrating a true British feeling for the underdog – showed themselves to be un expectedly sympathetic to the herbalists, and unwilling to have them hounded out of existence.

The herbalists of America at the turn of the century – the Eclectics and the Physiomedicals – could in no sense be described as underdogs. In 1909 it was calculated that there were perhaps 80,000 practitioners of what might be called the "dominant school", 10,000 homoeopaths, 8000 Eclectics, and another few thousand Physio-Medicals, osteopaths (newly arrived on the scene), chiropractors, hydrotherapists, and other practitioners. These figures were not necessarily accurate, but certainly the A.M.A.'s position was far from commanding, and they gazed across the Atlantic in some envy at the wealthy and confident British Medical Association.

The B.M.A. enjoyed one handsome source of revenue – its *Journal* – and in 1880 the A.M.A. had launched its own *Journal* in imitation. But although a fortune was dangled temptingly before its eyes by the huge and growing patent medicine industry, anxious to promote its products to the medical profession as well as the public, the *Journal* for years virtuously refused to accept advertising for secret or patent remedies. In 1899, however, the A.M.A. needed a new General Secretary and *Journal* editor, and the post went to forty-seven-year-old George Simmons, an English-born ex-homoeopath who in 1892 became a convert to allopathy and – like many converts – an implacable foe of the creed on which he had turned his back.

Simmons saw no reason why the A.M.A. should suffer for its virtue, and succeeded in engineering a complete rethinking of A.M.A. policy on this vital question. An editorial in 1905 declared warmly of its new-found friends: ". . . there are plenty of honestly made and ethically exploited proprietary prescriptions that are therapeutically valuable and that are worthy of the patronage of the best physicians":

henceforth the *Journal* would cheerfully accept advertisements for patent medicines, as long as their active ingredients were revealed to the A.M.A.'s newly formed Council on Pharmacy and Chemistry, which would vet them. Although the A.M.A. still frowned on those quack nostrums which were touted to the public with extravagant claims to cure this or that disease, it was perfectly prepared to allow such claims as long as they were only addressed to the medical profession in its professional journals.[14] "Thus", as Coulter concluded, "the A.M.A. allied with, and was conquered by, the patent medicine industry".[15]

Financially the results were instantly gratifying. *Journal* revenue rose from $33,760 in 1899 to $150,000 in 1909. Half a century later, it ran at over $9,000,000 and supplied more than half the A.M.A.'s revenue.

With its financial problems on the way to solution, the A.M.A. addressed itself with fresh energy and confidence to the other crisis facing it at the end of the nineteenth century: too many doctors and much too much competition from Irregulars. They had already tried unsuccessfully to deal with the homoeopaths by weeding them out of medical schools before they graduated. In 1878 Dr. Nathan Davis had proposed an addition to their Code of Ethics: "It is considered derogatory to the interests of the public and the honour of the profession, for any physician or teacher to aid, in any way, the medical teaching or graduation of persons knowing them to be supporters and intended practitioners of some irregular and exclusive system of medicine".[16]

Now the A.M.A. did an about-face, and in 1901 a completely new policy was adopted: far from having nothing to do with medical sectarians of any kind, the A.M.A. cordially invited them all to become members. They were more than welcome – as long as they were prepared to give up their formal allegiance to Babels and sects. And once inside the fold they could, of course, practise exactly as they pleased: ". . . when so elected, they are no longer homoeopaths or eclectics, but are promoted to be plain physicians like the other of us."[17]

Beguiled by this welcome, Little Red Riding Hood stepped confidently inside the cottage; throughout the United States, doctors deserted the local Irregular Institute and joined the Regular medical society. Tolerance was the new order of the day, and the Irregulars congratulated themselves on their conquest of prejudice. "The fact that there are ten to one against us in point of numbers", John Uri Lloyd told the Ohio Eclectics in 1905, "does not imply that there are ten antagonistic men against us now."[18] He could recall the bad old days when he had been "so aggravated and so worried, surrounded, persecuted, ostracised" that even this gentlest of men was hard put not to retaliate. Now things were very different: "Didn't we last night hear the Regular representative tell us there was now no feeling against us?"[19]

Even if much of the competition was being disarmed, it still left the root of the problem intact: too many badly-trained doctors, graduating from far too many low-grade schools. The obvious solution was to raise entry requirements and upgrade educational standards, so as to slow the influx of students, and filter out some of the less suitable candidates.

In 1896 the *Journal* began publishing a series of reports on the nation's medical schools, sharply criticizing those it considered to be no better than degree-shops, and in 1902 the A.M.A. formed a Council on Medical Education to consider this urgent question. National standards of medical education were appalling at the time, and those run by the Eclectics were in no way superior to most of the Regular ones: on the contrary, since the demand for Eclectic practitioners always outstripped the supply, their schools were even more tempted than the Regulars' to take in students without looking too closely at their scholastic credentials, and to hand out degrees that were not always honestly earned.

In 1907 the Council began visiting each of the 160-plus schools throughout the States, giving each a numbered rating according to a list of ten categories, which included such areas as preliminary education requirements, laboratory facilities, teaching equipment, and evidence of original research – if any – by the teaching faculty. The ratings were not at first published, though each school was told its own total. But the A.M.A. faced a difficulty. Though it could claim to represent the majority of American doctors, it had no actual powers to enforce the higher standards it believed necessary, and in the case of the Irregular schools, its criticisms were unlikely to carry much weight, if any, since it would inevitably be accused of bias. Moreover, the cost of the detailed door-to-door inspections was proving to be great.

At this point a *deus ex machina* appeared on stage: the Carnegie Endowment for the Advancement of Teaching, with all its millions, offered to take over the remaining expenses, and send its own experts around to confirm the A.M.A. ratings. It was agreed with the A.M.A. that "while the Foundation would be guided very largely by the

Council's investigation, to avoid the usual claims of partiality no more mention should be made in the report of the Council than any other source of information. The report would therefore be, and have the weight of, a disinterested body, which would then be published far and wide. It would do much to develop public opinion."[20] The man appointed by the Carnagie Endowment was Abraham Flexner.

Two years later, in 1910, the Flexner Report burst like a bombshell on the great American public. It revealed in lurid details the low standards, the poor equipment, and the inadequate or non-existent clinical facilities of many of the nation's medical schools. The Report spoke of a dissecting-room "indescribably filthy: it contained, in addition to necessary tables, a single, badly-hacked cadaver, and was simultaneously used as a chicken yard",[21] of a college whose laboratory facilities were limited to "a few small, undescribably dirty and disorderly rooms, containing three microscopes, a small amount of physiological apparatus, some bacteriological stains, a few filthy specimens, and meagre equipment for elementary chemistry, but no running water."[22] It detailed the night-school for students who could not afford full-time study, where the clinical facilities were limited to "looking on at surgical work . . . no children's diseases, no acute medical diseases at the bedside, no contagious diseases".[23] There was the "University" which, on being asked to show its laboratories, could only conduct the inspector to a large room, and claim "equipment" and "about ten oil-immersion microscopes 'locked-up' ".[24]

"A vast army of men" concluded the Report, "is admitted to the practice of medicine who are untrained in sciences fundamental to the profession and quite without a sufficient experience with disease. . . . For twenty-five years past there has been an enormous over-production of un-educated and ill-trained medical practitioners".[25]

The Carnegie Foundation was faithful to its word: although the Report referred in passing to the fact that its information had been "carefully checked with the data in possession of the American Medical Association", it went on to state that "the work has been so thoroughly reviewed by independent authorities, that the statements which are given here may be confidently accepted as setting forth the essential facts."[26]

Presenting the Report for the Foundation, Henry S. Pritchett issued an inspiring challenge: "Let us address ourselves resolutely to the task of reconstructing the American medical school on the lines of the highest modern ideals of efficiency. . . ."[27] He added a pious hope "that this publication may serve as a starting-point both for the intelligent citizen and for the medical practitioner in a new national effort to strengthen the medical profession."[28]

Thus the general impression received by the public was that of a princely public service rendered by an impartial millionaire philanthropist. In effect, it was also a death-sentence for the nation's Irregular schools.

Of the eight Eclectic schools, the Report declared that none had "anything remotely resembling the laboratory equipment which all claim in their catalogues". Three of them were under-equipped; the rest "are without exception filthy and almost bare. They have at best grimy little laboratories . . . a few microscopes, some bottles containing discoloured and unlabelled pathological material, an incubator out of commission, and a horrid dissecting-room". The Report found them more culpable than a Regular school for these inadequacies: ". . . the Eclectics are drug-mad; yet, with the exception of the Cincinnati and New York schools, they are not equipped to teach the drugs or the drug therapy which constitutes their sole reason for existence".[29]

In other important respects, too, the Eclectic schools were found wanting; none had "decent clinical opportunities", and three of them had no dispensaries at all. But the Report indicated a steady decline in Eclectic fortunes: there had been ten schools in 1901, and now there were only eight, and the number of graduates in 1906 had been 186 as against only 84 in 1909.

For years Scudder and King had deplored the low standards of Eclectic education, and done nothing about it, secure in the belief that they were no worse than many of the Regulars. Now they were to pay the price.

Physio-Medicalism did even worse: the Report dismissed it in a note. "It had three schools in 1907; only one, that in Chicago, is left. . . . There were 149 physio-medical students in 1904; there are now 52; there were 20 graduates in that year, 15 in 1909."[30]

Far more deadly, however, than any amount of adverse comment on this or that school was the Report's majestic verdict on the whole notion of sectarian medicine. Flexner invited his readers to look beyond the petty squabbling of the sects to the new dawn of modern, scientific medicine. "Is it essential" he asked "that we should now conclude a treaty of peace, by which the reduced number of schools shall be so pro-rated as to recognize dissenters on an equitable basis?"[31]

He answered his own question firmly in the negative: "medicine is a discipline in which the effort is made to use knowledge procured in various ways to effect certain practical ends. With abstract general propositions it has nothing to do. . . . Modern medicine had therefore as little sympathy for allopathy as for homoeopathy. It simply denies outright the relevancy or value of either doctrine". Sectarian schools were thus as unnecessary as they were undesirable: future practitioners must all start from the same scientific basis and the rest was up to them: "No man is asked in whose name he comes – whether that of Hahnemann, Rush, or of some more recent prophet".[32]

Having disposed of the sectarians, the Report gave its own ideas on what the new modern, scientific medicine needed as an educational base. The laboratory sciences were at the very heart of this concept – anatomy, pathology, bacteriology, physiology, pharmacology: ". . . the century which has developed medical laboratories has seen the death-rate reduced by one-half and the average expectation of life increased by ten or twelve years".[33]

Pharmacology was crucial: originally only negative "it rapidly pruned away exaggeration and superstition . . . [and] ascertained . . . the utter uselessness of dozens of concoctions with which the digestive capacity of the race has long been taxed". Now it faced at last a positive opportunity: "Given . . . this or that condition . . . cannot an agent be devised capable of combating it?" And among the answers with which it had already come up were "cocaine, the antipyretics, the various glandular preparations and serum therapy".[34] Pharmacology was vital to the budding doctor, since it would help him distinguish between good drugs and the worthless ones touted by unscrupulous manufacturers.

Botany was no longer necessary: "Materia medica, now much shrunken, need concern itself only with the pharmaceutical side, aiming to familiarize the student with drugs of proved power and the most agreeable and effective forms in which these may be administered."[35] Such an educational curriculum might have been specially devised to turn out enthusiastic clients for the big pharmaceutical companies. It focussed on disease rather than health, on cure rather than prevention. Nutrition figured only fleetingly, in passing, as an adjunct to drug therapy: "Therapeutics subsequently adds to these agents whatever resources the clinician has accumulated – baths, electricity, massage, psychic suggestion, dietetics, etc.".

In the words of a recent commentator: "The drive to improve medical cure to the neglect of medicine care carried the day. Flexner's views prevailed and the 'basic' sciences of medical education were declared to be biochemistry and physiology; the equally 'fundamental' sciences of epidemiology, economics and sociology were excluded from the curriculum."[36]

The Flexner report achieved more than the wildest dreams of the A.M.A. Within the next four years 29 schools went out of business, by 1927 the number had dropped to 80, and State licensing boards eventually closed all but the 66 medical schools approved by the A.M.A. The Physio-Medical school disappeared almost at once. Four of the eight Eclectic schools had closed by 1915; by 1920 there was only one left, and that, too, closed its doors in 1938.[37] Today, no U.S. medical school can exist without A.M.A. approval.

But the Regular schools were not left to struggle unaided: since 1910, the Rockefeller General Education Board and other Foundations have showered millions of dollars on allopathic educational institutions, with the General Education Board alone contributing about $600,000,000.[38] It has been estimated that nearly half the faculty members now receive a portion of their income from foundation research grants, and over sixteen per cent of them are entirely funded in this way.[39]

Disinterested philanthropy? Since it has eliminated all effective forms of alternative medicine, and promoted a monopoly medicine which is heavily drug-orientated, we may well wonder.

22

Magic
Bullets

Dioxydiaminoarsenobenzol dihydrochloride is a long name for a
miracle. But a miracle was what it sounded like to the medical world
when the remarkable achievement of this compound – "606" for
short – was announced to the Congress for Internal Medicine, at
Wiesbaden in April 1910. "606" was the discovery of a brilliant
young Prussian biochemist, Paul Ehrlich (1854–1915), who worked at
the State Institute for Experimental Therapy in Frankfurt.

In the aftermath of the work of Pasteur, serum and vaccines had
seemed like the most hopeful modern responses to infection – still the
chief medical problem – and Ehrlich had spent years studying the
performance of antitoxins inside the human body. He had become
fascinated by the way in which the body, as part of its natural defence
mechanism, manufactures its own antibodies which zero in on the
invading bacteria and render them harmless – "magic bullets which
strike only those objects for whose destruction they have been produced by the organism".[1] He felt that it ought to be possible to
manufacture such highly selective anti-bacterials in the laboratory –
synthetic "magic bullets", as it were.

Ehrlich's earliest original work had been done with the dyes then
used to stain tissues for the pathology lab. (The landlady of his student
days wrote years later to remind him of the time when every towel in
her house was dyed brilliant red or blue.)[2] Ehrlich was struck by the
fact that certain dyes had an affinity for certain specific types of cell,
and when searching for his magic bullets, therefore, he first experimented with different dyes, injected into animals who had been
infected with different types of disease. To his delight a dye later
christened Trypan red turned out to be astonishingly effective against

the germs responsible for trypanosomiasis or sleeping-sickness – a killer tropical disease. Trypan red was next tried on human subjects in Africa with gratifying success.

Ehrlich reasoned that other chemical compounds might produce even more dramatic effects on germs that affected human beings, and since chemical derivatives of arsenic were being examined in labs throughout the world with some highly suggestive results, he began work with this strong poison. A series of more than 600 different arsenical compounds were produced by him in the lab and tried on experimental animals. The microscopic organism shaped like a twisting rod which produces syphilis in human beings – the spirochæte – had been identified in Berlin in 1905. Rabbits infected with it were injected with one after another of the compounds: "606" killed the spirochætes. Cautiously, Ehrlich tried it on human syphilitics: the same thing happened.

It was the very best news, greeted with banner headlines in the world's press after its announcement at Wiesbaden. Syphilis was not merely a personal tragedy for hundreds of thousands of victims annually but the most widely used treatment for it – mercury – was, as we have seen, often ineffectual, always disagreeable, and occasionally as deadly as the disease itself. Moreover the supposed conquest of syphilis had other than individual implications: for three centuries the disease had been the biggest single headache of military commanders. Camp-followers were almost always diseased, and it romped merrily through armies, prostrating large numbers of the effective force.

As it turned out, one huge dose of Salvarsan – as "606" had now been officially christened – was not the simple answer Ehrlich had hoped, and over the next three decades, modifications to the compound and its mode of application – together with completely different therapies, such as the heat treatment – were tried one after another.*

With the wartime spread of syphilis in England it was illegal in 1917 for any but regular practitioners to treat cases, not that it was supposed

---

*In 1917 a Viennese psychiatrist found that some patients in the advanced stages of syphilis got better after being subjected to a high fever. He tried out different types of fever, and settled on a benign form of malaria as the most effective, after which the malarial treatment was widely used. It was then reasoned that perhaps the high temperature alone was responsible for the good results, and straight heat therapy was introduced. Some of the worse symptoms of late syphilis – resistant to all standard treatment – disappeared after a course of hot baths, thus providing – centuries later – a *rationale* for the prolonged sweat-treatment with guaiac.[3]

modern medicine had found the cure. The National Association of Medical Herbalists, in a protest to the government at this annexation of yet another stretch of their terrain, pointed out the official delusion: "While we view with alarm the increasing number of cases of this loathsome disease, we unhesitatingly declare that the present [allopathic] practice of medicine is quite inadequate, and unable to eliminate the disease. During the last fifty years, thousands of cases in all its stages have been treated successfully by members of this Association, and in hundreds of cases after the Registered Practitioners had failed to cure."[4]

In the passion of its feeling, the Association sent out a circular to Trades and Labour Councils on the subject – their first appeal to organized working-class interests – drawing their attention to the deadly side-effects that the arsenic treatment was producing. (These included jaundice, kidney disease, optic atrophy, anaphylactic shock – occasionally leading to death – and an appalling type of arsenical dermatitis, in the most severe forms of which the wretched patient became bloated and lost all his skin.)

In 1920 the Association again drew the Government's attention to this problem: "We the members of the National Association of Medical Herbalists are alarmed at the number of cases of Venereal Disease, increasing throughout Great Britain, due to the fact that the medical profession are unable to cope with it by the use of 606 or preparations containing arsenic or mercury. So-called cured patients are suffering from the disease, others by poisoning from arsenic and mercury."[5]

Had the Association had scientific expertise, members skilled in pathology and biochemistry, the money to pay for laboratories and costly animal experiments, they might have been able to run their own experiments to show whether, as they claimed, herbal treatment was more effective. They had none of these, not even a College for their own basic training, and their suggestions and criticisms were brushed contemptuously aside by a medical establishment which pinned its faith on strong wonder-working chemicals. Nobody, now, was much interested in plants.

In the American *Index Medicus*, an annual listing appearing since 1879 of those articles published in the world's medical journals which were thought to have more than fleeting interest, papers detailing the investigation of a medicinal plant were few and far between in the early years of the twentieth century. In 1907 there were papers on the passion flower (*Passiflora incarnata*), a homoeopathic favourite with a mildly narcotic action, useful in dysentery, and goldenseal (*Hydrastis canadensis*), the Eclectic favourite. And in 1914 the *Index* listed a paper on papaverine, an alkaloid of the opium poppy which was thought to have potential in cardiac problems. But the *Index Medicus* had a distinct allopathic bias – after 1932 when it was taken over by the A.M.A. – and not until 1934 were medicinal plants even given the status of their own separate sub-section. In the meantime they figured only slightly, and the overwhelming majority of early twentieth-century papers were devoted to such subjects as advances in surgical and anæsthetic techniques, radiotherapy, the completely new science of endocrinology, the discovery of vitamins, and transfusion and injection techniques.

In nearly every field, medical science was racing ahead, but in the field which affected every single doctor – that of materia medica – progress was disappointingly slow. Writing of his father's prescribing habits in the 1870s, the U.S. physician Dr. Pusey wrote fifty years later, in 1932, that there was "little difference between the use of drugs then and at the present time, so far as I can judge."[6] And although both academic and commercial laboratories were working feverishly to produce effective new drugs, the first "magic bullet" remained the only one for more than two decades.

An English pharmacologist, Dr. E. W. Adams, reflected in the *British Medical Journal* of 28 March 1936, that "considering the spate of new drugs which has in ever-increasing volume poured forth from the laboratories of the world, the number proved to be of real and permanent value has not been nearly so large as might reasonably have been hoped".[7]

The most urgent problem facing all doctors was still that of infection. "The common and sometimes lethal consequences of spreading bacterial infections were a constant spectre looming over the practising doctor", wrote one Canadian physician of his early twentieth-century practice. "There was not a doctor who had not lost one or more of his colleagues following an apparently inconsequential needle prick or scratch. . . . The most impressive and frightening . . . was . . . gas gangrene. A simple puncture wound would permit the entry of the bacteria. Within hours, the subcutaneous tissues would be swelling and audibly crackling as the gas formed under the skin. The spread was so fast it could be clearly observed, and when death ensued the body was a swollen mass, with the features distorted and movement visible and audible, as the gas-forming organisms continued their work".[8]

Confronted with such swift killers as pneumonia, puerperal fever and meningitis, the regular doctor felt helpless. The Dean of the Medical School at Manchester University, looking back in 1971 on his early days of hospital training, recalled the feeling vividly: "I was a house physician through the winter months; and I can still remember the anxiety of my night round, about midnight, when we might have two or three lobar pneumonias in the ward: strong, healthy men perhaps, fighting for their lives against the pneumococcus. One in four would die; and the houseman knew there was very little he could do except support the nursing staff in their efforts to give the patient rest and keep up his morale."[9]

The medical herbalist, faced with such cases, had a personal anxiety too: if his patient died, he might very well have to undergo the strain and expense of a Coroner's inquest.

For a long time it was hoped that vaccines and sera might prove to be the answer, and by the early 1930s there were several preparations on the market. But they were extremely expensive, dealt only with limited types of infection, and unless the exact strain was accurately typed in a pathology lab, the serum was worse than useless, often causing a distressing serum sickness of its own, with swollen glands and aching joints to add to the patients' problems. Thus if the patient was young and fit, with a chance of fighting off the disease with his own resources, serum was seldom administered. Some doctors even resorted to bleeding instead. As for vaccines, a doctor and pharmacologist writing in *The Practitioner* in 1936, described them as "one of the greatest delusions of a generation", and suggested that "few now . . . regard them as anything but a danger in the treatment of acute and generalized infections".[10]

In despair at their own failure to produce effective drugs, many houses began re-examining another favourite nineteenth-century poison – mercury. In 1914 an appalled John Uri Lloyd had already protested against the new, widespread use of the drug that had killed Rhazes' apes: corrosive sublimate. "Who could have imagined that when the Eclectic fathers of old fought calomel as a harmful drug, its near relative, corrosive sublimate, then scarcely used enough to be mentioned, would ever become, perhaps, the greatest scourge, the most monstrous drug enemy of the human race?" Then, as now, the Irregular practitioner often had to pick up the pieces after Regular medicine had failed, and had plenty of chances to study the baneful side-effects of a drug at first hand. Lloyd concluded that ". . . We should advocate the suppression, by state and national law, of every 'biochloride' that carries more than the maximum internal dose of corrosive sublimate."[11] He was equally critical of many other current drug offerings: ". . . illogical serums, repulsive animal extracts, death-dealing arsenical compounds . . . coal-tar synthetics."[12]

The animal extracts he mentioned were highly popular at this time, and a 1930s doctor, leafing through the current stack of promotional literature, must occasionally have wondered if he wasn't browsing in a seventeenth-century pharmacopœia. By 1936, as Dr. Adams noted in the *British Medical Journal*, ". . . tablets and solutions have been prepared from almost every tissue and organ of the animal body, regardless of whether those tissues and organs could reasonably be supposed to produce an internal secretion or not. Thus we have extracts of tonsil, kidney, prostate, spleen, heart, brain, mammary gland, and so on." Dr. Adams, a former lecturer in materia medica, was scathing about them. ". . . I know of no authentic evidence that such products are of the slightest use", he commented. ". . . such therapy rests on no sounder theory than that of the savage who eats his enemy's heart to absorb his courage."[13]

The most striking progress came, not from pharmaceutical laboratories, but from studies in physiology, which produced insulin for diabetes in 1923, and the discovery that eating liver cured pernicious anæmia, though it was not at first known why.

Then in 1935, as the result of renewed work with dyes, a group of German scientists and doctors, led by Gerard Domagk, and working for the chemical firm of I. G. Farbenindustrie, at last announced what sounded like another genuine "magic bullet": called Prontosil Red, it was the first of a series of drugs containing the sulphonamide group of chemical compounds, and effective against streptococcal and staphylococcal infections. Domagk and his team had spent three years carefully testing and re-testing Prontosil before they announced it, and its discovery is seen today as the start of what has been called "the great drug therapy era", when wonder-drugs poured on to the market in increasing numbers, and medical miracles came to seem like the order of the day.

Prontosil red was tried out the world over, and elated reports of its success in pneumonia, meningitis, septicæmia and other bacterial infections poured in. At Queen Charlotte's Hospital in London, it was shown to reduce deaths from puerperal fever from about 20% to under 5% – a specially happy achievement. The terror went out of autopsies:

now "a young pathologist could prick his finger at an autopsy; see the red lines of lymphangitis on his forearm by late afternoon; take a few tablets of sulphonamide; and as he expected, find himself completely recovered in 36 hours".[14] Thousands of similar compounds were produced and patented during the next few years, including May & Baker's M&B 693, produced in 1938, which saved among others the life of Winston Churchill.

In 1928 Alexander Fleming, about to throw away yet another culture-plate on which his carefully-grown organisms had been destroyed by that wretched mould that likes stale bread and rotting fruit, *Penicillium notatum*, suddenly stopped in his tracks. The lowly mould was *destroying* organisms, he reminded himself. What if . . .? Everybody knows the happy ending to this story: the substance was called penicillin, and in modern medicine penicillin, with its derivatives, is still the greatest and most reliable of all the drugs used against a range of overwhelming infection. What is less often pointed out is that such moulds were used in professional medicine in ancient Egypt to stop wounds becoming infected – a use mentioned in the Ebers papyrus. They have been used the same way in folk medicine for as long as there are written records, and probably considerably longer.

The production of penicillin in quantity turned out to be an almost impossible task, but by 1940 there was a war on, and the demands of war make many things possible which would never be so in peacetime. With the help of American money and research facilities, the problem was solved just in time to save the Allied Armies of Invasion, in 1944, from that perennial threat to soldier-power, venereal disease. After the war, V.D. was thought to have been almost wiped out by its use. The side-effects of penicillin could be fatal – but that was true of almost any drug doctors were using, and no other was as effective.

The discovery of penicillin suggested that other useful organisms might be lurking in mould, soil or similar hiding-places. The U.S. pharmaceutical company Merck looked at 100,000 soil samples between 1939 and 1943 and came up with streptomycin, which when combined with P.A.S. produced the answer to a persistent threat, tuberculosis. Lederle produced aureomycin from a Missouri soil sample in 1945; and in 1947 Parke Davis announced the discovery of yet another miracle from the soil, isolated from a small fragment of Venezuela and christened chloramphenicol, which remains the most effective drug in typhoid fever and some forms of meningitis to this day. Prolonged study of the glands had enabled scientists at the Mayo

Clinic in Rochester, Minnesota to isolate the hormone cortisone in 1930, and in 1949 they tried it in patients suffering the painful disease rheumatoid arthritis with, at first, spectacular success.

The public grew blasé about medical miracles. It was beginning to seem perfectly normal that somebody, somewhere, should come up with a pill, a powder, or an ointment, or an injectable liquid that could cure all the diseases of mankind. The unknown pundit who coined the slogan, "a pill for every ill", may have meant it quite seriously.

In an article written by Dr. David Moreau for the English edition of *Vogue* in October 1976 to record and celebrate the achievements of sixty years of medicine, it is still possible to catch occasional whiffs of that euphoric optimism so widely felt in the late 1950s. After Prontosil touched off "the chemotherapeutic revolution which reduced nearly all non-viral disease to the significance of a bad cold", wrote Moreau, the new antibiotics included "the extraordinary semi-synthetic penicillins which effectively disposed of the growing menace of penicillin-resistant staphylococci . . . drugs to treat the mentally sick . . . Chlorpromazine . . . [and] all the other psychic palliatives . . . such as Librium, Valium and Equanil." Among "the almost endless lesser breakthroughs in the period" were the "cortisones used in arthritic and other inflammatory diseases . . . the sex hormones . . . culminating in the oral contraceptive pill". In the field of heart drugs "great progress was made with coronary vaso-dilators, anginal drugs and ganglionic blocking agents for blood pressure such as methyldopa". "Malaria", continued Dr. Moreau, "was finally conquered with side-effect-free daily doses of drugs such as chloroquine and proguanil . . ." Antihistamines, with cortisones, took the suffering out of the most allergic diseases, and even in cancer, "there have been a number of significant advances."

"If", concluded Dr. Moreau decisively, "the competitive drug industry is allowed to continue the extraordinary achievements of the last sixty years, by 2036 nearly all the health obstacles to survival into extreme old age will have been overcome".[15]

The key word in the sentence is, of course, "competitive." Before World War I there were dozens of pharmaceutical companies in Europe and in the United States, but it was the war itself that triggered America's explosive development in the field of organic chemistry. Up to that time, Germany's commanding lead had been unchallenged: "We have blindly failed to see the wonderful possibilities in the similar protection and development of the chemical industries", admitted

Professor Kraemer in the *American Journal of Pharmacy* in 1918.[16] Over half of the plant-based medicines prescribed by American doctors were supplied by American firms who also exported extensively. But in one field they were far behind – "the manufacture of synthetic chemical drugs".

When the United States finally found herself at war with Germany in April 1917, however, several treasured German patents were handed over to American companies to exploit under Government licence, according to the provisions of the Trading with the Enemy Act, and soon barbital, novocaine and arsphenamine – as "606" had now been renamed – were being widely manufactured in the U.S. American eyes were opened to the staggering business opportunity they had been neglecting – and the pharmaceutical explosion at once became inevitable.

". . . our manufacturers have seen the importance of extending their research laboratories, and it is quite likely that scientific work will be greatly stimulated in the United States", commented Professor Kraemer. "Never before in our country have we seen the close relationship between the scientifically trained expert and the manufacturer and between the inventor and the inventor and the banker". And he added with honest patriotic pride in this most American shrewdness: "If the capitalist can be shown that laboratory work is likely to become a commercial success, he is at once interested and his investment is certain".[17]

Pharmaceutical companies – then as now – have very heavy overheads. As Ehrlich himself had shown, it could take years of patient teamwork before a promising therapeutic substance surfaced – and then more months of careful trials with experimental animals were needed before the drug could satisfy the requirements of the new Pure Food and Drug Act of 1906 and be safely marketed. If they were to recover the massive investment all this involved, they would first have to secure a patent for their drug and so make sure of cornering the market; secondly, they needed to be sure the market was as big as possible.

Considerations like these made it almost inevitable that pharmaceutical companies should leave plants alone. The vegetable world had in its time provided many wonderful drugs – digitalis, belladonna, stramonium – the narcotic and sedative, *colchicum* or autumn crocus, effective in gout, and a few others. More recently the coca plant had given the world the alkaloid cocaine from which many modern anæsthetics were derived. But except in the minds of a few prejudiced Irregulars, there was no automatic assumption that plants would continue to provide badly-needed drugs.

On the contrary, in the eyes of the regular medical profession, the vegetable kingdom had failed badly on two counts. First, it had never produced a reliable cure for syphilis – mankind had had to resort, first, to the mineral mercury, and then to synthetic chemicals. Secondly – although the Irregulars might have disagreed – it had produced no reliable remedy for acute infection. This was the golden fleece for which in the 1920s, the pharmaceutical industry was racing. It seemed perfectly reasonable to expect that this, too, would come out of a laboratory the way Salvarsan had.

An even more telling argument against plant research was that it was unlikely to result in a product that could be patented and profitably marketed. Even if some industrial pharmacologist happened, by a miracle, upon another digitalis, its active principle might prove impossibly expensive to synthesize. Worse still, it might turn out to be less effective than the whole plant – in which case the company could write off the cost of years of research, since nobody could patent a plant. This was a genuine risk of which digitalis itself was a perfect example: most physicians then preferred to use whole-leaf preparations rather than extracted alkaloids – as some still do today.

Thus the vast expanding pharmaceutical industry of the United States turned its back on the plant world and looked to synthetic chemicals as its future. The nation's pharmacy students – many of their research grants funded by Rockefeller and Carnegie – came to realize that none of the plum jobs were in plant investigation. A new generation of doctors read a professional *Journal* in which column after column advertised the glamorous new synthetic drugs – and underwrote the A.M.A.'s existence in the same breath.

"The desertion of the study of vegetable drugs soon became almost complete", noted a pharmacologist for the magazine *Science* in 1941. ". . . at the present time researches dealing with plant medicinals are relatively rare and are becoming more so. Today is the heyday for organic synthetic chemicals. Present-day medical scientists only too frequently are apt to look askance at those who would investigate the therapeutic possibilities of the vegetable kingdom".[18]

Even when a plant offered real hope in a major medical problem, the profession tended to close its eyes. "There is probably no more valuable drug mentioned in any pharmacopœia than *oleum allii*, the active oil of garlic; yet there is scarcely any so little known to our profession generally", lamented the Englishman Dr. W. Minchin, in a 1918 article for the *Practitioner*.[19] He had been excitedly investigating the properties of garlic for nearly twenty years, had written a pamphlet claiming its usefulness in two much-feared diseases, tuberculosis and lupus, had found it astonishingly effective against the equally dreaded diphtheria – "it robs this disease of all its terrors" – and considered it an antiseptic without a rival since, unlike any other known antiseptics, it was completely harmless to the body tissue. He quoted a clinical trial run by the Metropolitan Hospital in New York, when fifty-six modern treatments were tried over two years on 1,082 patients suffering from tuberculosis. The treatments included every known modern therapy, including arsenic and mercury compounds, vaccines, serums, antitoxins, surgical intervention – and garlic. The hospital concluded its report unequivocally: "Garlic gave us our best results, and would seem equally efficacious, no matter what part of the body was affected." Minchin went on to make the highly interesting suggestion that the low incidence of T.B. among practising Jews and on the Continent might be due to their garlic-eating habits.[20]

Had garlic been a brand-new chemical compound newly issued from a German or American laboratory, it would have been trumpeted throughout the world, and doctors everywhere would have rushed to try it. As it was, one or two adventurous doctors took a hint from Dr. Minchin, with great success, but his work and his passionate pleas that garlic should be widely tested were ignored by the profession as a whole, tuberculosis remained a dreaded killer disease for decades longer, and anybody today who suggested that a hospital should try experimenting on its patients with garlic would get some very funny looks, although numbers of research papers attesting its usefulness have been published over the last twenty years.

This orientation of the drug houses and their patrons, the physicians, away from the plants and in the direction of synthetic chemicals, required no great shift in established professional thinking, either in the United States or in Britain where much the same situation arose. Apart from the handful of plant-drugs which had been, as it were, "professionalized", plant medicine had all the wrong connotations to the average medical doctor.

It was messy, "unscientific", difficult to standardize and reduce to a neat little pill. Besides, it kept the lowest kind of company, such as "the promoters of patent medicines, which were composed largely of

complex mixtures of such substances – veritable vegetable soups",
as the American Dr. Morris Fishbein commented acidly in 1936.[21]
Typical of one such remedy was rudbeckia (*Echinacea angustifolia*), first
introduced, he claimed, as "the main ingredient of a remedy known as
Meyer's Blood Purifier . . . according to the label, powerful as an
alterative and antiseptic in all 'humorous and syphilitic indications,
old chronic wounds . . . ulcers, carbuncles, piles, eczema . . . gangrene
. . . adverted typhoid in two or three days, and cured malaria, diphtheria, rabies and bee stings' ".[22] Most nineteenth-century patent
remedies were actually based on a hint taken from either Thomsonian
or Eclectic practice, rather than the other way round, but according to
Dr. Fishbein, *Echinacea* was an exception, since it was only after this
marvellous cure-all was launched that it was "promptly adopted by
the medicoes of the Eclectic schools . . . [and] shortly afterwards
different proprietary concerns introduced it to the public under the
name of echtisia, echthol and echitone."[23]

Satirical comments of this kind successfully obscured from the
public a fact that Dr. Fishbein himself may not have known – that
Echinacea does in fact possess quite remarkable antiseptic and alterative powers, amply confirmed by research, which is why it is attracting so much attention in herbal circles today, and is widely used in
herbal and homoeopathic medicine.*

Decades of successful and intensive use of herbs by the Thomsonians, Eclectics and Homoeopaths of America, and by Coffin and his
followers in Britain were not now likely to recommend them to the
medical profession. On the contrary, patronage by such hopelessly
unscientific systems of medicine only damned herbs by association.

As for the Indian connection in North America, it had been so
thoroughly exploited and debased by the patent-medicine vendors of
the nineteenth century that the mere mention of Indian usage was
almost enough to sink the good name of a medicinal plant. By the
grimmest of ironies, this commercial boom in "Indian" medicine
coincided with the deliberate destruction of that Indian culture and
civilization from which it borrowed its trade-names. While the white
U.S. manufacturers of patent medicines made fortunes out of Zuni
stomach renovators and Seminole Cough Balsam, Comanche Blood

---

* *Echinacea* is the chief ingredient in two herbal products increasingly prescribed by family doctors for upper respiratory tract infections as alternatives
to antibiotics: Potter's Antifect, and the Continental Echinaforce from
Biohorma.

Syrup, Kickapoo Cure-All, and Bright's Indian Vegetable Pills, the Indian himself was being systematically uprooted from his homelands, largely exterminated in a series of battles, and corralled into reserves.

The Indian had not yet been resurrected as the anti-hero of a thousand cowboy films, nor had he yet arisen as the noble savage to haunt the conscience of the United States. He survived unattractively, sullen, idle and degenerate, living in reserves like wild animals in a safari park, dependent on white charity. When Indians occasionally figured in papers quoted in the *Index Medicus* of the 1920s and 1930s, they were no longer the members of a proud master-race: they were now a minority ethnic group with squalid medical problems – like congenital syphilis and chronic alcoholism.

Perhaps beyond all these factors – emotional, professional, and economic – that decided the future of medicine from plants, one more quantity in the equation must be weighed: the *hubris* of a generation that could still, genuinely, believe in scientific progress, and which merrily imagined itself the new Master of Creation, capable of producing in the laboratory a miracle superior to that of the plant itself, capable of more efficient chemistry than the staggeringly intricate processes initiated and completed every micro-second inside the meanest roadside plant, capable of producing better, purer, more powerful drugs.

Such a spirit dictated Morris Fishbein's approving comment on the speed at which plants were being dropped from the United States *Pharmacopœia*: ". . . all the signs and portents indicate that the great deluge of modern scientific chemotherapy is about to wash away the plant and vegetable debris."[24] Only a few years later, Dr. Fishbein was picked to edit the *Journal* of the American Medical Association.

23

Return to Nature

"One may still see in London, especially in the spring, a brightly painted cart driven round and making frequent stops for the sale of refreshing drinks with this flavour [sarsaparilla]. I understand that it is described, with certain other old–fashioned simples, by an agreeable and non–committal word – 'an alterative' ".[1] These words were written in 1925; the "alterative" in question was sarsaparilla, but its status had once been higher than that of a pleasant spring–time tonic. Introduced into Europe from the Caribbean in the sixteenth century as a cure for syphilis, its reputation had see–sawed for centuries, some specialists in syphilis greatly preferring it to mercury, others swearing that it was totally inert, others again using a combination of both.

An article in the *Practitioner* of May 1870 told of twenty–five years continuous use of it for the syphilitic patients of Leeds Infirmary. The writer, Dr. T. Clifford Allbutt, found that large doses of a decoction of sarsaparilla, more than a pint a day, worked wonders for "patients . . . who have gone through many courses of mercury, whose irritable mucous membranes will not bear any more iodide of potassium, and who are so sallow, so worn, so broken down, so eaten up by disease as to seem fit only for the grave. These persons clear up on such quantities of sarsaparilla . . . it will not supercede mercury and iodide of potassium in straightforward cases, but it has its place where these means have failed."[2]

Fifty years later, Leeds Infirmary was no longer using sarsaparilla for its syphilitic cases, and few doctors were still prescribing it. But it never lost its popularity with the general public, and Messrs Potter & Clarke, the leading British suppliers and manufacturers of botanicals, found it one of their best–selling spring herbs. Dr. Buchanan's Blood

Purifier containing seaweed and sarsaparilla sold in 9d. packets; Compound Red Jamaica Sarsaparilla cost 4½d. a packet; for 6d., you could buy a packet of Sarsax powder, which would make two gallons of sarsaparilla beer; and many an anxious man no doubt secretly dosed himself with their Extract of Sarsaparilla with Iodide of Potash – almost the Leeds Infirmary prescription for syphilis.

In the 1930s, Potter & Clarke's delightfully old-fashioned London shop in Farringdon Road, almost under the arches of Holborn Viaduct, attracted a wide cross-section of customers. Office-girls anxious to lose weight came in to have made for them a mixture containing bladderwrack (*Fucus vesiculosis*) – that black rubbery seaweed with the round pod-shaped bubbles which children love to pop – believed to counter obesity by stimulating the thyroid gland. Tired businessmen dropped in for a tonic made of kola, *Cola spp.* – as stimulating as caffeine – and damiana (*Turnera diffusa var. aphrodisiaca*), which as its official name suggests, is believed in Mexico to be especially good for tired businessmen.

Fresh-faced Miss Oakley, who presided over the shop, would also sell you some of the mud-coloured, green and red-speckled leeches kept in a large bowl. But leeches were only a sideline; herbs were what the customers were after. "Herbs are coming back," said Miss Oakley happily in the summer of 1938. "Our sales have gone up a lot recently".[3]

Even the popular press interested itself in this phenomenon. "More doctors are recommending herbal treatment", noted the *Sunday Dispatch* with evident surprise on 22 March 1936. "Scientific investigation has shown that herbal prescriptions once regarded as 'Old Wives' tales' are actually beneficial." A West End doctor said to the *Sunday Dispatch*: "Folk cures are the product of centuries of patient groping after healing knowledge, and many of them seem at least worth inquiring into".[4]

The phrase "old wives' tales" indicates another of the dismissive attitudes that herbal medicine has had to endure – and by which it is still hampered. It is a fact that for thousands of years, in almost every culture, the day-to-day use of herbs has been practised largely by women – the simplicity, the homeliness and the earthy practicality of such a medicine perhaps recommending itself more strongly to the feminine mind than that of the ambitious, out-going male. In many cultures, traditions of herbal medicine have only survived thanks to continuous use in this domestic way, while male-dominated professional medicine discarded them or largely replaced them with stronger, often poisonous drugs, and impressive healing techniques such as the hallucinogenic drugs of the witch-doctor. Thus it comes as no surprise to find that the gentle revolution which again placed medicinal plants firmly in front of the British public was largely the work of two women – Mary Grieve and Hilda Leyel.

Mary Grieve was a Fellow of the Royal Horticultural Society, green-fingered, a passionate gardener, with a lifelong interest in medicinal plants about which her knowledge was encyclopedic. At the outbreak of war in 1914, she was running Whin's Vegetable Drug Plant Farm and Medicinal Herb Nursery at Chalfont St. Peter, in Buckinghamshire. The war produced a crucial shortage of many vital medicinal plants, since at this time England, like America, relied almost entirely on the Continent for its crude drug supplies. Two months after the beginning of the war, the Board of Agriculture & Fisheries issued a pamphlet on "The Cultivation and Collection of Medicinal Plants in England", which made this need known to the general public.

The enthusiasm of the response took everyone by surprise. It resulted in "the indiscriminate cultivation and collection of all kinds of plants . . . with the result that the manufacturers were inundated with parcels of rubbish," while all over the country, "hundreds of small folk . . . cottagers, gardeners, women of modest means, began to ask how they could help in supplying the drug market with English-grown plants with advantage to themselves."[5]

Mr. E. H. Holmes, the Royal Horticultural Society's leading expert on medicinal plants, wore himself out answering queries, giving lectures throughout the country, and writing dozens of articles. In the meantime, a small group, the Herb Growers' Association, sprang into existence as an offshoot of the Women's Farm and Garden Union to guide and coordinate these amateur efforts. The demand for information was insatiable. To meet it Mary Grieve began running special courses at Chalfont St. Peter, and issued a series of pamphlets which made the cultivation of medicinal plants – an occupation which has bankrupted many a hopeful small-businessman – sound delightfully easy and profitable. "Daily we tread underfoot numerous weeds worth hundreds of pounds to any chemist versed in the process of extracting their juices. . . . Just now the saleable value of dried thistle [blessed] is 38s. a cwt . . . So great will be the demand both during the war and after that no garden owner need anticipate having a surplus herb stock on his hands".[6]

She was, it turned out, cruelly optimistic. Demand slumped drastically after the war as cheaper imported supplies again began flowing into the country. At the beginning of World War II – memories of hundreds of disappointed small-holders still vivid in official minds – the Ministry of Health established a special Committee on Vegetable Drugs which went out of its way to discourage amateur herb-farmers: ". . . while the development of organized collection of herbs growing wild is most valuable and should be encouraged, the *growing* of medicinal herbs is a highly specialized industry which is not without its dangers to the inexperienced."[7]

Another official body, the Medical Research Council, was more negative still: "Our advice to the amateur gardener or small-scale cultivator is not to embark on growing medicinal plants unless he has been officially asked to do so. He may well be wasting ground which would be better employed raising food for people or livestock."[8]

In 1939, however, far fewer medicinal herbs were actually being called for – or, indeed, much missed – by the medical profession, apart from the obvious ones like digitalis and belladonna, whereas in the World War I, numbers of herbs were used with regularity. Among them was the tiny fragrant lily-of-the-valley (*Convallaria majalis*), a cardiac tonic with a digitalis-like action which proved "most useful in cases of the gassing of our men at the front", according to Mrs. Grieve.[9]

The wartime popularity of garlic must have gladdened Dr. Minchin's heart: it was widely used in front-line casualty stations as an antiseptic dressing for suppurating wounds, and military doctors praised it to the skies. In 1916 the Government asked urgently for tons of the bulbs, offering 1s. a pound – a very high price indeed – for as much as could be produced.

The wartime shortage of cotton for surgical dressing was acute, so another folk remedy was employed – sphagnum moss (*Sphagnum cymbifolium*), the peasant's bandage, so incredibly absorbent that two ounces of it can absorb up to two pounds of moisture. An enterprising Army doctor, Lieutenant-Colonel Cathcart, had foreseen the cotton shortage at the beginning of the war, and experimented with sphagnum moss as a substitute so successfully that in 1916 it was put on the War Office approved list, and collected nationwide by volunteers. In mossy Perthshire, the Duke of Atholl lent several of his shooting-lodges to accommodate gatherers, and in the Shetland Isles, stern

Presbyterian ministers exhorted their congregation to spend the Sabbath gathering moss. Cleaned, dried, sterilized and loosely packed into muslin bags, the moss was sent to hundreds of front-line first-aid posts, to be moistened with garlic juice diluted with a little water and applied to wounds.[10]

Hundreds of miles from these grim scenes, Mrs. Grieve's students toiled, sweated, and absorbed a little of all she knew about what they had once considered weeds. In 1916 the *Pall Mall Gazette* published a tasteful account of the school, written in that whimsical prose which herbs so maddeningly often inspire. "Poetry and practical utility are most happily combined in that admirable form of war work for women – physic or herb gardening. . . . The garden, which is tucked away behind one of the beautiful Buckinghamshire hedges, even before it is seen, exhales a fragrance of enchanting complexity. . . . Lavender, balsam, myrrh, mint, meadowsweet, southernwood, wild thyme, and other aromatic herbs commingle in 'a most excellent cordial smell'. A white butterfly hovered over the head of a brown-haired girl in an amber tunic who was weeding a bed of chamomile. Near by a fair-haired 'flapper' was digging. An athletic student in a blue smock was wheeling a heavy barrow of weeds. . . . Each one of the three hundred-odd plants here cultivated are potential ministering angels."[11]

This revival of interest in medicinal herbs outlasted the war. It grew among the general public, and it encouraged other women to found, in 1927, the Society of Herbalists, with its headquarters at Culpeper House, Bruton Street, London W.1.

Hilda Leyel, who put her personal fortune into this venture, had grown up botanizing. "That famous headmaster, Edward Thring . . . first taught me botany when I was a baby", she wrote. "I still remember the pride I felt when he strapped the black japanned tin lined with green to my tiny back, and though at the time I was only four and much too young to enjoy searching in the heat for rare plants like Ladies' Tresses and Green Hellebore, the names of the plants, like the dates of the English kings, were impressed on my mind so vividly that it has been impossible for me ever to forget them."[12]

Hilda Leyel was attracted to medicine, but her first anatomy lesson repelled her for life, and she turned back to the more congenial study of medicinal plants, writing books, lecturing and eventually practising as a herbal healer herself. The Society, which was set up as a co-ordinating organization for healers, herb-growers and sellers, worked closely with the National Association of Medical Herbalists, and all her life Hilda Leyel battled energetically for the recognition of the qualified herbal practitioner.

For the millions who still believed that herbal medicine had not made much progress since Culpeper and his astrological references, she published in 1931 *A Modern Herbal*, based on Mary Grieve's pamphlets, which showed the full extent to which traditional plant lore had been investigated and confirmed by modern science.

If Hilda Leyel achieved nothing else, many modern fans would agree that in Culpeper House she founded one of the most uniquely appealing shops in London. Here generations of townswomen, buying deliciously scented soaps, sachets, and pot-pourri, also learned for the first time that there was nothing better for a sore throat than a gargle of red sage, while coltsfoot and horehound were almost magically effective for a nasty cough. More serious cases were seen by Mrs. Leyel herself, a true healer who often had a queue of patients extending out into Bruton Street, and was still seeing patients when she was bedridden with cancer at the age of seventy-seven. For hundreds of customers, this may well have been their first contact with a system of medicine they had not imagined was still being practised.

This rise of public interest in herbal medicine had breathed a new life into the National Association of Medical Herbalists. By 1922 there were 112 students taking their tutorial course, and with a Labour Government in power – likely to be more sympathetic to their cause than a Conservative one – they set about lobbying M.P.s for a Medical Herbalist Registration Bill which would finally give them official status. Over 130 M.P.s promised to help their new-found Parliamentary friend, Commander Kenworthy, to pilot through this Private Member's Bill, and they optimistically watched it receive an unopposed first reading.

But the Bill never reached a second reading, and when approached, the Minister of Health, Mr. Wheatley, remained coldly aloof. The Government would allow no time for the Bill; he could spare no time to receive their deputation. If they had anything important to say, perhaps they would let him have a note of the chief points in writing; "he would be happy to consider it".[13]

The Association dashed off an eloquent letter appealing for Government help in the passage of their Registration Bill. "It is our desire" they pointed out, "to compel a standard of Education and Registration so that the public shall be enabled to differentiate between Bona Fide

Herbalists and those who trade on the name". There was a real demand for their services, they added, "by a large and increasing number of the general public". The Minister wrote back that he could not see his way to recommend that Government help with the Bill should be forthcoming, although he had "carefully considered" the various points they raised.

The Association made a last effort: "We fully realise the tremendous influence brought to bear upon your Predecessors by our opponents" they began, and went on to point out that they, too, had important friends: ". . . our cause has always found favour in the eyes of the not inconsiderable section of the electorate that your party represents . . . a great number of Trade Unions connected with the Labour movement have sent up resolutions in our favour . . . at least half the members are favourable to our cause."[14]

It did no good, and when, in 1930, the osteopaths ran into the same stone wall of official indifference and antipathy, their new Parliamentary friend, Mr. R. J. Wilson, Member for Jarrow, advised the Association to change their tactics for the time being.

Put first things first, he told them: "My advice to you is to continue your educational policy. Make the Medical Herbal practitioner thorough and efficient. Make your diploma a hallmark of sound training. Eliminate the charlatan by the service that your members alone can give: probably the public will do this for you. . . . It should be the effort, from now onwards, of every follower of the various forms of treatment outside the conventional, to enter upon research vigorously."[15]

This letter, read to a Council meeting in September 1930, made a deep impression on them all – they had been attempting to find premises and start a school since the end of the war. In 1928 Lord Clifford of Chudleigh had actually offered the use of four rooms, including an extra large one which could have made a perfect lecture-hall, in a building he owned in Victoria Street. The rent was very moderate – £400 a year, plus something towards the electricity, 3s. a room weekly for cleaning, coal at 1s. a scuttle – and for a moment a vision had danced before the Council's eyes. They would "go out in all directions to obtain funds by means of concerts, dances and other forms of entertainments", while the spacious lecture-room – when not in use by the College, could be sublet to "various societies" as "another source of revenue". Wiser, colder counsels prevailed. At the Annual Conference that year – possibly the sight of the pitifully small number present, a mere twenty-six, was in itself a deciding factor – caution carried the day, and the Victoria Street scheme was turned down by fifteen votes to eleven.[16]

Two years later, Mr. Wilson's letter stiffened their determination, and when their Treasurer Mr. Jennings handsomely offered to pay out of his own pocket the rent for a couple of rooms in Bloomsbury plus the upkeep for the first year, and to provide equipment and a library into the bargain, this much more modest scheme was thankfully adopted. Formally opening the College of Botanic Medicine at 46 Bloomsbury Street, on 19 March, 1931, Mr. Wilson could congratulate them on taking his advice: the Association was on the right track to recognition.

Among the College's first lecturers was a relative newcomer to the Association, Frederick Fletcher Hyde, who in the best British Botanic tradition had followed his father, Council Member Frederick Jesse Hyde, into practice, after graduating in botany with first-class Honours at London University. He turned out to be as dedicated as he was hardworking, as single-minded as he was brilliant: in his twenties he was already planning basic courses in physics, chemistry, zoology and botany for the Association's tutorial training scheme, still run by Mr. W. H. Webb from Southport. In addition to helping his father run their successful practice in Leicester, he was also appointed Secretary of the newly formed Research Department in the mid-1930s, and threw himself into its development with energy. The Association became his life. But even with talent and enthusiasm of this order to staff it, the College was a heavy liability. There were never enough students to keep it solvent and it soon declined to the status of a mere night school. In 1940, under the strain of a staff depleted by mobilization, and heavy bombing in the area, it closed.

Over the years, the Association had grown so used to its lonely, friendless battle for existence, that early in the 1930s it came as something of a shock to members to realise that they were now only one of a number of similar organizations catering to a public which seemed curiously dissatisfied with laboratory medicine, and eager for a more positive approach to the question of its health. Across Europe alternative medicine boomed; fitness classes were crowded; yoga became popular; and homeopaths, osteopaths, naturopaths and herbalists were all busier than ever before.

In the Third Reich, Adolf Hitler's enthusiasm for all things Aryan raised folk traditions to near-religious status. Folk medicine became respectable, Germany's already lucrative drug-plant industry was encouraged as a patriotic duty, new chairs in pharmacognosy were created in universities, and learned papers explored the new significance of this "sunken culture".

In 1933 a law was passed granting to naturopaths and herbalists almost equivalent status with qualified doctors and surgeons, and Rudolf Hess remarked reverently: "I have had experience of the value of natural healing on my own body. Science admits that it is faced with failure. The natural remedy, it seems to me, is to return to Mother Nature".[17] By 1938 Dr. Weiss of Berlin University was noting disapprovingly in the *Deutsche Medizinische Wochenschrift*, "we are in danger of a veritable flood of new special preparations from all sorts of plants, and of popular literature on plant therapy".[18]

The unorthodox practitioners of Great Britain no doubt looked with envy at their colleagues across the Channel. But although almost all agreed in theory to the idea that they ought to join hands against the common foe allopathy, in practice this turned out to be unexpectedly difficult to accomplish. Two former Presidents of the Association resigned or were expelled in 1931, because of their support for the British Institute of Organic Medicine. They later formed the Botano-Therapeutic Institute which occasionally discussed reunion with the N.A.M.H., but never achieved it.

Differences of opinion led to the formation of yet another splinter group, the British Herbalists' Union. And among other unorthodox bodies which came and went in the 1930s were the British Health Freedom Society, the Society of Physical Medicine, and the Congress of Natural Healing.

Taking advantage of these divisions, the wartime Government – in a Parliament heavily populated by regular doctors (there were as many as sixty of them) – suddenly struck. In 1941 the Pharmacy and Medicines Act was rushed with indecent haste onto the Statute Book: the Association awoke to the fact that overnight they had become illegal practitioners, since one of its sections removed their right to supply herbal medicines direct to their patients. "It was," said Frederick Fletcher Hyde later, "one of the greatest shocks of my professional career".[19]

The Act aroused a much more hostile public reaction than the Government had anticipated, and the Association, with powerful support from Hilda Leyel, contested it vigorously. As far as the herbalists were concerned, it remained, in effect, without power. The

N.A.M.H. members continued to practise, while the Government was induced to promise that in any future medical legislation, the herbalists would be consulted.

When the time came, however, Aneurin Bevan – drafting post-war plans for the new National Health Service, turned out to be quite as unhelpful as his predecessor. He pointed out to the Association – now formally re-named the National Institute of Medical Herbalists – that even together with the British Herbal Union, they represented only some 500 of the country's 1,200 herbal practitioners, for whom they could thus hardly claim to speak, while their educational programmes simply were not good enough.

In anticipation of such criticisms, the General Council for Natural Therapeutics had already been set up to represent herbalists, osteopaths and naturopaths. Member organizations were urged to eliminate under-trained or part-time practitioners, and a register of properly qualified practitioners was being compiled. Like other bodies before and since, however, the Council soon gently fragmented itself out of effective existence.

In an effort to resolve their differences and speak with one voice, the Institute and the Union then held joint annual Conferences for three years running, at which the training of their members, and a name for a new joint body were hotly debated. The rock on which all their efforts foundered, however, was the question of the trading herbalist, operating on shop premises who had never taken any qualifying examination. Both organizations had numbers of such members; but they were raising their educational sights fast, at this time, attracting graduates and professional people, and the image of the backstreet herbalist was precisely the one they wished to play down.

Then, as now, there was a real need for some kind of training scheme for the trading herbalist, who is called on for his advice in just the same way as the corner chemist is asked to prescribe for passing customers. And there was no reason why the Institute and the Union could not have got together and worked out a two-tier system of membership which would cater both for such traders – the equivalent of the French *herboristes* – and those who wanted to become full-time practitioners, a working compromise which would have resulted in a single, much more powerful Herbal Association.

As so often in the history of Botanic Medicine, however, there were strong personal issues involved, neither side was willing to sink its individual identity, and the two organizations continued on their separate courses – as they have done to this day.

To resolve the training question for the British Herbal Union, its Directors then founded a company, the General Council and Register of Consultant Herbalists, incorporated in 1960: candidates must complete a basic course followed by a spell of clinical training, and pass a qualifying examination before being accepted for membership, after which they can describe themselves as "Registered Medical Herbalists". The Institute preferred to toughen up their membership qualification by stages. Today, the N.I.M.H. full-time and external courses last four years, and no new members are accepted unless they reach the exacting standards demanded by the Examination Board.

The attitude of the postwar Labour government was hardly encouraging to expensive educational schemes: some members argued that they had already undertaken to run full-time five-year courses and must stick to their plans, while others pointed out that after they had bankrupted themselves setting up the school, Mr. Bevan was perfectly capable of saying, "You have put this into operation upon your own responsibility, and in my view it is not sufficiently comprehensive".[20]

In the end the question resolved itself. Mr. Bevan finally offered the Institute participation in the National Health Service on terms which, while giving them the smallest possible income from N.H.S. prescriptions, would also have subordinated them to the regular medical profession. They opted to remain outside – and the immediate incentive for shouldering the almost impossible financial burden of the full-time school disappeared, although many members argued unhappily that they could not afford to go ahead without it.

Its counsels divided, its school still non-existent, its very existence legally in question, the Institute drifted through the 1940s and the 1950s; perhaps not since the last decades of the nineteenth century had its future seemed so bleak. Its members could, however, comfort themselves with the thought that in Britain, herbal medicine did at least still exist and had some kind of future.

In America the last Eclectic School, in Cincinnati, had closed in 1938, while the Physio-Medicals – for so long the friends and the inspiration of British herbal medicine – were heard of no more. Even after Flexner had swept the landscape bare of effective competition, however, the American Medical Association continued to fret about what it called the "Cultist Menace", and in 1921 it invited representatives from "many of the foundations prominent in the field of public health" (its old Rockefeller and Carnegie allies), to consider "the rise of

antivivisectionists, chiropractors, osteopaths, and non-medical cult-
ists". But the conclusion they all came to was that given enough
publicity, the nuisance might go away of its own accord. Since then
the A.M.A. has been indefatigable in its self-imposed duty of edu-
cating the American public about "quackery" of every persuasion,
while keeping tight control of all the medical schools in the United
States.

They came to believe their own propaganda: an Associate Professor
of Applied Physiology at Yale alluded scornfully, in 1934, to "the sad
fact that for fourteen or fifteen centuries after Galen's time sick men
and women and children were dosed with the useless 'herbs' that
Galen had recommended". They were, he went on, "the sort of
medicaments that old women in the country sometimes use even now
for home remedies – horehound water and onion syrup, sassafras tea
and tansy stew. . . . Even now herb drugs – and some few of them are
of course very valuable in medicine – are called Galenicals".[21]

This contemptuous attitude was, however, less common than it had
been a decade earlier. Slowly, the pharmaceutical companies were
coming round to the view that plants might be worth closer investigation after all. The distinguished British pharmacognosist, Professor
J. W. Fairbairn, speculated in 1953, in the *Journal of Pharmacy and
Pharmacology*, on some of the reasons for this change of heart: "The
impression had been growing, since the recent discovery of vitamins
and hormones, that future medical treatment would soon become
independent of the 'bottle of medicine'. . . . The spectacular results of
sulphonamide therapy, however, served to focus attention again on
the use of materia medica as a means of treating disease. The branch of
materia medica which received the greatest stimulus was naturally
concerned with synthetic organic chemicals but slowly the stimulating effect extended to natural products of vegetable and animal
origin . . . especially since the discovery of the antibiotics. I think it is
safe to say that there is now a greater scientific interest in the vegetable
materia medica than for the last decade or two."[22]

Even before the revolution sparked by the discovery of Prontosil,
however, at least one American pharmaceutical company had reason
to feel much more open-minded about plants. The little shrub Ma
Huang (*Ephedra sinica*) had been a standby in Chinese medicine for
centuries, its antispasmodic and stimulant properties recorded as early
as the sixteenth century. In 1887 a Japanese chemist isolated its alkaloid
ephedrine, and in the 1920s Eli Lilly's chemist Dr. K. K. Chen took

another look at it. Soon after, Eli Lilly began marketing it to the Western world as a highly useful therapy for asthma, and a stimulant to the central nervous system.

Apart from the huge antibiotic field, postwar research initially concentrated on drug-plants whose pharmacological activity was already well-known – such as senna, rhubarb, may apple (*Podophyllum peltatum*), and green hellebore (*Veratrum viride*). It turned out that some of the alkaloids in *Veratrum* were effective against high blood pressure. Podophyllum was another obvious choice for investigation, with its long history in folk and Indian medicine of use against skin cancer. Today the resin of podophyllum is still the drug of choice in the treatment of soft warts (*condylomata acuminata*) although the surrounding skin has to be carefully protected, and it is also being studied for anti-tumour action. A staggering field opened up to research chemists, in which the unimaginable prize might be the answer to cancer.

Then in 1947 chemists at the Swiss company Ciba began looking at a plant long popular in Indian folk medicine, *Rauvolfia serpentina*. Their attention had been drawn to it by published accounts of experiments in India, where researchers had registered definite drops in the blood pressure of hypertension patients who had been given crude extracts of the plant. While the Ciba chemists were still hard at work, a report describing even more promising results appeared in the *British Heart Journal*, and a Massachusetts heart specialist, Dr. Wilkins of Boston, following up this lead, gave the powdered root of *Rauvolfia* to fifty patients suffering from high blood pressure. Over the next eight months their blood pressure steadily dropped. With beautiful timing, Ciba were able to announce that they had isolated the alkaloid responsible for this action – reserpine – and soon they were marketing it as the drug Serpasil.

The saga that finally convinced pharmaceutical companies everywhere that they could no longer afford to ignore plants was that of the American research chemist, Russell E. Marker. This unpredictable genius, funded by a pharmaceutical company, had devoted his academic life at Pennsylvania State College to work on steroids. Steroid is the collective name for a group of chemical compounds inside the human body, which had been recently tracked down and studied by endocrinologists. Among these steroids are the body's hormones, chemical messengers sent out to other parts of the body of such glands as the pituitary, the thyroid, and the hypothalamus. The gonadotrophic hormones sent out by the pituitary gland of a woman in the course of her menstrual cycle stimulate a follicle within her ovary which then produces, in turn, two more hormones, œstrogen and progesterone. These two hormones were exceedingly interesting to the medical profession in the 1930s and 1940s, since if they could be produced synthetically, control of a huge range of gynœcological problems and disorders seemed within reach, while the male hormones testosterone and androsterone might have equally exciting possibilities.

But the hormones proved staggeringly expensive and complicated to extract from the obvious animal sources. The ovaries of 50,000 sows yielded a paltry 20 milligrammes of progesterone to one researcher in 1934, while a whole ton of bulls' testicles had given up less than 300 milligrammes of pure testosterone.[23] Marker became convinced that hormones could be more simply and much more cheaply produced by starting with a plant, some of which were known to contain steroid "precursors", which could be chemically transformed into synthetic hormones. He began looking at hundreds of plants, the most promising of which was the Mexican yam (*Dioscorea mexicana*). After lengthy studies, Marker concluded that he could convert one of its constituents, diosgenin, into progesterone by an efficient five-step process, which could easily be adapted for cheap mass-production: a further three-step process would then convert it into testosterone!

If a twelfth-century alchemist's apprentice had casually related to his master that he had, actually, discovered how to transmute crude carbon into pure gold, he could hardly have expected a greater degree of scepticism than Marker's cool announcement provoked in the pharmaceutical company funding his research. It was so much too good to be true that they simply did not believe him. Whereupon Marker walked out on both the company and the University, and moved to Mexico City, where he set up his own laboratory in a tiny rented cottage. There he calmly produced, from *Dioscorea*, four and a half *pounds* of progesterone – at that time, worth eighty dollars a gramme. A few weeks later, he set up a small Mexican firm called Syntex S.A. to market the new synthetic hormones, prices dropped worldwide, and the "Pill" suddenly became a commercial possibility.[24]

With plants making the headlines in this way, life suddenly looked brighter for the Cinderellas of the natural sciences, America's pharmacognosists banded together to assert their new importance in the American Society of Pharmacognosy, launched in a beer cellar in

Chicago in 1956, which subsequently took over publication of the monthly journal *Lloydia*, while in Germany another clearing-house for information in this field was set up in April, 1953. *Die Gesellschaft für Arzneipflanzenforschung und-Therapie* (The Society for Research into Medical Plants and Therapy) began to publish – as did *Lloydia* – in its monthly multilingual journal, *Planta Medica*, papers on research into medical plants from all over the world.

One after another pharmaceutical companies now became keenly interested in this neglected source of new products. They were not, however, interested in just any old plant that grew in their own backyards, as any really promising research would at once have all their competitors homing in on the same readily obtainable source. What they were after was some remote, exotic plant that nobody had ever heard of, and that they could have entirely to themselves. If a witch-doctor gave them the lead, so much the better: since *Rauvolfia*, folk medicine had mild scientific respectability, and modern drugs from the jungle made colourful copy for press handouts.

But U.S. companies now paid the price for Flexner's heavy emphasis on organic chemistry at the expense of pharmacology: there were not enough experts in the field. As a result, some extremely expensive mistakes were made – all of them detailed later with a certain satisfaction by the American pharmacognosist Dr. Norman Farnsworth.[25]

There was, for instance, the pharmaceutical company that set up a programme for which leads were to be supplied by combing works on medical botany, and concentrating on a selection of plants in some remote and primitive country. Around twenty promising plants were noted, and orders were given for collection of a kilogramme of each. Many of these plants, tested in the laboratory in the U.S., turned out to have highly intriguing pharmacological activity. Unluckily, very little of this could be duplicated in later tests with new supplies of plant material, because the company had failed to ensure what would have been elementary procedure to any trained pharmacognosist – correct identification of the particular species. Even in closely related species, activity can vary enormously.

A much more expensive mistake cost another firm nearly $500,000. A physician with a long experience of tropical conditions suggested to them that he should spend some time in a remote jungle, observing – as a doctor – what plants used by the local medicine-men were actually effective, then shipping consignments of them back to the company for study. The company delightedly agreed to his offer, congratulating themselves on a novel and superior approach to the whole question. The physician carried out his part of the programme most conscientiously. He collected some highly promising plants, made copious notes on them all, numbered them, and then prepared voucher specimens so that each could be identified back home. Unfortunately, he numbered these specimens by writing on a leaf of each with a ball-point pen. Worse yet, the specimen plants were so badly packed that many of the leaves crumbled to dust, and almost none of the numbers were still legible. The promising plants could not be identified – and the $500,000 the company paid the doctor for his research went straight down the drain.[26]

In the small world of research chemistry, stories like these made the rounds, pharmaceutical companies who felt they had made fools of themselves resolved to be wiser, and plant-research programmes sank back to the lowest level of priorities. Farnsworth hazards one more reason for their decline in popularity: a sceptical attitude among these workers was hardly likely to produce good results. That such scepticism was still common was noted in 1964 by a man who had made his career in pharmaceutical research, Stanley Scheindlin of Richardson-Merrell, Inc. ". . . One thing hasn't changed in the last twenty or twenty-five years," he wrote in the *American Journal of Pharmacy*. "Back in 1942 many scientists considered plant drugs the remnant of a dark age, from which we would soon be liberated by organic synthesis . . . and today, pretty much the same attitude prevails."[27]

Moreover, some of the economic prizes had turned out to be fool's gold after all. It often happened that some glamorous new plant-derived drug product – an alkaloid synthesized at vast cost, perhaps – turned out to be so demonstrably inferior to the whole plant extract when it came to be tried on patients that it was not worth marketing. The chemists who had been so proud of their achievement in synthesizing reserpine in 1956 might have saved themselves the bother. Some doctors continued using the powdered root – fewer side-effects, they claimed – and it soon turned out that reserpine extracted straight from the plant was cheaper anyway – seventy-five cents a gram as opposed to the synthetic version which cost $1.25.

One way or another, pharmaceutical companies had largely decided by the early 1960s that the plant game was not worth the trouble, and they happily returned to the molecular synthesis they had so many reasons to prefer. Soon, spinning the molecules of an already familiar compound, one German firm struck gold. It had produced, and was soon busily marketing all over Europe, what seemed like the perfect sedative, apparently so little toxic that even pregnant women could take it safely. They called it Thalidomide.

24

The
Price of Miracles

The measure of success of alternative medicine is the degree of public disillusionment with the orthodox medical system of the day. The quack's triumph is the doctor's failure, and the millions in the early nineteenth century who turned to homoeopathy and Thomson, to Beach, to Coffin, to Botanic Medicine, were not so much attracted by a theory, or lured by the idea of dosing themselves with herbs, as they were thoroughly dissatisfied with a therapy that killed as often as it cured, and was painful as well.

But the disillusionment with modern chemotherapy that in the early 1960s began filling the appointment books of herbalists and homoeopaths, osteopaths, naturopaths and acupuncturists went much deeper than this, because the hopes it had raised had been correspondingly higher. For years the public had been reading headlines that announced one therapeutic miracle after another. "Cortisone Breakthrough for Arthritis," "New Hope for Heart Patients," "Hormones to End Menopause?" carolled the newspapers. When the National Health Service was set up in Britain in 1947, it was actually believed that merely extending the benefits of medical care to the entire population would bring about a dramatic improvement in the public health: thereafter, much sickness would go away – and the nation's health-care bill would begin dropping steadily.

Setbacks like the Thalidomide tragedy were a cruel awakening. The public now learned – many of them for the first time – that there was a price to be paid for "magic bullets". It was called an "Adverse Reaction", it was unplanned, unwanted, unforeseeable – and sometimes fatal.

They learned that Ehrlich's dream of the "magic bullet" – the completely selective drug, homing in on its target while leaving intact the surrounding physical environment – was after all a dream. "Selectivity . . . is never absolute", said Professor René Dubos of the Rockefeller Institute, at a symposium on drugs in 1963. "Even a highly selective drug is . . . likely to react with some structure other than the one for which it has been designed. . . . Absolute lack of toxicity is an impossibility because absolute selectivity is a chemical impossibility".[1]

The public slowly realized, too, that quite often doctors had not the faintest idea how their drugs worked, how they might behave inside the body, or how other tissues – those not in the target area – might be affected by them. The comparison of an apprentice garage-hand tinkering with the engines of Concorde suggests itself.

Some of these adverse reactions are now being seen as allergic in character – the body reacting to an unfamiliar chemical structure which it cannot assimilate – according to Dr. Stephen Lockey, an American immunologist who has made a long study of such allergies. One of his patients had an allergic reaction to six different "chemical" diuretics, one after another. He finally put her on one a herbalist might have prescribed in the first place: an extract of *Taraxacum officinale* or common dandelion, and this time there was no allergic reaction.[2]

The toxicities produced by some drugs, according to clinician Dr. Dickinson Richards, are relatively easy to deal with: ". . . largely symptomatic and reversible . . . and . . . except in the very few serious or fatal reactions there appeared to be no lasting or inherent damage to the host".[3] Much more worrying, in his opinion, is another type of adverse reaction, produced by the modern generation of drugs that mimic the body's own functions: "With the advent of cortisone and the steroid series, the alterations were more profound and might be characterized as metabolic toxicities . . . a deep-seated and sometimes irreversible change involving the whole bodily mechanism." Another group of metabolic toxicities is evoked by "drugs which block at some stage or another some essential metabolic process, such as cholesterol synthesis."[4]

By the early 1960s, adverse drug-reactions of all these different kinds had become so common that they could be described as a new disease. And the new disease was given a name – "Iatrogenic" or doctor-induced – by Ivan Illich, who opened his attack on allopathy, *Medical Nemesis*, with the flat statement: "The medical establishment has become a major threat to health".[5] Iatrogenic disease was spreading like measles in a kindergarten: ". . . one seventh of all hospital days is devoted to the care of drug toxicity, at a yearly cost of $3,000,000,000", reported a U.S. Government Task Force on Prescription Drugs in 1969.[6]

Many of these adverse reactions were so slight as to pass almost unnoticed in the people suffering them – mild headache, a skin rash, upset stomach, temporary blurring of vision. Other reactions were a great deal worse.

In 1970 the British Imperial Chemical Industries marketed a new drug for the treatment of angina patients, called practolol or Eraldin. Soon the little blue pills were being prescribed as a "breakthrough" in the treatment of heart cases, since unlike many of its competitors the drug seemed not to affect the air passages, making it particularly suitable for those angina patients who also suffered from asthma or bronchitis. Four years later I.C.I. began warning doctors of two side-effects that had begun to show up. One of these was damage to the eyes: the worst cases went blind, others found that their tear-ducts had dried up, and they suffered miseries all day long from dry, gritty eyes. The other side-effect was a curious form of peritonitis, in which layers of tissue in the abdomen fused together. As more and more reports came in, I.C.I. finally withdrew the drug from the market, and paid over substantial sums in compensation.

Dry eyes are less horrific than limbless babies, and while the case of Eraldin was much less dramatic than that of Thalidomide, in some ways it was much more disturbing. I.C.I. had complied with every single test designed to secure the safety of a new drug. Eraldin had been tested exhaustively on animals – in none of whom had either of these reactions appeared. It had been tried on more than 2,000 patients, most of them closely supervised, over three years, without any such reactions being reported. And I.C.I's research director at the time, Dr. Garnet Davy, admitted that he had regarded Eraldin as the nearest thing to "the perfect drug".[7]

A committee of drug experts, meeting after the Eraldin incident in 1976, made a public statement pointing out that even more extensive laboratory testing could not have prevented this misfortune. "Medicines can never be entirely safe", they said. "Despite extensive testing and monitoring, unforeseen and unpredictable adverse reactions will continue to occur".[8] The accuracy of this statement was grimly underlined more than a year later. In December 1977 the *Lancet* told of six Eraldin victims who had been discharged after treatment for various side-effects, and then months later – long after they had stopped taking the little blue pills – had all begun to suffer from increasing shortness of breath. The drug had caused a thickening and stiffening of the lung and chest-cavity lining.

Other disquieting aspects of the glorious drug revolution began coming to light. Doctors were supposed to report on drug side-effects that they noticed to the appropriate monitoring authority – in Britain, the Committee on Safety of Medicines, or C.S.M. But as an article on the Eraldin story in the *Observer* pointed out in September 1976, the C.S.M. regularly claimed in its annual report that doctors were under-reporting, and it is easy to see why.[9] No doctor wants to believe that a drug he has himself prescribed can be making his patient worse, not better. Some of the Eraldin victims were ignored by their doctors even when they reported quite serious side-effects. A survey on prescribing habits in *Woman's Own* in May 1978 showed that sixty per cent of women who noticed side-effects after taking a drug – including "fairly serious" ones – told their doctors about them, but nearly three-quarters were told to go on taking the drug.[10] American doctors have an extra reason to be reluctant to report a side-effect: if it is a really serious one, they could be amassing evidence against themselves in a malpractice suit.

In *A Dictionary of Drugs*, published in 1971, the authors Dr. Richard Fisher and Dr. George Christie had some reassuring words for their readers: "Your doctor will prescribe only what he believes will help you; he knows your make-up, your illness and the drug, and he will warn you about possible untoward reactions if he thinks a warning is necessary."[11]

This cautious and well-informed physician is sadly rare, as the Eraldin saga itself showed. Doctors were repeatedly warned of the drug's dangers in 1974, but 290,000 prescriptions for it were written the following year by doctors in England and Wales; and even after the drug had been officially withdrawn in 1976, another 2,900 prescriptions were issued to unsuspecting patients. How did this happen? Forgetfulness, pressure of work, too much information to digest about too many drugs are all possible explanations for such carelessness. The most likely one, though, is the fact that far too many prescriptions are not written out by doctors at all: they are repeats written by unqualified auxiliaries – usually a helpful receptionist trying to save the doctor – and patient – time.

If drugs are magic bullets, it now appeared many of them get aimed at the wrong targets. The antibiotic chloramphenicol was discovered by the U.S. company Parke-Davis, and marketed in 1949 as Chloromycetin. Doctors were enthusiastic about its powers against typhoid and other fairly rare diseases caused by gram-negative bacteria – there still is no better antibiotic in these cases – but reports began coming in quite soon of side-effects which included severe, and even fatal blood disorders. By 1953 the F.D.A. had issued strong warnings, recommending that it should only be used for the original small range of serious diseases. Fourteen years – and several warnings – later, the dangers of chloramphenicol were given enormous publicity in the U.S. press following a Senate hearing on drugs, and sales at last began to drop. But when the A.M.A.'s Council on Drugs studied the case-histories of chloramphenicol victims, it found that in less than ten per cent of these ought the drug to have been resorted to at all. Like antimony three centuries earlier, a powerful and dangerous drug had been irresponsibly prescribed for a host of totally unsuitable conditions – including sore throat, asthma, mild unidentifiable fevers, iron-deficiency anæmia, earache – and the common cold. And antibiotics generally – which are effective against bacteria – are still widely prescribed today for virus infections like mild flu or heavy colds against which they are inappropriate.

As with antimony and mercury, many doctors appear curiously indifferent to the damage drugs can do. In the wake of the Thalidomide tragedy, the prescribing of drugs for pregnant women dropped sharply. The *Medical Letter* – an impartial, non-profit American periodical that publishes regular assessments of drugs – recommended that only urgently-needed drugs should be prescribed, "especially during the first trimester or close to the time of delivery".[12]

"I am four months pregnant, and taking drugs for nervous tension and migraine", wrote a reader to the British magazine *Woman's Own* in May 1978. "I worry about taking them now I'm expecting a baby, but my doctor doesn't seem to understand these worries".[13] Very likely not: since Thalidomide, the proportion of pregnant women taking drugs prescribed by their doctor, and the average number taken by each, has not gone down in Britain, and in the U.S. it has actually gone up slightly according to a survey published in 1977.[14]

It would be nice to believe that all the companies marketing and making fortunes out of drugs are well aware of their heavy responsibility to the public, and high-principled in their marketing techniques. More often, the evidence suggests that they are well aware of their responsibility to their shareholders, and their marketing techniques are those of any large corporation. In *The Drugging of the Americas* (1976) the author Milton Silverman showed that "multinational drug companies say one thing about their products to physicians in the United States, and another thing to physicians in Latin America". In promotional literature sent out to these countries – where there is no F.D.A. to police them, and proprietary drugs are often bought over the counter without a prescription* – Silverman showed that some very well-known U.S. companies were glossing over the hazards and exaggerating the usefulness of the drugs they were exporting. Parke-Davis in the 1970s was marketing its Chloromycetin in the United States as suitable only for a limited range of life-threatening infections. But for Mexico and Central Latin American countries, they were promoting it for use in dysentery, tonsillitis, ear infections, phlebitis, ulcerative colitis and syphilis, among others.[15]

Public disenchantment with drugs today is both fuelled by, and reflected in the press coverage they receive. Increasingly, this is highly critical, with many newspapers and magazines rightly taking the view that if the public cannot be adequately protected from such risks, they are at least entitled to be made aware of them. Today, when the public reads about drugs over breakfast, they are more often wonder-drugs that have gone wrong. "Valium, the most commonly prescribed drug in Britain, may accelerate the growth of cancer. It has this effect in rats", began a *Daily Mail* story in 1979.[16] " '100 per cent risk' for women on Pill", said the headline in the *Evening Standard* in summer 1979.[17] The French weekly *L'Express* ran a story in 1975 on medicine-madness – "La Folie des Médicaments."[18] The startling cover picture showed a transparent human head stuffed with a multicoloured variety of pills, and the story was heavily critical of excessive prescribing by drug companies. " 'Cures' that make the aged ill", was the *Sunday Times* headline for a 1976 story on the elderly who were suffering, simply, from over-medication.[19] In an earlier article in the same newspaper criticism of the widespread use of tranquillizers was headlined "Is it time to stop taking the tablets?"[20] A 1977 *Daily Express* feature that enquired in its title "Does it have to be drugs with

---

*As late as 1975 I myself bought over the counter, in a pharmacy in southern Spain, some suppositories that had been warmly recommended by a Spanish friend for my daughter's bad cough. They were specially formulated for children, and the pharmacist, too, was equally enthusiastic about their usefulness in a cough – they contained chloramphenicol.

everything?", concluded that "Potent and toxic drugs are now scattered so widely about by careless doctors that internal pollution is nearly as desperate a threat as the external kind".[21]

If the Thalidomide story had happened ten years earlier than it did, when the myth of scientific progress still seemed faintly credible, its impact might have been softer. But by the mid-1960s a generation was turning its back on progress and proclaiming flower-power instead. By the 1970s the cult of nature was no longer limited to the young. Health-food shops were booming, health magazines doubled their circulations, the public couldn't get enough books on nutrition, and "country" and "natural" became the two most overworked words in advertising copy – as in "natural country goodness".

Concern for the environment replaced the former careless assumption that it was there to be exploited: in America Barry Commoner, its self-appointed champion, became almost a cult figure. A decade earlier Rachel Carson's *Silent Spring* proclaimed the massive damage that chemical pollutants were inflicting on the environment, and it was inevitable that people also should begin to wonder about the damage that chemicals might be doing to the internal human environment.

Hardly surprisingly, herbal medicine began once more to enjoy an enthusiastic following. This time, there was no Thomson to lead the revolt against orthodox medicine, but this time, no such figure was necessary. In Britain, Culpeper House began opening new branches all over the country, and health-food shops extended their range of herbal remedies. New editions of Culpeper and Gerard appeared; Penguin Books issued a paperback version of the Mary Grieve's 1931 *Modern Herbal*; and dozens of new "herbals" appeared. Most of them were slim paperbacks that contained little more than a rehash of popular herbal writing, but for the first time since the 1830s, the herbal achieved coffee-table status. Instead of going off to their National Health Service doctor and getting prescriptions for next to nothing, more and more people began seeking out their local herbalist – if there was one to be found – and paying for his herbal prescriptions and advice.

"Natural" herbs must be best for you after all, reasoned large numbers of the general public: much better than all those dangerous chemicals. By "natural" they meant something taken straight from a plant – God-made, as it were. By "chemical" they meant a substance concocted in a laboratory – very definitely man-made. In any discussion about herbal medicine, it is difficult to avoid using these two terms to express a distinction between two kinds of therapy, but strictly speaking, the distinction cannot be expressed as simply as this, and it is important to an understanding of the real issues at stake to be perfectly clear what the word "chemical" actually means.

A chemical compound may be defined as a particular structure composed of molecules arranged in a set pattern. There are hundreds of millions of such structures scattered through the natural world, endlessly recurring with a million minor variations. Every plant is an elaborate complex of such structures: amino acids, steroids, sugars, alkaloids, salts, traces of minerals.

Among the hundreds of chemicals packaged in a single plant are many which exert a therapeutic effect on the human body when it is sick. For millions of years, mankind had tracked down and swallowed these plants in order to feel better, without having the remotest idea why they should have this effect. Later and more sophisticated ages studied and classified these effects: a plant might be, among other things, *antipyretic* or fever-reducing; *vulnerary*, good at healing wounds; *diaphoretic* or perspiration-promoting; *purgative*, helpful in emptying the bowels; *narcotic*, sleep-inducing; or *demulcent*, soothing to irritated tissue.

In the last hundred and fifty years, many of the chemical constituents of plants that were responsible for these different types of activity have been isolated, identified, produced synthetically in a laboratory, and their action closely studied in experimental animals.

When we talk of "chemical" as opposed to "natural" medicine, therefore, we are actually talking nonsense: all medicine, from the greenest witch-doctor brew to the most potent substance concocted in a pharmaceutical laboratory is composed of "chemicals". The difference is in the way they are produced; and in the way they are packaged.

In traditional herbal medicine, and in most of the more recent Western forms of this – Thomsonism, Coffinism, and modern British herbal medicine – the "chemicals" used are those elaborated inside a plant in the natural course of its growth, and presented to a patient in their original "package", suitably treated. The herbalist – like the traditional medicine-man – makes use of decoctions, infusions, distillations, expressed oils, or alcoholic tinctures made from a particular part of the plant – bark, root, leaf, flower, or fruit. What he does not do is break out this or that single chemical compound and use it on its own. (The Eclectics tinkered about with their plants to bolster a particular action or eliminate an undesirable one, but even they never used active principles on their own.)

Modern medicine still makes use of some whole-plant extracts: digitalis-leaf preparations are still preferred by some doctors to the extracted glycosides such as digoxin; a hospital casualty department always has plenty of syrup of ipecac on hand to induce vomiting in patients who have swallowed certain types of poisons; and some doctors still rely on senna or castor oil.

But the assumption of modern medicine – and one eagerly endorsed by the pharmaceutical companies – is that the particular chemical in a plant that has been pinpointed as responsible for its therapeutic action is the only bit of the plant worth bothering with, the rest being not merely worthless rubbish, but an obstacle to the production of that indispensable adjunct of modern medicine, the standardized, "purified" quality-controlled drug.

The drugs mainly used in modern medicine, accordingly, fall into one of four categories. They may be single chemical compounds extracted from a plant and used on their own – such as the reserpine from *Rauvolfia*. They may be synthetic versions of a plant chemical. compound – its molecular mirror-twin, with the identical structure, but prepared in a laboratory from coal-tar instead of occurring naturally in a plant. They may be chemicals based on a metal or mineral such as mercury, bismuth, antimony or sulphur – the "dangerous mineral drugs" against which the nineteenth-century botanic doctors inveighed so eloquently. Or they may be completely novel structures apparently invented by the pharmacist – usually by juggling with the molecular structure of a known chemical compound – which has been shown to give a desired action in, first, experimental animals, and then in human beings.

Rick Carlson has described* how the medical stage came to be set for this pharmacist's dream, the standardized drug: ". . . as medical techniques evolved, their delivery could be systematized. Disease was not an idiosyncratic reaction. Disease was a malfunction in the human machine, either through an internal disorder or through the activity of an external agent. The most effective way to treat disease was first to classify it accurately, and then to apply a like set of techniques designed to produce a like cure in like patients. . . . Today . . . medicine has compartmentalized the body into finer and finer machine parts".[22]

*In the chapter "A New Paradigm?" in *The Frontiers of Science and Medicine* containing the May Lectures of 1974 which were devoted to such controversial aspects of science today as biofeedback, plant response, and healing.

The magic bullets of today are increasingly sophisticated weaponry compared to Ehrlich's original crude missiles. They are not designed to restore general health, or to stimulate the body's own natural healing powers: they are ingeniously devised to suppress this or that painful syndrome of which the patient complains, by blocking or suppressing a bodily function which is seen as undesirable.

Thus allopurinol inhibits the body's production of excessive uric acid – the tiny crystals of which, lodged in joints, produce the burning, throbbing agonies of gout; while cimetidine, prescribed as Tagamet for sufferers from gastric acid, works by greatly reducing the excess production of gastric acid, which does the damage in the first place. To this point, we are in the realm of undisputable fact. In discussing the relative safety and efficacy of different types of a drug the arguments begin to rage.

Opponents of "chemical medicine" argue that the blocking or suppressive action of modern drugs may remove the distressing symptoms of, say, a peptic ulcer or gout, but does not touch the cause. The production of excess amounts of uric acid, as in gout, or of gastric acid, as in cases of peptic ulcer, is not in itself the disease, merely the symptoms of an underlying bodily malfunction, and it is this malfunction which must be attended to before the patient can be fully restored to health. Merely suppressing excess production will certainly alleviate the great pain and discomfort, but does not touch the root cause of the disease. Such suppression may have to be paid for in a trail of side-effects, and although some may be minor inconveniences, others may be life-threatening. Thus rheumatic patients, treated with phenyl-butazone derivatives, may suffer from drug-induced reactions ranging from giddiness and rashes to gastric ulcers, hepatitis, renal failures and acute blood disorders such as aplastic anæmia.

By contrast, argues the herbalist, plants act gently but surely to stimulate the body's own self-healing mechanisms. Medicinal substances packaged in a plant, he maintains, can be safely assimilated by the body, since plants are its natural food. Even if the body is deficient in minerals such as iron, copper or zinc, the easiest way for it to absorb them is, as it were, predigested in a plant. Man and plant are close biological kin: the lifeblood of the plant, its green chlorophyll, has a chemical structure almost identical to the hæmoglobin which is the central constituent of human blood; where chlorophyll has a molecule of magnesium in its structural pattern, hæmoglobin carries a molecule of iron.

Primitive people have a strong sense of this kinship, seeing men, animals, plants as children of the same parents: the sun and the earth. "All living creatures and all plants derive their life from the sun" an old Sioux Indian explained once: "If it were not for the sun, there would be darkness and nothing could grow – the earth would be without life. Yet the sun must have the help of the earth . . . and the action of the sun and the earth together supply the moisture that is needed for life."[23]

The nineteenth-century Botanic Doctors insisted strongly on the biological affinity between plant and man. John Skelton was arguing it forcefully long before the modern science of nutrition was developed: "Is there a deficiency of lime . . . iron or any of the substances, no matter of what kind? There is disease; common sense must tell us, if we can supply the deficiency, that we do all that is requisite to remove the disease; but can it be done by the application of any mineral or metallic substance? Most certainly not, for until that substance has passed through the vegetative state, it cannot be made to assimilate with the 'living fibre'."[24]

Frederick Fletcher Hyde sums it up: ". . . the whole biogenetically elaborated complex in the plant tissue . . . may include active principles . . . together with complex proteins, enzymes, trace elements . . . inorganic salts and ions, chlorophyll and Vitamin C, terpenoids, polycelluloses and pharmacologically potent alkaloids, glycosides and phenols in minute amounts. Such a complex which has been produced in the context of a living cell is found by clinical observation to be more readily assimilable and to elicit far fewer undesirable side-effects than the isolated principle."[25]

Modern herbalists maintain that plants are not only the safest way to administer medicine – but also the most effective. They point out that apart from their active principle, a plant contains other substances which may enhance its therapeutic action or reinforce the healing powers by a synergistic process not always fully understood. Digitalis provides a perfect example of both phenomena: digitoxin and verodoxin are both glycosides found in foxglove, but unlike digitoxin, verodoxin on its own is valueless as a tonic for the heart. Add four parts of useless verodoxin to six parts of digitoxin – which does have a tonic action – and the resulting mix will have the same therapeutic effect as ten parts of digitoxin. Moreover, the resulting brew will be less toxic than ten parts of digitoxin alone would be.

There is some evidence, too, to support another strongly-held belief of herbalists: that extracted active principles on their own – lacking these built-in safety factors, may be substances much too potent for the human body to deal with. Dr. Alec Forbes, a Plymouth doctor who has become one of the strongest advocates of alternative therapies within the ranks of allopathy, mentions *Rauvolfia*, as an example. "It has been in use for thousands of years in Ayurveda as a sedative. Mahatma Gandhi used to drink rauvolfia tea as a nightcap. Yet it has only taken twenty years for its most active alkaloid, reserpine, to start to go out of fashion because, although good for lowering blood pressure and sedation, it can cause severe depression."[26]

Pharmacognosists will concede the relative safety of the whole plant in such cases, as opposed to isolated chemical compounds because this is a difference that they can measure by fairly simple toxicity testing in animals or humans. But talk about "natural affinity" makes them deeply uneasy, and they are inclined to dismiss it as hopelessly unscientific rubbish. "To my mind" remarked one young British pharmacognosist when we discussed the question, "there is no difference at all between allopathic and herbal medicine. You're taking a chemical substance or substances and giving it to a body, and they are exerting an effect. So why raise the red herring that plants are living things and therefore interrelate with and affect the body in some peculiar way? I don't see that it's necessary".

Neither side, however, is likely to convince the other in this particular heated argument. The herbalists' belief that the whole plant is both safer and more effective medicine than isolated bits of it or manmade chemical compounds may be rooted in instinctive faith as much as reason, and reinforced by years of contrasting their own mild plant medicine in practice with what they see of the other kind. But this will not do for the scientist, who is trained to deal in facts rather than general observations: for him, a whole plant is a fact that can never be measured satisfactorily for the purposes of this argument, since it is made up of so many dozens of different chemical compounds, each of which would have to be tested alone or in combination with each of all of the others, separately and in combination – in itself, a long lifetime of research.

Even more heretical to the modern scientific mind trained to deal only with material phenomena is the suggestion that there could actually be any difference between a chemical compound extracted from a plant, and the same chemical structure created synthetically in the laboratory out of coal-tar. The two are chemically identical – there is no more to be said.

Until recently, there was indeed no more to be said, since scientists are not interested in statements about the instinctive belief of primitive people – or, indeed, any statement at all that cannot be verified in the laboratory. But a growing body of perfectly respectable scientific research suggests that there may, after all, be plenty more to be said, and that we are only at the beginning of a new knowledge of what plants and men and life itself are about, and how intricately man and plant interrelate.

It is suggested that plants, in common with all living beings, have a non-physical energy field which may react directly on the "energy field" of people they may be used to treat. Such a concept would not seem in the least strange to primitive people, many of whom act instinctively from such a conviction. The Chippewa Indian medicine-men, for instance, used to make an offering of tobacco to the medicinal plant when they gathered it, solemnly begging it to do its best for them. And most of us believe that there really are people with "green fingers" who are better than the rest of us at growing plants, not because of any technical superiority but because of a sympathetic affinity with the plants in their care.

The average pharmacognosist would probably dismiss such notions out of hand as mere primitive mumbo-jumbo. And he would certainly feel the same way – as indeed would most herbalists, if it comes to that – about the theories of Edward Bach (1886–1936), a gentle Welsh-born bacteriologist, who gave up a lucrative London practice to devote himself to researching healing plants. He became convinced that sun-warmed dew absorbed the vital healing powers of the plant on which it rested, and that this power could be transmitted to pure spring water standing in a glass bowl in full sunlight, in which were placed specific herbs. "His cure was not to attack the disease but to flood the body with beautiful vibrations from wild herbs and flowers, in the presence of which 'Disease would melt away as snow in sunshine.' "[27]

Call it beautiful vibrations, an energy-field, bio-plasma, etheric cosmic forces, bio-dynamism, or what you will, but the evidence for its existence has been fascinatingly reviewed by Peter Tomkins and Christopher Bird in their study, *The Secret Life of Plants*. And when at an international consultation on the use of plants in cancer organized by the World Health Organization in November 1978, Dr. Alec Forbes suggested that this "energy-field" was a factor which deserved careful scientific consideration, he was listened to with attention by the assembled plant experts who later agreed that there should be "open-mindedness" towards such ideas.[28]

Whether or not we accept that there is a biological distinction to be made between man-made chemicals on the one hand, and the medicine extracted from a living plant on the other, the human body often behaves as though there is, and the terrible toll of side-effects exacted by "chemical" medicine is the most eloquent argument possible that such a distinction can legitimately be made.

Until recent times, it would also have seemed a matter of sheer common sense. Oliver Wendell Holmes certainly thought so: "Whatever elements nature does not introduce in vegetables, the natural food of all animal life – directly of herbivorous, indirectly of carnivorous, are to be regarded with suspicion", he told his Harvard medical class in 1861. "Arsenic-eating may improve the condition of horses for a time . . . but it soon appears that its alien qualities are at war with the animal organization. So of copper, antimony, and other non-alimentary simple substances: every one of them is an intruder in the living system, as much as a constable would be, quartered in our household."[29]

The same conviction perhaps lingers unconsciously in the mind of the general public. If so, it would account for the vague but widespread impression that while plants may not be particularly powerful medicine, they cannot do you much harm either. Many plants most certainly can and do: there is no magical guarantee that because they can heal they cannot also slay. Indeed, for years the presumption was that the more powerfully poisonous a plant, the more likely it was to yield useful drugs. Among the outstanding examples of this are henbane (*Hyoscyamus niger*), a useful sedative for long used to induce twilight sleep, overdoses of which can cause dimmed vision, delirium, and death; meadow saffron (*Colchicum autumnale*), the plant successful in gout cases which – incautiously used – causes violent purging and eventually death; and blue flag (*Iris versicolor*), a useful liver stimulant which can produce nausea, vomiting and colicky pains.

But herbal medicine does have one indisputable advantage in safety terms over "chemical" medicine, and that is the fact that almost all its drugs have been in clinical use for centuries of recorded use, often administered by doctors competent enough to notice a particular pattern of side-effects showing up. As pharmaceutical companies, doctors and patients all know, side-effects do not have to be looked for, they have an unpleasant habit of announcing themselves. It seems reasonable to assume that any plant drug with a centuries-long reputation for being perfectly safe as well as effective has probably earned that reputation.

25

Herbs and the Law

The medical *cause célèbre* of the nineteen-sixties and seventies was the Thalidomide Affair. This drug was vigorously marketed as a safe sedative, and widely prescribed for women in the early stages of pregnancy. By the early sixties, an alarming correlation became apparent between the use of Thalidomide in its various forms and the birth of babies with gross physical deformities, of which the most characteristic was the absence, or vestigial development, of the limbs. The drug never received F.D.A. approval in America, and was withdrawn from sale in Britain in 1964, but the tragic consequences could not be reversed and the process of interlocking lawsuits and claims for compensation dragged on into the late nineteen-seventies.

In the wake of the Thalidomide sensation, it became obvious to everybody involved – Government health departments, doctors, drug companies – that the public needed both reassurance and more protection from prescription drugs. In America the Kefauver-Harris Amendment to the Food & Drug Act was rushed through in 1962, giving the F.D.A. powers to demand that in the future drugs be proved effective as well as safe: all drugs would now face much stiffer tests before they could be marketed. (So stiff, someone pointed out, that if aspirin or penicillin were new products they would never qualify.)

In Britain the Ministry of Health, as it was then called, began tentative drafting of a new Medicines Bill in 1964. Fresh in their minds, however – as recorded by Hansard – was the storm that the National Association of Medical Herbalists and the Society of Herbalists, with their high-placed friends, had brought crashing down on their heads in 1941. So this time they nervously sent a memorandum outlining the

Government's proposals to both bodies – who promptly sent copies to everyone involved, including Frank Power, a director of Potter's – the makers of herbal remedies.

Until this time there had been no restriction on over-the-counter sales of proprietary medicines to the public other than those listed in the Poisons Schedule. Potter's – along with several other herbal manufacturers – had a strong business going in this small field which was doing particularly well as demand for non-chemical medicine increased. Power had already heard unofficially that a new Medicines Bill was likely to change all this, and had called a meeting of some of the parties involved. Now, as he read the Ministry proposals, he realized that herbal practitioners and manufacturers alike faced possible ruin. The Ministry proposed to set up scientific committees, with medicine and pharmacy strongly represented on them, to evaluate all medicines on the grounds of safety and efficacy. Grimly, Power convened another, much larger meeting of herbal interests, including Frederick Fletcher Hyde, then President of the National Institute of Medical Herbalists, and representatives of the Society of Herbalists, manufacturers, and retailers. Almost unanimously, this group became the British Herbal Medicine Association. The new Association now approached the Ministry, explaining that they spoke for all the herbal interests likely to be affected by the new Bill. To their relief and delight, they were warmly received: ". . . we were informed that far from there being any desire to injure or kill off herbalism, *the Minister had instructed them that measures must be found to preserve the rights of persons who wished to undertake herbal treatment or to purchase herbal remedies.* We were told that there was still stored in the memory of the Ministry, the furore in Parliament on the passing of the earlier legislation which made them realize the strength in number and in desire of those who wanted the liberty of medicine other than the orthodox which was fast becoming a State department."[1]

The Association at once came to the point which had most alarmed them: was the Ministry really going to demand the same proofs of efficacy and safety for herbal remedies as for modern chemical drugs? If so, neither the herbal industry nor the herbalists themselves could survive, since there was no way by which they could possibly hope to raise the huge sums necessary to finance testing. They waited anxiously for the answer, and heard it with a deep sigh of relief: the Ministry "would accept as proof or safety and efficacy the fact that a herb had been in use for a long period without giving any ill-effect and presumably producing results to satisfy the consumer. We were further told that a herb for which a monograph appeared in any standard reference book and was not poisonous would be acceptable."[2]

This declaration was historic. Like the other great landmark in the history of British herbal medicine, the 1548 statute of Henry VIII, it was made in response to pressure from influential people and in recognition of deep public feeling. But it put the Association in a spot. What "standard reference book" could they possibly produce to the medical and pharmaceutical gentlemen of the probably-hostile scientific committee, which they would consider acceptable? Excellent monographs on many of the American herbs they used had appeared in American works of pharmacognosy such as those of John Uri Lloyd. But some of the herbs most relied on in British herbal practice appeared in no up-to-date reference book although papers on them were scattered through the literature. They could hardly put forward Mary Grieve's *Modern Herbal* – nearly a quarter of a century out of date – nor Potter's own delightful *Cyclopedia of Botanical Drugs*, written largely for the general public.

There was only one possible answer: to produce their own, up-to-date reference work. A scientific committee was established, with Fletcher Hyde as Chairman, which had as its object the compiling of a new *British Herbal Pharmacopœia*, containing monographs on every botanical agent in general use. The scientific committee eventually included four distinguished pharmacognosists, Professor E. J. Shellard, Dr. T. J. Betts, Dr. F. J. Evans and Dr. Betty P. Jackson; Florence Fletcher Hyde, a botanist and chemist; Dr. M. J. R. Moss and Mrs. M. B. Robinson as its pharmacist members; and Harry Hall of Potter's as its overworked secretary. Among its medical members was Dr. C. E. R. Winer, a physician who happened to be unusually knowledgeable about herbs, Dr. J. B. Williamson, and Dr. B. Howarth.

The *Pharmacopœia* came out in stages, the first part dealing with 115 herbs appeared in 1976, the second with 83 monographs in 1979, while the third and final part is still in preparation: at intervals monographs are revised and updated. Much of its material was drawn from papers published in the swelling tide of new scientific journals about medicinal plants, but much more was original, based on research specially carried out for this publication, and each draft was written and re-written after careful review at the Committee's meetings. The new *Pharmacopœia*, unlike Mary Grieve's herbal, is not designed for the lay reader, who probably would be unable to make head nor tail of the technicalities. It lists useful references, indications, contra-indications, combinations of herbs which have been found successful, standards and dosages.

While the scientific committee toiled on, the Government produced its Bill. To the consternation of the B.H.M.A., and despite Ministry promises, it would have made practice completely impossible for the consulting herbalist. He or she was no longer allowed to make house calls and only to prescribe for patients who called in person. Refill prescriptions could only be collected by the patient in person – even if extremely ill and supposed to be in bed. Only crude or powdered herbs could be used, either with or without water: there were to be no more of the useful concentrated extracts, solid extracts, tinctures and tablets which herbalists purchased ready-made and standardized by suppliers like Potter's; no more ointments or distilled waters or lotions, no more pills and suppositories. No non-herbal ingredients of the simplest kind could be used in the preparation of medicines by the practitioners for their patients. And the number of herbs they were allowed to use was drastically curtailed – "scores of active and useful herbs would have been withdrawn from us" said Fletcher Hyde.[3]

The British Herbal Medicine Association lobby swung into action. Fletcher Hyde at once wrote a letter to *The Times* pointing out the impossibility of their position under the proposed Bill. *The Times* published it – and every M.P. was sent a copy. Fifty thousand letters of protest were also printed and sent to all consulting herbalists, herbal shops and health-food stores for their clients and customers to sign and send to their M.P.: Mrs. Joyce Butler – a lifelong supporter of alternative medicine – tabled questions in the House of Commons, and Lady Meade Fetherstonehaugh, then President of the Society of Herbalists, lobbied the Peers. No M.P. could remember such a flood of letters of protest, and the Ministry men, Fred Hyde recalled with satisfaction, "were shocked to find out the strength of backing for herbal medicine".[4]

Over the years, point by point, plant by plant, the B.H.M.A. pressed its case home. Finally, in April 1978, the N.I.M.H.'s professional journal, the *New Herbal Practitioner*, was able to celebrate "the culmination of fifteen years of patient negotiations with Parliament and the Department of Health and Social Security; the result of the determination of a handful of men and women who refused to allow herbal medicine to be obliterated from the United Kingdom".[5] It published the Orders under the 1968 Medicines Act affecting the herbs the now licenced practitioners might prescribe; those only to be used up to a certain dosage – these included *Lobelia inflata*, *Atropa belladonna*, and *Colchicum autumnale*; those which might only be used externally – such as *Arnica*; and those which herbalists might no longer use. These last included some potent allopathic favourites – ergot of rye (*Claviceps purpurea*), used to hasten childbirth; may apple (*Podophyllum peltatum*); Savin (*Juniperus sabina*), so dear to the back-street abortionist; and foxglove (*Digitalis purpurea*). Few herbalists would in fact have prescribed any of these.

Herbal practitioners could relax, up to a point, although they still suffered from the old disabilities inflicted on them over the years by an antagonistic medical establishment – and from a ten per cent V.A.T. charge on fees for both their services and their prescriptions the Government had imposed in 1973.

The herbal manufacturers had less reason to be happy. The B.H.M.A. had managed to secure important concessions for them in the final draft of the Bill – under its first proposals many of their products could only legally have been sold at a pharmacy, cutting out their most important customer, the health-food shop. But in the future they would only be allowed to continue in business if they applied for, and got, a manufacturer's licence, and the Ministry inspectors who went around to see that each firm was conforming to its new standards of documentation, tight control over manufacturing processes, and quality control, made it plain that in their eyes, Potter's making herbal remedies and Smith Kline & French turning out potent chemicals were as one.

Some of the smaller herbal firms went out of business as a result; one or two amalgamated with larger companies. Potter's alone spent around £250,000 rebuilding, extending laboratory facilities for extra testing, and hiring more staff. Under the 1968 Act, every proprietary medicine on the market received a Licence of Right, until it could be individually evaluated, but they all had to be registered, new licences applied for in each case, and labels reworded. The free over-the-counter sale of aspirin – which no government in its right mind would dare to limit – probably poses a far greater threat to the public's health than all the herbal remedies and herbalists' prescriptions put together, and many practitioners felt that they were a totally inappropriate target for Government action.

But in practice, the 1968 Medicines Act has done herbal medicine in

Britain a signal service. It has compelled all those concerned to become more scientific, it has imposed higher standards for manufacturers, which in turn can only serve to increase public faith in the product, and it has, if unintentionally, fathered a *Herbal Pharmacopœia* which is the first of its kind in the Western world. And in recognizing that traditional herbal medicine is a special case, which, within limitations, should not be dealt with in the same way as the modern laboratory-produced drugs, the British Department of Health and Social Security has set a precedent which other Western countries may feel they can follow.

Herbal interests are also represented in official legislative bodies such as the Committee on the Review of Medicines, and the Committee on Safety of Medicines.

On the whole, the British patron of herbal medicine can consider himself fairly lucky. But orthodox prejudice against herbs remains as deeply entrenched as ever. The director of one herbal manufacturing company told me "We're always aware of scepticism and hostility – usually quite bluntly expressed. And when we apply for licences for new herbal remedies, we come up against a general brick wall of prejudice – even when they've used the same ingredients in traditional medicine for hundreds of years".

Fred Pestalozzi of Zurich will wryly confirm this. In the early 1950s Pestalozzi was a successful young executive in the family machine-tool business. At the age of thirty he fell ill, the doctors told him he had Menière's disease, and he resigned himself to a short life of decreasing activity. Then someone told him of a marvellous herbal yeast tonic made by an inspired scientist. Pestalozzi went to see him, tried it, and, today, in his late fifties is a highly impressive personal advertisement for the tonic he began to manufacture himself. He called it Bio-Strath Elixir, and in the preparation procedure which he finally settled on, the herbs in the recipe are not simply mixed and bottled. They are fed to *Candida utilis*, living yeast cells – "nearer to a human cell than a plant cell, because it needs oxygen", points out Fred – which in turn ferment a mixture of honey, orange juice and malt. As well as the original Elixir, nine other Bio-Strath remedies have been formulated based on medicinal herbs; among them a Heart Formula containing hawthorn (*Crataegus oxyacantha*); a Kidney-Bladder Formula with dandelion (*Taraxacum*), and bearberry (*Arctostaphylos uva-ursi*); and a Rheumatism Formula containing cowslip root (*Primula officinalis*).

In Switzerland, with its long tradition of herbal medicine, such preparations are not usually subjected to clinical trials to test their efficacy and safety; registration with the appropriate Intercantonal Office for the Control of Remedies is enough. But Pestalozzi was aiming at a much bigger market, including the U.S., and was well aware that there, especially, he was likely to run into problems. He determined that from the outset the Bio-Strath operation should be as super-efficient and as scientifically "respectable" as he could possibly make it. In addition to creating in his Zurich plant a model of stream-lined order, he set about organizing a series of clinical trials which would leave nobody in any doubt of the worth of his product.

The results of some of these were startling, to put it mildly. In double-blind trials with 123 mentally retarded children in the Netherlands, assessors agreed that there was a marked improvement in the ability to concentrate and the power of self-expression of the children who had been taking Bio-Strath.[6] Another trial, carried out on white mice by the Department of Radiobiology at Zurich University, demonstrated that Bio-Strath had a measurable protective action on the fertility of white mice receiving X-ray treatment – the mice being fed Bio-Strath had larger litters after whole-body irradiation, the baby mice were bigger, and they produced more litters.[7] In yet another test, sixty medical practitioners assessed the effect of each of the Bio-Strath preparations on 1,140 patients: the overwhelming majority were so impressed by the improvement produced that they said they would prescribe it again.[8]

Since Bio-Strath contains herbs already in common use, Pestalozzi and his British agent at the time, Michael van Straten, applied fairly confidently for a licence to the Committee on Safety of Medicines, set up by the Department of Health following the 1968 Medicines Act. The appeal was twice turned down. The Committee at length told van Straten that no licence would be issued unless they could produce the standard acceptable evidence that the Bio-Strath preparations were both effective and non-toxic. Pestalozzi then arranged for his products to be tested in a commercial laboratory both for chronic toxicity and for possible teratogenic (fœtus-damaging) effect – perhaps the first time that a herbal remedy had been subjected to the same battery of costly and extensive tests as an ordinary ethical drug.

No adverse effects were seen in any of the preparations in any of the tests. Further trials to prove efficacy showed results that would have fascinated the medical world – if they had been produced by some newly-launched pharmaceutical product instead of by common herbs in an over-the-counter dietetic supplement. Van Straten summed up the impressive findings: "Bearberry . . . is a powerful antibiotic; dandelion is a safe and effective diuretic; thistle increases the flow of bile; hawthorn is a cardiac stimulant; passion-flower increases the strength of the heart contraction but not the rate; primula is a powerful anti-inflammatory agent, especially in arthritic conditions, and is more effective than aspirin without the gastric side-effects".[9]

By the time these tests were concluded, Pestalozzi and van Straten could produce the results of an even more dramatic study: at a leading Swiss cancer hospital, the Inselspital at Berne, a double-blind trial was carried out on patients convalescing from surgery, and receiving radiation therapy. Bio-Strath produced dramatic improvements in appetite, physical activity and general condition: the patients taking it gained an average of around seven pounds more than the control patients.[10]

Eventually, after hearings that lasted a whole day, the Medicines Commission recommended to the Committee that Pestalozzi be granted licences for six of the nine special Formula preparations. "The irony is that none of the ingredients in any of the three that were turned down is actually banned from general sale in Britain", commented van Straten.

The Bio-Strath story is depressing on several counts. The side-effects of X-ray treatment are one of the biggest problems in cancer therapy, since such treatment not only lowers the bodily resistance and general stamina of patients, but is itself potentially carcinogenic. Further tests in rats and mice have indicated that Bio-Strath actually had a tumour-reducing effect, as well as an impressive protective action, and these findings have appeared in such impeccably respectable publications as *Radiologica, Clinica et Biologica*, the *European Journal of Cancer*, and *Hippokrates*. Bio-Strath would thus seem an excellent and completely safe way to protect cancer patients undergoing X-ray treatment, and improve their general condition. Yet its astonishing performance in such cases has been virtually ignored by the medical world. The Inselspital doctors were asked by Pestalozzi to continue their trials for five years, at his expense: after originally agreeing, they changed their minds a month later, and stopped the trials without explanation. Neither Pestalozzi nor van Straten has been able to persuade a single hospital to run similar trials.

The effectiveness of the preparations – using herbs which have been employed in folk medicine for recorded centuries – might have been thought to merit them general medical interest. Aspirin, which can produce gastric complications, is the most widely used drug in arthritic cases today: ought not doctors to be interested in a safe remedy that is even more effective without the gastric problems? Or a safe and effective diuretic? Or an impressive cardiac tonic? Sir Derrick Dunlop, Chairman (1969–1971) of the Medicines Commission, was once reported as saying: "Show me a safe medicine and I will show you an ineffective medicine".[11] But when many doctors were shown medicine that was safe and effective they didn't want to know.

As for the Committee itself, its wary attitude, when faced with preparations containing only familiar herbs, which had passed stringent safety and efficacy tests with high marks, contrasts oddly with its behaviour when dealing with certain modern drugs. In the late 1960s and early 1970s, for instance, hundreds of thousands of women in the U.S.A. and Europe were taking hormone pregnancy tests: several companies marketed this profitable spin-off from the contraceptive pill. As early as 1967, research by Dr. Isabel Gal in an English children's hospital suggested that the use of such tests might be associated with abnormalities in the babies that resulted from these pregnancies. The Swedes banned their use in 1970, the Finns followed suit in 1971, and in January 1975 the F.D.A. put out a powerful warning: drugs containing sex hormones should never be used in early pregnancy since they might "seriously damage the fœtus . . . including heart and limb reduction defects." In April 1975 two of the Committee's own staff published data which showed the tragic link between birth deformities and the taking of this drug. And only after the *Sunday Times* published strong criticisms of the Committee's feet-dragging attitude did it send out a warning to doctors – followed by a second warning in 1977. It could not even be claimed that there was a pressing medical need for the drug: since the early 1960s, the much simpler and completely safe urine pregnancy test had been available.[12]

Had a herbal remedy been even faintly suspected of producing such consequences, there would certainly have been outraged cries from the medical press, and nation-wide publicity. As Fred Pestalozzi once remarked with a shrug, "It is hard work to work for nature".

If it is hard work in Europe, in America it is next to impossible. Bio-Strath was freely marketed for some time in the United States with the approval of the Food and Drug Administration – and then suddenly banned. Four years of correspondence, endless harassing questions and demands for trials followed, at the end of which the F.D.A. ruled that Bio-Strath could no longer be imported. Pestalozzi took the case to court and won. Finally, the F.D.A. banned it on safety grounds – but refused to reveal their reasons.

As a last resort, Pestalozzi asked the Swiss Consul to telephone the F.D.A.: "I have a responsibility for the health of the Swiss people", he told them. "If you have found anything harmful in Bio-Strath, then you must tell me". The F.D.A. finally admitted they could produce no negative evidence, and today Bio-Strath is once more on sale in the United States.

To students of F.D.A. history this story would be commonplace. The F.D.A. has probably done a better job policing dangerous drugs than the equivalent British authority – but it often appears even more zealous in its self-appointed task of cracking down on "health quackery" – a task in which it is enthusiastically assisted by the A.M.A. To both organizations, the health quack is a dangerous and unscrupulous fellow who goes around telling people that if they eat the right food, avoid food additives as much as possible, and take vitamin supplements if necessary, they will improve their chances of staying healthy.

To the evident dismay of the U.S. medical establishment, the American public has turned health-food shops – with their lines of vitamins, dietary supplements like Bio-Strath and packets of dried herbs – into a booming business, and it would be strange if there were no rogues and charlatans involved. But in its zeal to protect the great American public from this supposed gang of crooks, the A.M.A. has spent fortunes on running impressive national congresses on health quackery, which the A.M.A. President claimed in 1968 cost more each year than the entire cost of health education plus the cost of all medical research done in the U.S. And the F.D.A., for its part, has even been known to confiscate a consignment of honey shipped to a health-food store on the grounds that the presence of a book for sale nearby in which honey was described as particularly valuable nutritionally constituted "labelling". Indeed, on 19 January 1973, the F.D.A. actually proposed new regulations which would have made it illegal, among other things, to claim that there is a relationship between diet and disease, or that cooking or other processing of foods may cause nutritional losses, while many of the best-selling health-store lines such as individual B vitamins, rutin, and bioflavonoids would require a doctor's prescription.

Senator William Proxmire, who fought the F.D.A. on the vitamins issue, claimed that "The F.D.A. and much, but not all, of the orthodox medical profession are actively hostile against the manufacture, sale and distribution of vitamins and minerals as food or food supplements. They are out to get the health-food industry and to drive the health-food stores out of business. And they are trying to do this out of active hostility and prejudice."[13]

Herbal medicine in the United States arouses much the same prejudice and hostility – and for exactly the same reason: it is taking customers away from the multi-billion dollar prescription drug industry which underwrites the very existence of the A.M.A., and which has successfully brainwashed generations of doctors into believing that outside drug-oriented orthodox medical thinking lie only the grey realms of quackery.

In the United States, herbal medicine offers a temptingly easy target, despite its rapid growth in public esteem. Officially, it can hardly be said to exist, since most of the medicinal plants that are on permitted sale in dried form, for self-medication in the form of a "tea" or infusion, are so permitted as "food additives" and not as medicine.

When the 1958 food additives amendment to the F.D.A. statutes was passed, numbers of additives and ingredients were exempted from stringent new testing requirements because they had a long history of safe use. Thus, together with herbs and spices used almost entirely as flavouring or perfuming agents, such as cumin, caraway seeds and cinnamon, numbers of herbs used almost exclusively for medical purposes also crept into the haven of the Generally Recognized as Safe (GRAS) list; among them were benzoin (*styrax benzoin*) – the principal ingredient of Friar's Balsam – chamomile, dandelion, elecampane, horehound and marsh mallow root.

But no category was ever established for medicinal plants as such, many of the most common and useful of which, such as agrimony, mugwort (*Artemisia vulgaris*) and plantain, do not appear on the GRAS list, and technically may not be sold for food or drug use.

This Alice-in-Wonderland situation arose because at the time the new regulations were drafted in 1958 it was high noon in the new age of the wonder-drugs and herbal medicine was considered – by both the F.D.A. and the pharmaceutical industry – to be no more than a quaint folkloric survival; and in the United States – unlike Britain – there was no voice to speak up for the herbal practitioner, manufacturer or client. So herbal medicine in the U.S. continues to exist only in a legal limbo, permitted to be sold as a "food additive". Any claims, by any firm, that a herbal product is medicinal, or any labelling which suggested how it should be used medicinally, would at once remove it from this culinary category, and transfer it to the "drug" category – where it would at once be required to satisfy F.D.A. requirements costing millions of dollars and taking 5–7 years. Asked in an interview in 1979 whether they might consider establishing a special category for herbs, neither "food" nor "drug", the F.D.A.'s Joseph Perrat, a lawyer in the GRAS division, firmly rejected the idea.[14]

This lack of legal status has left the herb industry highly vulnerable to sudden onslaughts such as the notorious sassafras case.

Tea made from the root-bark of the sassafras tree has been widely drunk for over 200 years in the U.S., with no reports of adverse reactions. But in 1960 the F.D.A. fed massive amounts of safrole, a constituent of the essential oil of sassafras, to a number of rats, and noted that it resulted in liver cancer. They promptly banned sales of sassafras tea, although it has been pointed out – by Norman Farnsworth among others – that since safrole is highly insoluble in water, only traces of it would be found in a cup of sassafras tea. It was further pointed out that logically, the F.D.A. should also ban sales of nutmeg, star anise, pepper and ordinary tea, since all contain varying amounts of safrole. Sassafras tea, however, remains on the F.D.A. Unsafe list, and stocks of it may theoretically be seized at any time, along with other herbs that a British herbal practitioner would need constantly.

But in the United States there are no carefully-trained herbal practitioners who belong to a recognized organization with decades of experience behind it, and a well-informed public opinion on its side. The handful of establishments running courses in herbal medicine cannot offer their students a professional status that would command respect or credibility in scientific circles. And it does not help their image that the most enthusiastic protagonists of herbal medicine in the States tend to be young, denim-clad and anti-Establishment.

As for the herbal trade, no one would be more delighted to see it organized, scientifically respectable and powerful than Dr. Norman Farnsworth – and no one feels more real regret that it is nothing of the kind.

"There are some firms making a quick killing" he said, "and every year, two or three of the smaller firms go out of business, usually ruined by the legal fees involved in tussles with the F.D.A. They have no one to blame but themselves. To the best of my knowledge, there isn't a picogram of technical expertise in the whole of the organized herbal industry that can be brought into play to assure the consumer of the authenticity and safety of the products they sell.

"It should be mandatory that all herbal products be properly labelled, with their scientific and common names, the country of origin, the plant part(s), and a quality control number: and the F.D.A. should periodically check these products for the safety of the public. The F.D.A. rightly contends that the industry is doing virtually nothing itself to prove the safety of the herbs it is selling. Well, they probably can't do everything the F.D.A. wants, but they could make some attempt to improve their own standards. A few years ago, they did begin to make some effort along these lines, but interest soon petered out. I have a hunch that the industry knows that for the most part the F.D.A. will leave them alone, and they are willing to sit back and rake in the profits until such time as the F.D.A. is mandated by public pressure to take action".

He is equally critical of the F.D.A.'s attitude: "they don't want to know, don't want to get involved and are unresponsive to suggestions. They admit that Congress has not given them funds to regulate the herb industry, and from my experience with the F.D.A., their current personnel have little understanding of the inherent toxicological and technical aspects of herbs. They are primarily interested in interpreting current laws in a way that will cause them the fewest problems".[15]

In 1974 the American Society of Pharmacognosy set up a Botanical Codex Committee, chaired by Farnsworth, to consider the preparation of a "Botanical Codex", similar to the British Herbal Pharmacopœia it was hoped might aid the F.D.A. in making rational decisions in the regulation of herbal preparations.

Instead, the F.D.A. suddenly issued in 1977 a new Compliance Policy Guide listing 27 herbs as "unsafe" – which, as Farnsworth pointed out, was itself riddled with scientific inaccuracies. As one instance, morning glory (*Ipomoea purpurea*), was listed, on the grounds that its seeds contained amides of lysergic acid. Farnsworth pointed out that this was untrue of the *purpurea* species, and that presumably the F.D.A. meant *Ipomoea violacea* = *I. tricolor*. There are 175 horticultural variants of this species, he added, only seven of which have been shown to contain trace amounts of L.S.D.-like compounds. He calculated that an adult would need to consume about 350 seeds of the right variant to get any pharmacological action at all. Since the average morning-glory seed packet contains around ten seeds, the odds against achieving such an effect were thus high.

Farnsworth proposed to the F.D.A. that the Codex Committee could produce mini-reviews of 400 or so of the most commonly used herbs, drawing on the combined expertise of the members of the Codex Committee. "I imagine it would probably work out at about 200 being banned from over-the-counter sales – herbs are not by any means the innocuous little green things so many people imagine, and pokeroot (*Phytolacca americana*) – which contains an immuno-suppressant and can cause rectal bleeding – would certainly be on that list, for instance.

"Another 100 or so herbs would be ruled absolutely okay for unrestricted over-the-counter sales, and perhaps another 100 would need more work to be done on them. The F.D.A. has pigeonholed this proposal, on the basis that they themselves have not yet decided on a policy relative to how herbs should be regulated".[16]

Farnsworth's own solution would be for the F.D.A. to establish a new category for regulating herbal teas, drawing on the plentiful data already published to establish their safety and efficacy, rather than continue the absurdities of the present GRAS situation; and to insist on proper standards of labelling and quality control. But there are no signs at present of the F.D.A. adopting this sensible solution – similar to that of the British Department of Health and Social Security.

Herbal medicine may offer an easy target to orthodox medicine in the United States – but that certainly does not save it from attack, and even the most respectable promoters of herbal medicine tend to look nervously over their shoulders at the A.M.A. and the F.D.A.

In 1970 Paul M. Kourennoff published a fascinating book called *Russian Folk Medicine* crammed with accounts of herbal cures and popular remedies. Kourennoff reminded his readers that "American herbalists are forbidden by law to give any medical advice or suggest any of their wares in connection with any specific affliction", and went on to say of the treasury of folk remedies he had gathered together ". . . we do not recommend the use of any of them – unless no medical help can be obtained".[17] Ironically, a qualified doctor contributed a foreword to the book, in which he added wistfully, "It could give us a profound insight into the hidden powers of nature if we were able to use the contents of this rich literary work in our medical practice".[18]

Even the American Herb Society – which is as primly respectable as any village church fête committee – is so terrified of being tainted by the herbal-quackery label that it sends out notes with its brochures and literature disclaiming any active involvement in this dangerous area.

In the absence of qualified herbal practitioners, Americans who want to treat themselves herbally are restricted to dosing themselves with infusions made from herbs bought loose, or ready-packaged in ordinary tea-bags. Thus herbal medicine in the U.S. is largely a do-it-yourself herb-tea business, and a booming one at that. But having tried for years without success to convince the public that they were wasting their money on useless herbs when they could be spending their dollars on really powerful, effective drugs instead, both the A.M.A. and F.D.A. have now switched tactics. Today, the talk is of the appalling threat to American health that these herb teas may represent.

In 1976 the *Journal* of the A.M.A. carried a Special Communication (reprints were available as separate sheets) headed "Sassafras and Herb Tea – Potential Health Hazards." Referring to the fact that the consumption of "not only sassafras but herb tea in general has increased in accord with the current public interest in natural products", the article went on to warn that "In addition to the known and potential toxic properties of a number of commonly employed herbs used in making tea, one should also recognize that the consumption of herb tea generally may result in changes in the bioavailability characteristics of concomitantly administered drugs. We plan to publish evidence showing that herb tea is rich in tannins which can complex with, inactivate, or prolong the absorption of certain drugs. Consequently, to ensure safe and effective drug therapy, it would seem appropriate for physicians to evaluate their patients in terms of extemporaneous herb tea usage and to discourage these practises whenever feasible".[19]

The logical inference is that doctors should tell their patients that on no account should they drink ordinary tea – rich in these ominous tannins – when they are taking drugs. Or, if the action of complex modern drugs can be distorted by one simple biological factor, maybe patients taking drugs should stop eating and drinking altogether?

More recently, the *Medical Letter* ran an anonymous story headed "Toxic Reactions to Plant Products Sold in Health-Food Stores". This article contained strong suggestions that chamomile tea could cause anaphylactic shock, that tea made from devil's claw root (*Harpagophytum procumbens*) should be avoided during pregnancy because it has oxytocic properties, and that ginseng contained small amounts of œstrogens, and was recently reported to cause swollen and painful breasts in women.[20]

The scientific "evidence" for these disturbing statements was dismissed as both dishonestly presented and near-worthless by Farnsworth in a long careful study of the sources quoted. He pointed out that the basis for the alarming suggestion about chamomile tea rested on a single report of a thirty-five-year-old woman who suffered an anaphylactoic reaction after drinking a cup of chamomile tea. "To the best of my knowledge," added Farnsworth, "this represents the first and only report in the medical literature attributing this effect to chamomile tea. However, my search of the literature on the subject only extends back to about the year 1850."[21]

In the four years 1972–1975, there were 16,121 deaths due to accidental ingestions in the United States: only twenty-two of these were attributed to "noxious foodstuffs and poisonous plants. The increasing use of herbal teas in the United States has not been paralleled by increased incidences of adverse effects", concluded Farnsworth.[22] This statement could certainly not be made about prescription drugs.

26

East and West

"Chinese traditional medicine and pharmacy are a great treasure-house, and vigorous efforts should be made to explore them, and to raise them to a higher level".[1] This statement by Chairman Mao in 1958 changed China almost overnight from a country where medicine had been fast becoming Westernized to one in which herbal medicine and acupuncture – previously looked down on as hopelessly "un-scientific" – would now occupy a prominent and honoured place in the state medical scheme.

Mao was certainly not exaggerating when he spoke of his country's treasure. For thousands of years the Chinese have not only cherished and developed their own traditions of medicine, but have also period-ically recorded them with the utmost care and clarity. About 2,000 years ago the Chinese medical classic *Nei-ching* appeared, an 18-vol-ume work with 162 chapters, in which were elaborated, among other knowledge of the time, the detailed points of acupuncture. Soon after, the companion to this work, the *Shen Nung Pen Ts'ao*, or book of materia medica, was published, which listed over three hundred medicinal plants with descriptions of their therapeutic properties. In A.D. 657, during the Tang dynasty, the government ordered a major revision and updating of this work which occupied 2,000 scholars for the two years. Nearly a thousand years later, in 1578, the *Pen Ts'ao Kang Mu*, or Chinese Pharmacopœia, appeared. Its author, Li Shih-chen, was the son and grandson of physicians in the Yangtse basin and devoted his life to the study of ancient medical texts. He travelled throughout China interviewing scholars and peasants, from whom he collected hundreds of prescriptions. Many are still in use, and his book is still considered a standard reference for any research on plants.

This long tradition was interrupted early in the twentieth century when the Kuomintang Government decided that traditional medicine was unscientific and barred it from hospitals; in 1929 a law made its practice illegal. Traditional doctors, confident of huge popular support, continued defiantly to practice, and home remedies continued to circulate among the people.

Mao's decision to overturn this ban was not based solely on a peasant desire to do honour to his class traditions. At the time China faced a medical crisis, since there were not remotely enough Western-trained practitioners to treat a population of 800,000,000, while the cost of imported Western drugs was an intolerable burden on the economy. Under Mao's new directive, those practitioners already trained in Western methods were to be given further training in traditional methods, while traditional practitioners, for their part, were given a crash course in Western methods. To fill the huge health-care gap, a new class of paramedical practitioners was created – the Barefoot Doctors, part-time auxiliaries who received a short basic training (by Western standards it would be considered startlingly inadequate) so that they could treat patients – with herbs, acupuncture or Western-style drugs. There are now nearly 2 million such individuals.

The goal of China today is to develop a body of medical knowledge that combines, quite literally, the best of both worlds – traditional and Western. A patient calling at the out-patient's department of a big Chinese hospital will be seen, first, by a traditional practitioner, who may recommend surgery, acupuncture or give him a prescription. If the latter, it is likely to be herbal: of the 4,000 prescriptions dispensed daily in the pharmacy of the Lung Hua Hospital in Shanghai, in 1974 about 3,000 were for herbal mixes. Every Chinese hospital has its own "decoction room" containing thirty or so huge copper pans in which the infusions of mixed herbs are heated over steam, before a day's supply of warm decoction is handed to the patient in a thermos bottle. (Refrigerators are scarce in China – which is why it's a one-day supply – and the Chinese like to drink their medicines warm.)[2] If the prescription is more complicated – and many of them contain up to twenty different plants – the patient takes it to the drug room where the herbs will be weighed into a little package for him to make into infusion at home.

There is no antagonism between the two systems of therapy: indeed the Chinese often combine them in one treatment – herbal tonics are often administered to patients who are facing Western-style chemo-therapy to improve their general health and resistance. Such drugs as streptomycin and penicillin are now mass-produced inside the country, which is already almost completely self-reliant in drugs, and indeed exports them to other countries.

The Chinese have devoted themselves with enthusiasm to the development of their herbal materia medica – there are fifty research institutes studying traditional herbal drugs – and their approach is pragmatic. Chronic bronchitis is almost as common in some parts of China as the common cold is in England, so in 1971 the Government initiated a crash programme to find a remedy. Some 290,000 medical workers were sent to the countryside, factories and mines to study the disease and different treatments for it, and over 100 traditional remedies were collected for study. A number of plants frequently used in traditional medicine were studied: one of the most popular finally yielded a simple chemical substance which was named rori-fone, and this was subsequently shown in animal and human studies to be the active ingredient. Rorifone is now widely used in hospitals throughout China to alleviate the symptoms of chronic bronchitis.[3]

The Chinese approach to medicinal plant research is almost the exact reverse of that favoured by the big Western pharmaceutical companies. In looking for a new medicine, the Chinese begin the hunt for it where the traditions of folk medicine are strongest, and try it in the traditional form, a decoction or infusion made from the whole plant – root, leaves, bark or whatever. Only when it has been proved empirically to work do they start analysing it, taking it apart, and studying its individual constituents to see what makes it tick thera-peutically. Usually, they put it right back together again before they use it in medical practice. In Chinese traditional medicine, perhaps eighty-five per cent of treatment takes the form of herbal preparation.

This sensible approach has already paid off handsomely. Among other herbal drugs now being tried out is one that may be useful in the prevention of malaria, Ch'ing Hao, derived from a species of worm-wood (*Artemisia apiacea*); a highly effective treatment for diseases of the coronary artery is Tan shen (*Salvia miltiorrhiza*), related to our own sage (*Salvia officinalis*), long reputed in traditional medicine for its efficacy in stimulating the blood circulation; while another promising herbal treatment for coronary cases is Mao-tung-ching (*Ilex pubes-cens*) – in ninety-five out of ninety-eight patients testing it, it was claimed that agonizing chest pain disappeared or was much reduced.[4]

Cases that in a Western hospital would be referred at once to surgery are often treated herbally in China: more than eighty per cent of cases of acute appendicitis are routinely treated with herbs instead of being dealt with surgically.

Most significantly, in two areas of urgent and agonizing worldwide interest – cancer and birth-control – the Chinese are coming up with herbal answers. One such is a fungus, *Polyporus umbellata*, which has been used for centuries in traditional medicine. It is now being investigated, and the results are promising: "Significant symptom improvement and enhancement of immune fuction and/or survival times increase are recorded in over 300 patients with a variety of different types of cancer during a two-year study. During this evaluation period, very few side effects were noted, especially lack of bone marrow, depression and leukopenia."[5]

Cephalotaxus fortunei, a plant related to the yew, has yielded a potent anti-cancer agent named harringtonine which is currently being tested in humans in China, with promising results. (In the United States, a related compound, homoharringtonine, is being studied in cancer patients: it is obtained from *Cephalotaxus harringtonia*, which grows in the States).

Even when Chinese cancer patients receive conventional Western chemo-therapy, they are very often prescribed herbal treatment as well, as supportive or adjunctive therapy, or to cope with side-effect problems.

The Chinese approach to their overwhelming population problem has been sociological as much as medical: marriage is discouraged for women under twenty-five, and men under thirty, and while the first child of a marriage receives a government subsidy, subsequent children do not. They have made contraceptive advice freely available, and they have been searching hard for alternatives to the pill. A male anti-fertility agent, gossypol, isolated from cottonseed oil – it is not a steroid – begins to take effect about four to five weeks after daily oral doses start.

Before 1949, schistosomiasis, V.D. and drug-addiction, as well as ordinary infectious diseases, killed millions of Chinese annually. The staggering improvement in the national health, and the universal availability of reasonable health care – judged by competent observers to be at least equivalent to U.S. standards of effectiveness – would in itself be an impressive achievement, earning it the admiring interest of the Western world. But the Chinese medical system today fascinates the Western world for a quite different reason: the low cost, by Western standards, at which it has been achieved.

This has been possible partly because in the People's Republic the government has mobilized national effort and dictated individual behaviour to a degree which would be inconceivable is a Western society; because the Chinese have kept bureaucratic overheads trimmed to the bone; because so much medical care is delivered by practitioners who have received little of the long and expensive training that burdens Western medicine so heavily. For most minor illnesses, the Chinese go to their community pharmacy, where the pharmacist is more often than not a traditional doctor who has received no formal Western-style training at all, and who is himself training other pharmacists in the old apprenticeship style.

But it is in the area of drug costs that the contrast between the West and China is so striking. The annual drug bill of the Western world runs into billions of dollars, and is constantly rising. In 1980, Britain's prescription drug bill was around the £900 million mark. Another huge item on the drug bill is the rising cost of treating its unintended victims. As long ago as 1974 it was estimated that in the United States, iatrogenic disease was probably adding around $4.5 billion to the national medical bill.[6] Moreover, the resources on which the pharmaceutical industry is based – oil and coal – are dwindling: whether we like it or not, we shall have to cut our drug use, or pay increasingly higher prices. And even if biotechnology solves this problem, it's unlikely to lower costs.

Increasing numbers of doctors recognize the limitations and defects of drug-oriented modern Western medicine, and some of the most profoundly critical studies of the system have been written by doctors themselves. In 1977, an American physician, Dr. Hywel Davies, predicted: "I believe that drug abuse by the medical profession will subside until it becomes nothing but a historical curiosity which pertained to the era between World War II and this decade. The profession will adapt itself to the real, rather than the neurotic needs of society, and rationalize itself into another sort of symbiosis, which is more concerned with health than disease, with nature rather than the chemical laboratory".[7]

Dr. Percy Brown, a British doctor who runs a group practice in Gravesend, has limited his own drug list to a basic twenty, reviewed annually. He had so impressed the British Medical Association with his first-hand accounts of medicine in China that the B.M.A. held their

1979 annual conference in Hong Kong – from where Dr. Brown led several parties of British doctors into China. "We simply cannot go on as we are," comments Dr. Brown. "The cost in cash, and the cost in iatrogenic disease is unsupportably high".[8]

No nation, not even wealthy America, can afford to go on squandering enormous sums on health care when the returns are so disproportionately small. The British Health Service staggers from one crisis to another, while the rocketing cost of health care is a major political issue in the United States. What is more, the huge sums spent have not even bought higher standards of health. On the contrary, according to one critic, "A recent World Health Organization study has shown, in fact, that in a number of industrial countries the life expectancy of people over the age of sixty has actually started to fall. In the United States, where expenditure on health care is enormous, life expectancy for men and women of all ages is falling. Infant mortality rates are rising in many developed countries."[9]

While the United States and Western Europe can still afford to throw their money around on fancy drugs while failing to tackle medical problems at the grass-roots level, the rest of the world can't. In the Third World, there simply is not money enough to pay for Western-style technological medicine, an advanced pharmaceutical industry, hospitals staffed with costly gadgets, and legions of doctors trained at great expense. And if there were, money spent this way would be money misspent much of the time.

But the Third World has pressing medical problems: schistosomiasis or bilharzia, as it used to be called, is one of them. Schistosomiasis is a debilitating and slow-killing disease that affects more than 300 million people – perhaps one in eight of the world's population – living in tropical and sub-tropical countries: it is spread by a parasite that lives in water-snails. Since its victims – and the countries where it is endemic – are among the poorest of of the world's poor, it does not get much attention from the pharmaceutical companies, and there are few effective drugs for the management of the disease itself. But the Egyptian High Institute of Public Health may have come up with a better and cheaper answer. A tiny plant, *Ambrosia maritima*, has been found to contain in its leaves a chemical so toxic to snails that an infusion of one part in a thousand of water will kill them all. *Ambrosia maritima* is one more plant that makes it harder for anyone investigating the plant world not to believe in a benevolent providence: the little plant so fatal to snails is especially plentiful near snail-breeding grounds, safe to handle, and apparently harmless to fish, livestock and human beings, though snags may show up in more detailed studies. What is more, it even matures during the summer – at the peak of the snail-mating season.[10]

The World Health Organization, which has successfully eradicated smallpox from the world, has now set up a Special Programme on Tropical Diseases: one of its targets will be the control or eradication of the snail that transmits schistosomiasis, and it is intended to develop such plant materials for this purpose; the chemicals currently being used to kill the snails are expensive, and the snails soon develop resistance to them.

Another tropical disease in the W.H.O. programme is malaria, which presents much the same problems. In the early 1960s, it was optimistically believed that modern technology had almost wiped it out. India cut cases from a 1947 high of 75 million to a mere 125,000 by 1965. But Pakistan, down to 9,500 cases in 1961, was back to 10 million by 1975.[11] And in May 1978 the World Health Organization was told that thirty to forty times more cases of malaria were being reported than in the late 1960s.[12] Why? The disease seems increasingly resistant to the most widely available drug – the synthetic chloroquine – though this problem is much slighter with the plant-derived quinine. Even if spraying and drugs were the answer, however, the Third World cannot continue to foot the bill for this increasingly costly approach to the malaria problem.

Considerations of this kind had earlier prodded the World Health Organisation into an epoch-making decision. In 1974 banner headlines publicized it to the world: "W.H.O. gives the green light to Witch Doctors". After a lengthy study of world health needs, made jointly by UNICEF and the W.H.O., it had been concluded that if the world was to reach the goal of adequate health care for everyone by the year 2000 – surely one of the most noble projects mankind has ever set itself – Western-style technological medicine could not possibly serve the health and financial needs of the developing countries. The realistic alternative – which the W.H.O. has now adopted as its official policy – was to encourage all Third World countries to develop their own traditional systems of medicine: in other words, to build upon the rich traditions they already possess, as the Chinese are doing. As a logical extension of this policy, the Thirty-First World Health Assembly made an equally historic recommendation in 1978 which urged all countries to begin systematic scientific study of their medicinal plants, with the accent on galenicals or "whole-plant" drugs.

The W.H.O.'s first pronouncement had already promoted medicinal plants to what Farnsworth describes as "a high degree of visibility, to the whole world, including the established scientific community".[13] A programme later established by the W.H.O., in which he is closely concerned, is likely to intensify the spotlight.

In January 1976 the W.H.O. set up a Task Force on Indigenous Plants for Fertility Regulation. Their brief: to find a plant that could be used as a "morning-after" or an "after-one-missed-menses" aid to family-planning programmes. An active and safe plant extract might be acceptable, or a purified active compound. Only orally effective and safe substances would be considered. The programme was also interested in orally effective and safe contraceptives, for use by the male, that are plant-derived. The W.H.O. Special Programme was not interested in finding another relative to the "pill", which must be used continuously over long periods of time: it was predicted that agents used only infrequently would have less possibility of long-term side-effects.

To attain this goal, four collaborating W.H.O. research-centres – in the United States, Sri Lanka, Hong Kong and South Korea – are hard at work.

The Anti-Fertility project could have taken years to set up, but for Farnsworth's unique computerized index of medicinal plants. Since 1970 Farnsworth and his students have systematically collected and computerized every new piece of scientific information on medicinal plants, as well as much that had already been published: at the flick of a switch, they can now get a print-out of all the available data – kept continuously up to the minute – on any one of around 25,000 species. Some 3000 new plants are added to the computer's inventory annually.

For the W.H.O. Task Force project, it was also decided to include information on traditional medicine among the leads to be followed up: and after the computer had been programmed accordingly, it came up with a total of 4000 plants. A further refinement of the programme narrowed the field to around 350. The scientists in the programme are now enthusiastically confident that they have identified a number of highly promising compounds, which are being closely studied.[14]

In November 1978 the Ghanaian-born Dr. Henry Bannerman, then in charge of the W.H.O. Traditional Medicine programme, called another Geneva meeting, to consider another critical world health problem – and this time one that chiefly afflicts the affluent developed countries: cancer. "Cancer today strikes one out of every four Americans" noted a U.S. writer in 1976, "two out of every three families. . . . This year alone, more than a million of us will begin treatment for malignancies."[15]

Cancer presents twentieth-century medicine with its most urgent – and its most baffling problem. Since Congress passed the National Cancer Act in 1970 at Nixon's instigation, the United States has poured billions of dollars into research into this many-headed hydra of a disease. The annual budget of the National Cancer Institute alone runs at around $1 billion annually, and huge sums are being spent by most Western countries. Yet these vast sums have not been matched by comparable therapeutic advances: we are still far from knowing why or how cancer strikes, or how to save its victims. And many experts in the field are coming to believe that we should be devoting more of those huge resources to cancer-prevention, rather than to pursuing the distant pharmaceutical cure of a complete cure.

After studying the cancer question in depth the W.H.O. experts meeting in Geneva concluded that the Western approach to finding this cure had been largely unsuccessful. The most effective drug used in Western cancer therapy is still one derived from a plant – the alkaloid vincristine, from the Madagascar periwinkle (*Catharanthus roseus*) discovered by an Eli Lilly research chemist. Since that time, the National Cancer Institute has screened thousands of plants for anti-tumour activity. Yet as speakers at the conference pointed out, results have been negligible, perhaps since, as one of them suggested, the search has been "to a large extent. . . random", instead of focussing on leads from folk medicine.[16]

The W.H.O. Anti-Fertility Task Force may demonstrate the striking success that could be the result of using modern scientific methods to follow up traditional medicine leads. And in many countries around the world, the United States and Britain excepted, the W.H.O.'s forceful lead has stimulated a mild resurgence of interest in their own traditional medicine. The W.H.O. is doing all it can to encourage this by organizing educational projects, producing cash to pay for research, and setting up award schemes. One of these projects was carried out by a Guatemala medical school; they had noticed that village practitioners appeared to be not only treating diabetic patients but even curing them using local plants. The Guatemala project is being supervised by U.S.-trained doctors, who've put the herbal "cures" through the hoop of thorough lab tests: they concluded that patients actually "seem able to regain the capacity to manufacture their own insulin and to metabolize carbohydrate".[17]

This and other stories are heartening signs that Western doctors may possibly be beginning to see some value in the native practitioners they have despised for so long, and this is especially true of international aid and relief agencies. For instance a number of the Western doctors and nurses working in Thailand with Cambodian, Laotian and Vietnamese refugees are now actively enlisting the help of the local traditional healers, who to uprooted and emotionally shell-shocked patients offer the comforting reassurance of the familiar.[18] This change of heart is as welcome as it is overdue.

Willingness to learn from witch doctors, however, is rare in Western medical circles. Even in countries with a desperate need to mobilize their own native resources in this way, the contempt for traditional medicine that years of Westernized medical training has bred into the most educated sections of the population – including, usually, all its politicians – cannot be eradicated overnight, or even, perhaps, in this generation.

In the *British Medical Journal* of 15 September, 1923, an editorial contemplated with astonishment the decision of the Madras Government to encourage indigenous systems of medicine. The *Journal* then devoted two-and-a-half dense pages to a withering expose of ayur-vedic medicine – the traditional medicine of India – and concluded sternly that "if the Madras Government has the interests of the Indian people genuinely at heart, it will expend its energies in planting modern science in the country, by the agency of scientists and teachers trained in Western methods, instead of endeavouring to stimulate the belated indigenous systems into renewed activity".[19] These senti-ments were warmly applauded in a later issue by a retired army medical man: ayurveda was dismissed by him as "a so-called system of medicine for which a man trained in Western methods can have nothing but pitying contempt".[20]

After years of such indoctrination, there are many countries where once-rich traditions of native medicine have died out, and knowledge accumulated over centuries has gone to the grave with the last of its practitioners. North America itself offers the most striking instance of this process. When the Indians were uprooted and scattered over the continent in the last half of the nineteenth century, the end of the trail for many of them was totally unfamiliar terrain, where the medicinal plants they chiefly relied on were not to be found, and at the same time the chain of oral tradition had been broken by forced migration and death. By the early years of this century, most of the Indians were relying on the white doctoring made freely available to them – usually in the person of a physician with a thorough contempt for Indian medical practices. Gladys Tantaquidgeon of the Mohicans thinks that by the early 1900s, no more than a dozen or so of her group were still using traditional remedies.[21]

Here and there Indian herbal practitioners survive, like seventy-eight-year-old Ella Besaw of Bowler, Wisconsin, who was taught Indian medicine by her great grandmother, a full-blooded Oneida from New York State: Ella claims particular success in treating asthma, emphysema and diabetes, and has white patients coming to her.[22]

But the handful of Indians still practising the medicine of their ancestors are very much aware that they are probably the last of their line. Nora Thompson Dean, a Lenape herbalist of the Delaware tribe, told me that few of her people still practise Indian medicine, and although there is some interest in tribal traditions, none of the younger members really want to apply themselves to learning Delaware medicine.[23]

Other rich sources of traditional medicine knowledge are drying up fast. The wanton destruction of vast tracts of the Amazonian rain forests, with the break-up and dispersal of the Indian tribes living there, will certainly mean the permanent loss of invaluable information about local medicinal plant species, which are also doomed to wholesale obliteration. Yet it was from Indian tribes living in just such settings that the West has learned of some of its most valuable drugs – ipecac, cocaine, and quinine are three that spring to mind.

In almost every native tribe, moreover, the most important medical knowledge is a jealously guarded secret, traditionally passed on by the medicine-men only to their eldest son or some other trustworthy person. Jo Kokwaro, in the preface to his *Medicinal Plants of East Africa*, admitted that he had to resort to bribes and perjury to extract much of the information in it from unwilling informants, adding that even so, to the best of his knowledge, "not all the information about the local drug plants is in this book since a few people categorically refuse to reveal their secrets".[24] Kokwaro notes that "we often hear of our leaders disapproving of the use of local plants, and advising people to use modern medical facilities".[25]

Such attitudes are widespread in the West. When an enterprising young doctor at London's Dulwich hospital cured an intractable post-operative infection in a kidney-transplant patient by laying strips of paw-paw (*Carica papaya*) across the wound – a remedy he had seen successfully used by South African native doctors dressing dirty wounds – every reporter in Fleet Street at once reached for his pen and started writing. "The witch-doctors' paw-paw cure – cut-price from Fortnum and Mason" said the *Daily Mail*,[26] while the doctor himself was reported as admitting sheepishly to *Evening Standard* reporters: "It's not awfully scientific, I have no idea why it works."[27]

If this excellent instance of applied observation is "unscientific", so was William Withering's treatment of heart patients with extract of foxglove. It was Withering, we should remind ourselves, who said: "We must not disdain to learn the Medicinal uses of Plants from the meanest of Mankind; especially when they use their remedies in an uncompounded form."[28]

27

The
Green Sweep

The current surge of interest in herbal medicine began in the 1960s, and the "Green Sweep", as it has been called, has been gathering momentum ever since. The statistics are startling: World consumption of medicinal plants was rising by 1977 at a steady 7.7 per cent annually, and in the United States, sales of herbal products have shot from nearly-zero a decade ago to a market value in 1979 of at least $150 million, a 35 per cent increase over 1978 sales.[1]

All over Western Europe herbs are best-sellers today whether in glossy new pine-decorated herbal boutiques in inner cities, or sold in market stalls from fragrant sacks labelled "For the Blood" or "Against Insomnia". For those without the faintest idea how to medicate themselves in this novel and delightful way, there are a hundred new herbals to advise them – in at least one case, that of the celebrated French Maurice Mességué, backed up by a brisk herb-retailing business. And in countries with centuries-long traditions of herb doctoring, the old herbalists are coming out of retirement to preside over crowded consulting-rooms.

Herbal medicine today does not even need this base of local tradition to establish itself strongly, as the Dutch have proved. Unlike neighbouring Germany, Holland has few folk-medicine traditions of its own. Yet a single company, Biohorma, producing pure herbal and homoeopathic medicines under license from the Swiss firm of Bioforce, was able to notch sales of forty-five million guilders in 1979 – a figure which was itself up fifty per cent from their previous year's trading. The home-doctoring guide written by the firm's founder Dr. Vogel – a modern Culpeper – sold nearly half a million copies in Holland alone.[2]

As with other "alternative" therapies, the rising popularity of herbal medicine has turned it into a force to be respected by any democratic government with an eye to its voters. In France, where the trained *herboristes* were threatened with extinction as their numbers dwindled, the government was compelled by public outcry to reinstate the old two-year course in herbalism for these over-the-counter practitioners, which had been abolished by the Vichy regime in 1941 – under pressure, it is thought, from the big German pharmaceutical companies.

In Italy, despite strong and active opposition from the pharmacists who alone, under present law, are permitted to sell herbs as medicine, the government is likely to bow to public wishes in the near future and set up similar full-scale university courses in herbal medicine, instead of the ludicrously inadequate month-long course allowed at present. If this happens, the *herboristeria* with a diploma will then be permitted to advise as well as to supply, as in France.

Successive Dutch governments since 1945 have evaded the issue of what to do about "alternative" therapies by adopting the time-honoured ploy of appointing a state commission to consider the matter instead. The fourth of these, appointed in May 1977, was recruited almost exclusively from the ranks of professional doctors. Dutch public opinion, however, is used to making itself felt, and since a poll in January 1980 showed that seventy-five per cent of the Dutch wanted alternative therapies included in their National Health Service, the current commission is more than likely to recommend a modified version of this course – whatever their own feelings.[3]

Even when herbal medicine is denied legal status, it is being legitimized through the back door, as it were, all over Europe. Legislation outlawing it is not enforced; court sentences imposed for flouting existing laws are not served; assistants in herbal establishments who are not permitted to give advice freely do so; and official bodies charged with issuing – or withholding – licences for herbal medicines wave them through or let them pass unlicenced.

In the United Kingdom there are at present over 3,000 different herbal medicinal products on the market, using some 400 different herbs. Many of these are being manufactured under old of-right licences due to expire soon, and strictly speaking, the Committee on Safety in Medicines, to which applications for renewed licences must go, is entitled to insist on the same costly efficacy, safety and toxicity tests for a garlic cough mixture as it would exact for an "ethical" drug from a big manufacturer. In practice, it seems likely that as long as the product is an old-established one, containing familiar herbs which don't figure on the official restricted list, and as long as the makers can prove suitable manufacturing standards of hygiene and quality control, they will get their licence without too much of a fuss.

The further threat such products faced as little as two years ago – that of punitive Common Market requirements before licensing – seems unreal today. It is hard to imagine any Western European government having the courage to defy the clearly-expressed opinion of its electorate by backing such proposals.

The deep disillusionment with orthodox medicine which has powered this herbal boom is not confined to Western Europe or the United States. Eastern bloc countries, too, are producing their Culpepers. Bulgarian folk-healer Peter Dimkov learned herbalism from his mother, then travelled all over the countryside asking people about the local herbs they used for medicine. In his nineties he then compiled a three-volume work entitled *Bulgarian Folk Medicine* which is being published by the Bulgarian Academy of Sciences.[4]

Dimkov's compatriot Dr. Dimiter Pamukov runs a herbal consultancy practice in a big Sofia hospital with the blessing of the State Ministry of Health. Patients book appointments for weeks ahead, and he and his three colleagues claim to see 10,000 patients a year. They are particularly consulted by sufferers from non-malignant uterine tumours, asthmatic bronchitis, chronic ulcers, endocrine disorders and cardiac problems. Dr. Pamukov is about to launch on the market a "Home Pharmacy" kit of thirty-two herbs, with a guide to their use singly or in one of 140 combinations.[5]

The medical profession itself, meanwhile, is suffering a crisis of confidence, though few would go as far as the celebrated Dr. Julius Hackenthal of Hamburg, scourge of the German medical establishment, who declared on television his conviction that "our medical profession makes more people sick than healthy".[6]

Cautiously, discreetly, doctors are beginning to prescribe treatments and medication at which they would have raised their eyebrows ten years ago. When Biohorma of Holland ran a one-day seminar of their products specially for doctors, about 80 came, and although many of them were openly sceptical, most were visibly impressed.

But open-mindedness, a willingness to admit errors, and a readiness to learn from whatever source have never been hall-marks of the medical profession. Even if a handful of doctors are prepared to give an honest trial to those alternative techniques or therapies which have made such an impact on the public, the vast majority are not.

A mountain of prejudice stands between today's doctors and the use of simple plant medicine, while the hostility, the amused contempt, or even the outrage that the very idea of doctoring people with plants evokes in medical circles has to be experienced to be believed.*

There are a number of obvious reasons for this prejudice. Herbal medicine is damned by association in medical eyes because it belongs to medicine's dark and discreditable past, when doctors were so often ineffectual; because it is practised by people they consider inadequately trained, if at all; because it is practised by lay-people trying to doctor themselves; and because it is practised by peasants and primitive people the world over. There is, moreover, a major communication problem between the orthodox and the herbal practitioner to be overcome, with years of mistrust, suspicion, scepticism or hostility on both sides threatening the possibility of a good working relationship.

Much more of the professional prejudice against medicinal herbs comes from ignorance. The Western doctor today grows up in an atmosphere of extreme scepticism about the value of plants in his materia medica – a scepticism which the big drug companies certainly do nothing to dispel. The doctor has probably had little or no experience in their direct use, and may find it genuinely hard to believe that an infusion of chamomile tea could lull an anxious patient to sleep just as effectively as a little white pill.

He is almost certainly unaware of how many times a day he himself writes a prescription for a plant-based drug; he might be amazed to learn that one quarter of prescribed drugs sold in U.S. pharmacies contain constituents derived directly from real green plants.[7] He might be equally amazed to learn that it is to primitive peasant use of plants that medicine today owes its most important cardiac drug (digitalis); some of its most important painkillers (the opium poppy); the most reliable cure for amoebic dysentery and the most widely-used vomit in poison cases (*ipecacuanha*); the model for most local anaesthetics (cocaine from the coca tree); the model for all anti-malarials and itself the most successful (quinine from Peruvian bark);

---

*Following successful trials with Bio-Strath in Switzerland, Michael van Straten suggested to the Marie Curie Foundation in London that they should run trials of it, too; after months of preparation, the projected trials were dropped at the last moment. In explanation, the Chairman said it was felt that some doctors in the Foundation would object to working with herbs.

the most widely used anti-inflammatory and painkiller (aspirin); and the most successful anti-cancer drug (the alkaloids vincaleukoblastine and leurocristine from the Madagascar periwinkle, *Catharanthus roseus*).

Below these layers of prejudice and ignorance, there runs a much deeper and more violent objection to the use of herbs which can be summed up in one word: unscientific. In the clean, clinical mathematically-ordered context of modern medicine, there is no place for the disorderly living plant. Western medical students spend years and years learning to be doctors, and painfully cramming their skulls with an endless procession of facts. They are aware that others around them are busily accumulating more facts still, and they believe that striking medical advances will come about as a result. They grow up with an exaggerated respect for facts, figures, graphs, and numbers. They are, literally, blinded by science. Just as they imagine that those diseases about which the sum of medical knowledge is greatest will be most curable, so also they assume that a standardized chemical medicine whose action has been thoroughly studied for years, and every one of whose constituents is known, must be the most effective.

For this sin fell the angels. Not surprisingly they find it almost impossible to believe that someone who knows nothing of a disease mechanism could still be capable of curing it, or that a plant whose chemical structure is an unelucidated riddle can be effective medicine. Such assumptions would not be made in the East, but they rise easily in the Western mind, which has become preoccupied with information at the expense of wisdom and experience.*

It must be conceded even by doctors, however, that if a great deal of knowledge may solve our medical problems, a little knowledge has created a great many of them. Most modern pharmaceutical drugs are based on enough detailed research to show that this or that specific chemical process in the human organism appears to trigger a patient's malady; and enough expertise to devise a drug that will suppress or inactivate that process, thus removing the disagreeable symptoms of which the patient complained.

---

*In an interview on German T.V., Dr. Willy Richstein, press spokesman for the Bavarian Chamber of Doctors, was asked his views on the unorthodox cancer treatment being administered to patients in his Ringburg clinic by Dr. Joseph Issels. Dr. Richstein had never visited the clinic, nor studied the mass of documented clinical evidence available, but he commented ". . . when the best brains in the world are looking for a cancer cure, could two Bulgarian peasants find one? It is not possible."[8]

We are still very ignorant about the way the human organism works. We are not only at the beginning of our knowledge of immunology, for instance, we are only at the beginning of our knowledge of even a single cell. We do know that the human organism is made up of hundreds of thousands of delicately interlocking parts, and the more we know about the millions of intricately inter-related chemical reactions that keep it all ticking over, the more clumsy modern drug therapy comes to seem.

This picture of the body as a complex and delicately balanced organism has only begun to emerge from applied biochemical studies within the last century, and more particularly in the last few years. Yet the notion of an essential balance and harmony which is disrupted by disease is central to every form of "alternative" therapy, just as it is to every known form of traditional medicine, from Hippocrates and his Four Humours, to ayur-vedic practitioners whose three *Dosas* must be kept in balance, to the Chinese who view human health as a delicate equilibrium between *yin* and *yang*.

Ironically, research into the chemistry of the body not only shows up more and more the defects of modern chemo-therapy, it also provides a rationale for herbal medicine. A modern British herbalist, Mrs. Ann Warren-Davis, puts it this way: "Every cell in the human body contains a series of balancing mechanisms of stimulation or relaxation, controlled by complicated feedback balances. These intricate balances require a constant supply of nutrients, lack of any one of which over a limited time can be compensated for via some secondary pathway, but over a long period will create a chronic condition which is sometimes irreversible, but which can usually be corrected even in the most seemingly hopeless conditions with the use of the correct balance of nutrients." She points out that these nutrients come ready-packaged in plants, which contain "many biodynamic constituents in a form easily and rapidly absorbed by the human body . . . proteins, sugars, carbohydrates, minerals and trace elements, antibiotic agents, vitamins . . . fatty acids, mucilage, tannins and many other substances such as hormone and prostaglandin precursors."[9]

As a case in point, Mrs. Warren-Davis has been treating patients suffering from multiple sclerosis with oil extracted from the evening primrose (*Oenothera biennis*). It contains, she explains, "a high proportion of linoleic acid, plus another vital fatty acid, the gamma linolenic factor which is essential for sufferers from multiple sclerosis who for some reason not fully understood . . . become unable to form a vital prostaglandin known as PGE2. This oil, combined with the use of a special diet, helps to rehabilitate some of the sufferers over a long period of time."[10]

The oil may also help prevent the formation of blood-clots, which could make it a useful addition to the diet of those heart patients at risk from coronary thrombosis, or for women on the Pill. But it is unlikely that doctors will ever write a prescription for the oil in this form. Instead, they will wait for the standardized, synthesized version which several drug companies are reported to be working on at the moment, in the hope of a profitable, patentable product. If so, they will wait a long time before it can reach the market in this form, since it must undergo years of testing. And they may wait for ever: "it has seldom been found feasible or even economical to produce drugs of plant origin by synthesis," Dr. Farnsworth reminds us.[11]

Drug companies can hardly be blamed for wanting to show a profit: that, after all, is why they exist. But it is the commercial interests of this particular slice of big business, combined with the vast prejudices of the medical profession – the baneful conspiracy of physician and apothecary against which Paracelsus raged – that have together produced the tragic reality of Western medicine today. And the medicinal plants which constitute the most valuable, the most reliable, and by far the most promising source of new and effective drugs for our ills are little considered in the West today, while in the United States they are more completely neglected than at any other time in their history. The "Green Sweep" which looks so brightly promising to the general public has in practice made hardly a penny's worth of difference to the direction in which the public funds spent on medicine are channelled. In the United Kingdom, probably more public money is spent subsidizing the Members' Dining-Room in the House of Commons than on researching medicinal plants.

In the United States, the research and development budget of the pharmaceutical industry is probably in excess of $1 billion annually. Of this, it is estimated a pitiful $200,000 is budgeted for plant research.[12] And other than the plant-screening programme of the National Cancer Institute, which has had its budget severely cut back over the last few years, I know of no major U.S. medicinal plant research programme being paid for out of public funds.

In both countries – as in most of Western Europe – the protagonists of herbal medicine are not even wealthy enough to put their case squarely before the public: it takes money, unfortunately, to lobby governments, make useful contacts in the right places, advertise, promote, defend cases in a court of law or build head offices and staff them with enough secretaries to answer all letters.

Since Government health departments will not, and pharmaceutical companies do not spend money in this direction, who will? In the light of current legislation, nobody. And small herbal manufacturers will not take the risk since even if regulatory bodies like the F.D.A. or the Committee of Safety in Medicines are not cracking down on existing branded herbal medicines already on the market, that is far from a guarantee that they will not insist on the full panoply of safety, toxicity and efficacy tests for any new herbal product that comes before them for licensing. The costs of such testing are so high – between $5 and $10 million in the United States – that only major drug companies can contemplate them.

Apart from the sheer cost of screening and testing new plant drugs, there is another stumbling-block: the habit Western research establishments have of insisting that a plant must be broken down, its active ingredient "purified," and all testing done on this compound alone. Little white crystals with a fine new chemical name are more impressive than a muddy extract, and the practice has a clean scientific ring to it. But the reasons for testing the compound rather than the whole plant are in fact strictly commercial, since only the isolated compound offers any hope of a profit, and it is not "scientific" in the truest sense at all. The complex action of a plant often eludes such crude investigation, and many of the most effective plants known to herbalists would show up as either toxic or relatively inert if tested this way, so Western scientists probably discard hundreds of plants of real value.

For all these reasons the prospects for medicinal plant research in the United States and Western Europe look bleak. There will be little or no scientific investigation of many of the plants used by herbalists or traditional healers, which could be major gains to the Western pharmacopœia if their activity were confirmed in human beings under experimental conditions: zoapatl (*Montanor tormentosa*), widely used in Mexico in menstrual problems, and devil's claw (*Harpagophytum procumbens*), giving ease to thousands of arthritis sufferers, are just two which suggest what we may be missing. And doctors will continue to ridicule the idea that a plant can not only cure you, but actually do you good, like ginseng and its powerful cousin Siberian ginseng (*Eleutherococcus senticosus*). Yet in trials carried out in Russia with hundreds of human volunteers, this latter plant has turned out to have so wide a range of beneficial activity that a new name has been coined for it: it has been classed as an "adaptogen", since it improves the subject's performance or powers of endurance to a degree which has recommended its use to Russian cosmonauts and athletes.

No modern drug could ever hope to equal its range of beneficial effects, although pharmacists have had a stab at producing a man-made adaptogen. And if any kind of laboratory version could be produced, it would certainly exact a heavy toll in side-effects, as do stimulants like caffeine or the amphetamines. No such side-effects have been reported for *Eleutherococcus*, other than a slight and passing rise in blood-pressure, which makes it – by Western medical standards – a wonder-drug if ever there was one. Yet officially United States doctors will get no chance to try it themselves, since the F.D.A. has already refused it GRAS status, and it can only be imported illegally.[13]

What makes *Eleutherococcus* particularly interesting is that it is a completely novel plant drug, unknown in traditional medicine, and discovered by fairly recent research when the Russians were hunting for a homegrown substitute for the expensive ginseng they were importing from China and Korea. Screening other members of the same Araliaceae family, they put this dark-berried plant through their standard mouse-stamina test and noted that mice fortified with it swam nearly half as far again as the control mice.

Interest sharpened, more tests were done at the U.S.S.R. Academy of Science's Institute of Biologically Active Substances, and the decisive test was personally supervised by the Institute's Director, Professor I. I. Brekhman. He watched the performance of a large group of athletes running a 10-mile race, and saw that those who had taken the plant drug clocked up an average time of 5 minutes less than the runners who had only swallowed a placebo. By 1962, *Eleutherococcus* was officially entered in the Russian pharmacopœia.[14]

Two centuries ago the herbalist John Hill sensibly asked "why should he, who has not yet informed himself thoroughly of the nature of the meanest herb which grows in the next ditch, ransack the earth for foreign wonders?"[15] Do similar adaptogens grow in our own back-gardens? To our shame, and to our loss, we are in no position to find out.

Sooner or later the Western world, too, must open its eyes to the value of this vast natural treasury which through pride or through greed we have neglected for centuries.

"It is impossible," wrote John Skelton "for the most indifferent to have their attention directed to the vegetable kingdom without becoming convinced of the economy and provision ever existing within, and . . . the dependence of every creature upon its productions for security, either in health or disease".[16]

"Chymia egregia ancilla medicinae; non alia pejor domina."

Bibliography

The complete list of books, journals, papers and pamphlets that I have read through, skimmed, or dipped into in the course of researching this work would be tediously long. I have listed here only those which I found particularly interesting, informative or thought-provoking. Medical journals and other sources drawn on will be found detailed in the reference notes.

Unpublished Sources

Archives of the National Institute of Medical Herbalists. Private correspondence, as listed in the Reference notes.

Published Sources

Abithel, John Williams, (ed.), *The Physicians of Myddvai* (London, 1891).

Allport, Noel S., *The Chemistry and Pharmacy of Vegetable Drugs* (1944).

Arber, Agnes, *Herbals: Their Origin and Evolution* (Cambridge, 1912).

Archer, John, *Every Man his Own Doctor* (London, 1673).

Ashburn, P.M., *A History of the Medical Department of the US Army* (Boston, 1929).

Aubrey, John, (ed. Anthony Powell), *Brief Lives* (London, 1949).

Banister, John, *A Storehouse of Physicall and Philosophicall Secrets* (London, 1583).

——, *The Workes of that Famous Chyrurgian, Mr. Iohn Banester, By Him digested into five Bookes* (London, 1583).

Baldry, Peter, *The Battle against Bacteria* (Cambridge, 1965).

Barton, Benjamin Smith, *Collections for an Essay towards a Materia Medica of the United States*. (Philadelphia, 1804).

Beach, Wooster, *The British and American Reformed Practice of Medicine* (Birmingham and London, 1859).

Bézanger-Beauquesne, Lucienne, Pinkas, Madeleine, and Torch, Monique, *Les plantes dans la therapeutique moderne* (Paris, 1975).

Bigelow, Jacob, *American Medical Botany*. 3 vols. (Boston, 1817–1820).

Biggs, Noah, *Mataeotechnica Medicinae Praxeos* (London, 1651).

Blanton, Wyndham, *Medicine in Virginia in the Eighteenth Century* (Richmond, Va., 1931).

——, *Medicine in Virginia in the Nineteenth Century* (Richmond, Va., 1933).

Blythe, Peter, *Drugless Medicine* (London, 1974).

Bonser, Wilfrid, *The Medical Background of Anglo-Saxon England* (London, 1963).

Böttcher, Hellmuth M., trans. Einhart Kawerau, *Miracle Drugs: A History of Antibiotics* (London, 1963).

Bowle, John, *Henry VIII* (London, 1965).

Bowness, Charles, *The Romany Way to Health* (1970).

Breckon, William, *The Drug Makers* (London, 1972).

Brunton, T. Lauder, *A Textbook of Pharmacology, Therapeutics and Materia Medica* (London, 1893).

Buchan, William, *Domestic Medicine, or, a Treatise on the Prevention and Cure of Diseases by Regimen and Simple Medicines* (London, 1797).

Buret, F., *Syphilis in Ancient and Prehistoric Times*. 2 vols. (Paris, 1891).

Burill, Ives, *La Marquise de Sévigné* (Paris, 1932).

Burton, Elizabeth, *The Jacobeans at Home* (London, 1962).

Carlson, Rick J., (ed.) *The Frontiers of Science and Medicine* (London, 1975).

Chambers, John D., *A Pocket Herbal* (London, 1800).

Chapman, Stanley, *Jesse Boot of Boots the Chemists* (London, 1974).

Cockayne, Rev. Oswald (ed.), *Leechdoms, Wortcunning and Starcraft of Early England*, 2 vols. (London, 1864).

Coffin, Albert Isaiah, *A Botanic Guide to Health* (London, 1866).

——, *Botanical Journal and Medical Reformer* (London, 1849–1859).

Colden, Cadwallader, *Letters and Papers* 8 vols, 1711–1775 (New York, 1918–1923).

Coleman, Vernon, *Paper Doctors* (London, 1977).

——, *The Medicine Men* (London, 1975).

Conway, David, *The Magic of Herbs* (London, 1975).

Cook, William H., *Womans Herbal Book of Health* (Southport, England, 1866).

Corbett, Thomas H., *Cancer and Chemicals* (Chicago, 1977).

Coulter, Harris L., *Homeopathic Influences in Nineteenth-Century Allopathic Therapeutics* (Washington, 1973).

——, *Divided Legacy*, 3 vols. (Washington, 1973–1977).

Craton, Michael and Walvin, James, *A Jamaican Plantation* (London, 1970).

Culbert, Michael L., *Freedom from Cancer* (Seal Beach, Cal., 1974).

Culpeper, Nicholas, *The Complete Herbal* (1973).

——, *A Physicall Directory, or, A translation of the London Dispensatory Made by the Colledge of Physicians in London.* (London, 1649).

Curtis, D. Alva, *Discussions Between several Members of the Regular Medical Faculty and the Thomsonian Botanic Physicians on the Comparative Merits of their Respective Systems.* (Columbus, Ohio, 1836).

——, *A Fair Examination and criticism of all the medical systems in vogue.* (Cincinnati, Ohio, 1855).

Davies, Hywel, *Modern Medicine* (London, 1977).

Debus, Allen, *The English Paracelsians* (London, 1965).

Deguéret E., *Histoire Medicale du Grand Roi.* (Paris, 1924).

Dennie, Charles Clayton, *A History of Syphilis* (Springfield, Ill., 1962).

Dewhurst, Kenneth, *John Locke: Physician and Philosopher* (London, 1963).

Dixon, Pamela, *Ginseng* (London, 1976).

Doe, John, *The Healers* (London, 1967).

Drinker, Cecil K., *Not so Long Ago* (New York, 1937).

Duffy, John, *The Healers* (New York, 1976).

Dunn, Richard S., *Sugar and Slaves* (London, 1973).

Eliot, George, *Middlemarch* (London, 1965).

Ellis, John, *Directions for Bringing Over Seeds and Plants from the East Indies* (London, 1770).

Elyot, Sir Thomas, *The Castel of Helth* (London, 1541).

Felter, H.W., *History of the Eclectic Medical Institute, Cincinnati, Ohio, 1845–1902* (Cincinnati, Ohio, 1902).

Fergusson, William, *Notes and Recollections of a Professional Life* (London, 1846).

Finkel, Maurice, *Fresh Hope in Cancer* (Health Science Press, England, 1978).

Fishbein, Morris, *A History of the AMA* (Philadelphia, 1947).

——, *Fads and Quackery in Healing* (New York, 1932).

Fisher, Richard B., and Christie, George A., *A Dictionary of Drugs* (London, 1975).

Flexner, Abraham, *Medical Education in the United States and Canada. A Report for the Carnegie Foundation for the Advancement of Teaching* (New York, 1910).

Fluck, Professor Hans, *Medicinal Plants and their Uses* (London, 1976).

Forbes, Dr. Alec, *Try Being Healthy* (Plymouth, England, 1976).

Forbes, Sir John, *Of Nature and Art in the Cure of Disease* (London, 1858).

Fox, William, *The Working Man's Model Family Botanic Guide* (Sheffield, 1904).

Fulder, Stephen, *The Root of Being* (London, 1980).

General Medical Council, *Report of the Committee on Professional Education* (London, 1869).

Gerard, John, *The Herbal* (facsimile edition) (New York, 1975).

Gesner, Conrad, *The Newe Iewell of Health* (London, 1576).

Gibbons, Euell, *Stalking the Healthful Herbs* (New York, 1966).

Gill, Harold B. Jr., *The Apothecary in Colonial Virginia* (Williamsburg, 1972).

Glasser, Ronald J., *The Greatest Battle* (New York, 1976).

Goldwater, Leonard J., *Mercury: A history of quicksilver* (Baltimore, Maryland, 1972).

Good, John Mason, *The History of Medicine so far as it relates to the Profession of the Apothecary* (London, 1795).

Goodall, Charles, *An Historical Account of the Colledge's Proceedings against Empiricks* (London, 1664).

Graham, Thomas J., *Modern Domestic Medicine* (London, 1835).

Greene, Graham, *Lord Rochester's Monkey* (London, 1974).

Greene, R., *Indianopathy or Science of Indian Medicine* (Boston, 1858).

Grieve, Mary, ed. Hilda Leyel, *A Modern Herbal* (London, 1931).

Griffin, Edward G. *World Without Cancer* (Westlake Village, Cal., 1974).

Grigson, Geoffrey, *A Herbal of All Sorts* (London, 1959).

Haggard, Howard W., *The Doctor in History* (New Haven, 1934).

Hamilton, James, *Observations on the Use and Abuse of Mercurial Medicine in Various Diseases* (Edinburgh, 1919).

Hand, Wayland D. (ed.,) *American Folk Medicine* (Berkeley, Cal., 1976).

Harcourt, Raoul d', *La médecine dans l'ancien Perou* (Paris, 1939).

Harriman, Sarah, *The Book of Ginseng* (1975).

Harris, Ben Charles, *The Compleat Herbal* (New York, 1972).

——, *Kitchen Medicines* (New York, 1968).

Harris, Lloyd J., *The Book of Garlic* (San Francisco, 1974).

Harvey, Gideon, *The Family Physician and the House-Apothecary* (London, 1678).

Hayes, John, (ed.), *The Genius of Arab Civilisation* (Oxford, 1976).

Henry, Samuel, *A New and Complete American Medical Family Herbal* (New York, 1814).

Hermannus, Philippus, *An Excellent Treatise teaching howe to cure the French-Pockes. Drawne out of the Bookes of that learned Doctor and Prince of Phisitians, Theophrastus Paracelsus* (trans), John Hester, in the Spagiricall Arte, practitioner (London, 1590).

Hertzler, Arthur E., *The Horse and Buggy Doctor* (New York, 1941).

Hill, A. Wesley, *John Wesley among the Physicians* (London, 1958).

Hill, Sir John, *The Useful Family Herbal* (London, 1789).

Hobhouse, R.W., *The Life of C.S. Hahnemann* (London, 1933).

Holbrook, Stewart H., *The Golden Age of Quackery* (London, 1959).

Hole, Christina, *The English Housewife in the Seventeenth Century* (London, 1953).

Holland, Henry, *Medical Notes and Reflections* (London, 1840).

Holmes, Oliver Wendell, *Medical Essays 1842–1882* (London, 1891).

Hooker, Worthington, *Rational Therapeutics: or The Comparative Value of different Curative Means, and the Principles of their Application.* Publications of the Massachusetts Medical Society, (Boston, 1860).

Hughes, William, *The American Physician* (London, 1672).

Huxley, Anthony, *Plant and Planet* (London, 1978).

Hylton, William H., (ed.) *The Rodale Herb Book* (Emmaus, Pa., 1974).

Illich, Ivan, *Medical Nemesis* (London, 1975).

Inglis, Brian, *Fringe Medicine* (London, 1964).

——, *A History of Medicine* (Cleveland and New York, 1965).

——, *The Case for Unorthodox Medicine* (New York, 1965).

——, *Natural Medicine* (London, 1979).

Jameson, J. Franklin (ed.), *Narratives of New Netherland* (New York, 1909).

Jensen, Merrill (ed.), *American Colonial Documents to 1776* English Historical Series IX (London, 1955).

Josselyn, John, *New England's Rarities Discovered* (London, 1672).

Kaufman, Martin, *Homeopathy in America* (Baltimore, 1971).

Kent, Joan, *Binder Twine and Rabbit Stew* (1978).

Kett, Joseph F., *The Formation of the American Medical Profession* (New Haven, 1968).

King, John, *The American Dispensatory* (Cincinnati, Ohio, 1859).

King, Lester, *The Medical World of the Eighteenth Century* (Chicago, 1958).

Klass, Alan, *There's Gold in them thar Pills* (London, 1975).

Kloss, Jethro, *Back to Eden* (Woodbridge, Cal., 1975).

Kokwaro, Jo, *Medicinal Plants of East Africa* (East African Literature Bureau, 1976).

Kourennoff, Paul M., *Russian Folk Medicine* (London 1970).

Kreig, Margaret, *Green Medicine* (London, 1965).

Kremers, Edward, and Urdang, George, *History of Pharmacy* (Philadelphia, 1976).

Kutumbiah, Dr. P., *Ancient Indian Medicine* (Bombay, 1962).

Langham, William, *The Garden of Health* (London, 1578).

Lasagna, Louis, *The Doctors' Dilemmas* (New York, 1962).

Laurence, D.R., and Black, J.W., *The Medicine You Take* (London, 1978).

Law, Donald, *The Concise Herbal Encyclopedia* (Edinburgh, 1973).

Lawall, Charles H., *Four Thousand Years of Pharmacy* (Philadelphia, 1927).

Lee, Edwin, *Observations on the Principal Medical Institutions and Practice of France, Italy and Germany* (London, 1843).

Le Roi, J.A. (ed.), *Journal de la Santé du Roi Louis XIV* (Paris, 1862).

Lestrange, Richard, *A History of Herbal Plants* (London, 1977).

Levy-Valensi, J., *La Médecine et les médecins français au XVIIe siècle* (Paris, 1933).

Lind, James, *A Treatise of the Scurvy* (Edinburgh, 1953).

Lloyd, G.E.R., (ed.) *Hippocratic Writings* (London, 1978).

Lloyd, John Uri, *Origin and History of all the Pharmacopeial Vegetable Drugs* (Cincinnati, Ohio, 1929).

——, *Drugs and Medicines of North America* (Cincinnati, Ohio, 1884–1885).

Longmate, Norman, *King Cholera. The Biography of a Disease* (London, 1966).

Lust, John, *The Herb Book* (New York, 1974).

Mabey, Richard, *Plants with a Purpose* (London, 1977).

Macdonald, Duncan, *The New London Family Cook* (London, 1811).

McGrath, William R., *God-Given Herbs for the Healing of Mankind* (1970).

McKechnie, Robert E., *Strong Medicine* (Vancouver, British Columbia, 1972).

MacKinney, Loren, *Early Medieval Medicine* (Baltimore, 1937).

McLachlan, Gordon (ed.), *Medical History and Medical Care: A Symposium of Perspectives* (Oxford, 1971).

McLuhan, T.C. (compiled), *Touch the Earth* (London, 1973).

Maclean, Una, *Magical Medicine* (London, 1971).

Malleson, Andrew, *Need your Doctor be so useless?* (London, 1973).

Maple, Eric, *Magic, Medicine and Quackery* (Cranbury, New Jersey, 1968).

M(arkham), G(ervase), *The English House-wife*, in *A Way to Get Wealth*. (London, 1638).

Marti-Ibanez, Felix, (ed.), *History of American Medicine; A Symposium* (New York, 1958).

Maxwell, Nicola, *Witch-Doctor's Apprentice* (Boston, 1961).

Melmon, Kenneth L., and Morrelli, Howard F., *Clinical Pharmacology* (New York, 1972).

Mességué, Maurice, *C'est la nature qui a raison* (Paris, 1972).

——, *Of Men and Plants* (London, 1970).

Miller, Amy Bess, *Shaker Herbs* (New York, 1976).

Millspaugh, C.F., *American Medicinal Plants* (Philadelphia, 1887).

Mitchell, G. Ruthven, *Homoeopathy* (London, 1975).

Monardes, Nicholas, (ed. S. Gaselee), *Joyfull Newes out of the Newe Found Worlde* (London, 1925).

Needham, Marchmont, *Medela Medicinæ* (London, 1665).

Newman, Charles, *The Evolution of Medical Education in the Nineteenth Century* (Oxford, 1957).

Newton, Robert S., *An Eclectic Treatise on the Practice of Medicine* (Cincinnati, 1861).

Newton-Fenbow, Peter, *A Time to Heal* (London, 1971).

Pachter, Henry M., *Paracelsus: Magic into Science* (New York, 1951).

Packard, Francis R., *Life and Times of Ambroise Paré* (London, 1922).

Packard, Madge E. and Buley, R. Carlyle, *The Midwest Pioneer* (New York, 1946).

Pagel, Walter, *Paracelsus: An Introduction to Philosophical Medicine in the Era of the Renaissance* (Basle, 1958).

Palaiseul, Jean, *Au-dela de la médecine: tous les moyens de vous guérir interdits aux médecins*. (Paris, 1957).

Paracelsus, (ed. J. Jacobi), *Selected Writings* (London, 1951).

Paracelsus (ed. Dr. Bernhard Aschner), *Samtliche Werke* (Jena, 1926–1932).

Paracelsus (ed. Karl Sudhoff), *Samtliche Werke* (Munich, 1929–1933).

Pascal, James Imperato, *African Folk Medicine* (Baltimore, 1977).

Pereira, Jonathan, *The Elements of Materia Medica* (London, 1854).

Petulengro, Leon, *The Roots of Health* (London, 1971).

Phillips, Eustace D., *Greek Medicine* (London, 1973).

Pilpoul, Pascal, *La querelle de l'antimoine* (Paris, 1928).

Pollak, Kurt, *The Healers* (London, 1968).

Pouchet, F.A., *Histoire des sciences naturelles au moyen age*. (Paris, 1853).

Poynter, F.M.L., (ed.), *The Evolution of Pharmacy in Britain* (London, 1965).

Pusey, William Allen, *A Doctor of the 1870s and 1880s* (Illinois & Maryland, 1932).

Reece, Richard, *The Medical Guide*. (London, 1824).

——, *A Practical Dissertation on the means of obviating and Treating the Varieties of Costiveness* (London, 1826).

Revolutionary Health Committee of Hunan Province. *A Barefoot Doctor's Manual* (London, 1978).

Rodale, J.I., *The Hawthorn Berry for the Heart* (1971).

Rohde, Eleanor Sinclair, *The Old English Herbals*, (London, 1974).

Rosebury, Theodor, *Microbes and Morals*, (St. Albans, 1975).

Ross, A.C. Gordon, *Homoeopathy* (1976).

——, *The Amazing Healer: Arnica* (1977).

Rubin, Stanley, *Medieval English Medicine* (Newton Abbot, 1974).

Salmon, William, *Seplasium: The Compleat English Physician* (London, 1692).

Sherwood Taylor, F., *The Alchemists* (London, 1976).

Silverman, Milton, *The Drugging of the Americas* (Berkeley, Cal., 1976).

Silverman, Milton, and Lee, Philip R., *Pills, Profits and Politics*. (Berkeley, Cal., 1974).

Sjostrom, Henning and Nilsson, Ribert, *Thalidomide and the Power of the Drug Companies* (London, 1972).

Skelton, John, *The Family Herbal and Botanic Record* (Leeds, 1855).

——, *The Epitome of the Botanic Practice of Medicine* (Leeds, 1855).

——, *The Family Medical Adviser* (Leeds, 1852).

——, *A Plea for the Botanic Practice of Medicine* (London, 1853).

——, *The Science and Practice of Medicine*. First published 1870, reissued by the National Association of Medical Herbalists (London, 1904).

——, *A Treatise on the Venereal Disease and Spermatorrhoea.*

Smith, J. Dickson, *A Few Facts in Relation to the Lobelia and Pepper Practice: Its Prospects and Policy as Challenged by "Professor" M.S. Thomson in his Recent Pamphlet* (Macon, Ga., 1859).

Stearns, Samuel, *The American Herbal or Materia Medica* (Walpole, USA, 1807).

Stillman, J.M., *Paracelsus* (Chicago and London, 1920).

Stokeham, Wm., *Medela Medicorum* (London, 1768).

Sulblé, Docteur H. *Quelques charlatans célèbres au XVIIe siècle.* (Toulouse, 1922).

Talbot, C.H., *Medicine in Medieval England* (London, 1967).

Taylor, Norman, *Plant Drugs that Changed the World* (New York, 1965).

Teetgen, Ada B., *Profitable Herb Growing and Collecting* (London, 1919).

Theobald, Robert M., *Homoeopathy, Allopathy and Expectancy* (London, 1859).

Thompson, C.J.S., *Magic and Healing* (London, 1947).

——, *The Mystery and Art of the Apothecary* (London, 1929).

——, *The Quacks of Old London* (London, 1928).

Thompson, Flora, *Lark Rise to Candleford* (Oxford, 1945).

Thomson, Anthony Todd, *The London Dispensatory* (London, 1831).

Thomson, George, *Galeno-Pale: or, a Chymical Trial of the Galenists* (1665).

Thomson, Gladys Scott, *Life in a Noble Household (1641–1700)* (London, 1937).

Thomson, Samuel, *A Narrative of the Life and Medical Discoveries of Samuel Thomson* (Boston, 1825).

Thomson, William A.R., *Healing Plants: A Modern Herbal* (London, 1978).

——, *Herbs that Heal* (London, 1976).

Thornton, R.J., *A New Family Herbal* (London, 1810).

Timbs, John, *Doctors and Patients* (London, 1873).

Tobe, John H., *Proven Herbal Remedies* (New York, 1977).

Toguchi, Masaru, *Oriental Herbal Wisdom* (New York, 1973).

Tompkins, Peter, and Bird, Christopher, *The Secret Life of Plants* (London, 1975).

Treve, Wilhelm, *Doctor at Court* (London, 1958).

Turner, E.S., *Call the Doctor* (London, 1958).

Turner, William, *A New Herball* (London, 1551).

Underwood, E.A. (ed.), *Science, Medicine and History: Essays . . . in Honour of Charles Singer* (London, 1953).

Venzmer, Gerhard, *Five Thousand Years of Medicine* (London, 1972).

Vogel, Virgil J., *American Indian Medicine* (Norman, Oklahoma, 1970).

Wagner, Frederick, *Popular Methods of Natural Healing* (Mexico City, 1940).

Wagner, H., and Wolff, D. (ed.), *New Natural Products and Plant Drugs with Pharmacological, Biological or Therapeutic Activity.* (Proceedings of the 1st International Congress on Medicinal Plant Research 1976) (Berlin, Heidelberg, New York, 1977).

Wall, C. Cameron, and Underwood, E.A., *A History of the Worshipful Society of Apothecaries of London* (London, 1963).

Waller, John Augustine, *The New British Domestic Herbal* (London, 1822).

Wallis, Roy and Morley, Peter (ed.), *Marginal Medicine* (London, 1976).

Wallis, Thomas E., *A Textbook of Pharmacognosy* (London, 1960).

Watson, Gilbert, *Theriac and Mithridatium* (London, 1966).

Weeks, Nora, *The Medical Discoveries of Edward Bach, Physician* (Rochester, 1959).

Weiner, Michael A., *Earth Medicine – Earth Foods* (London and New York, 1972).

Wesley, John, *Primitive Physic, or an Easy and Natural Method of Curing Most Diseases* (London, 1781).

Westlake, Aubrey T., *The Pattern of Health* (Berkeley, Cal., and London, 1973).

Wheelwright, Edith D., *The Physick Garden* (London, 1934).

Whitlaw, Charles, *The Scriptural Code of Health, with Observations on the Mosaic prohibitions, and on the principles and benefits of the Medicated Vapour Bath* (London, 1838).

Whittle, Tyler, *The Plant Hunters* (London, 1970).

Williams, Guy, *The Age of Agony* (London, 1975).

Wingate, Peter, *The Penguin Medical Encyclopedia* (London, 1972).

Withering, William, *An Account of the Foxglove* (Birmingham, England, 1785).

——, *A Botanical Arrangement of all the Vegetables Naturally Growing in Great Britain* (Birmingham, England, 1776).

Wood, William, *New England's Prospect* (London, 1934).

Woodall, John, *The Surgion's Mate* (London, 1617).

Woodville, William. *Medical Botany*. 5 vols. (London, 1832).

Wren, R.C. (ed.), *Potter's New Cyclopædia of Botanical Drugs and Preparations* (London, 1975).

Yemm, J.R. (ed.), *The Medical Herbalist* (1977).

Young, J.H., *The Toadstool Millionaires* (Princeton, N.J., 1961).

Zee, van der, Henri and Barbara, *A Sweet and Alien Land* (New York, 1978).

Ziegler, Philip, *The Black Death* (London, 1969).

Notes

NOTE. In researching this book I have been particularly indebted to the authors of the three following standard works, each indispensable to anyone studying the subject, and on which I have drawn extensively, as the detailed reference notes which follow will show: Virgil J. Vogel, *American Indian Medicine*; Wyndham Blanton, *Medicine in Virginia in the Eighteenth Century* (also his *Medicine in Virginia in the Nineteenth Century*); Harris L. Coulter, *Divided Legacy*. References to books listed in the bibliography are given by author only at the first mention. Titles of articles and books not listed in the bibliography are given in full on the first occasion and abbreviated thereafter.

ABBREVIATIONS: AJP *American Journal of Pharmacy* (Philadelphia); AMH *Annals of Medical History* (New York); BHM *Bulletin of the History of Medicine* (New Haven); BMJ *British Medical Journal* (London); CBJ *Coffin's Botanical Journal* (London); DSBR, *Doctor Skelton's Botanic Record* (Leeds, England); EMJ *Eclectic Medical Journal* (Leeds, England); LLB *Lloyd Library Bulletin* (Cincinnati); JAMA *Journal of the American Medical Association* (Chicago); JAPA *Journal of the American Pharmaceutical Association* (Washington D.C.); JHM *Journal of the History of Medicine* (Baltimore); MH *Medical History* (London); NIMH Unpublished archives of the National Institute of Medical Herbalists, London; p.c. Private communication to author; Pract. *The Practitioner* (London); PRSM *Proceedings of the Royal Society of Medicine* (London).

Epigraph: James I, cited in Ross, *Homoeopathic Green Medicine*, 1978.

CHAPTER 1 The Medicine of Mankind
1. Solecki, "Shanidar IV, a Neanderthal Flower Burial in Northern Iraq", *Science*, 28 Nov. 1975, pp 880–1. 2. p.c. Mrs Ann Warren-Davis. 3. Norman R. Farnsworth, "Rational Approaches to the Search for and Discovery of New Drugs from Plants", paper presented at the first Latin-American and Caribbean Symposium on Naturally Occurring Pharmacological Agents, Havana, Cuba 23–28 June 1980, pp. 7–8. 4. *Ibid*, pp. 28–9. 5. Maxwell, p. 262 and pp. 344–6. 6. Mbuti, *African Religions and Philosophy* (New York, 1969), pp. 166–7. 7. Kourennoff, *Russian Folk Medicine*, p. 116. 8. Mitchell,

Homoeopathy, p. 120. 9. Ross, p. 13. 10. Fulder, *The Root of Being*, pp. 138–140. 11. Stannard, "The Herbal as a Medical Document", *BHM* XLIII, 1969, pp. 214–5. 12. Jackson, "From Papyri to Pharmacopoeia", in Poynter (ed.), *The Evolution of Pharmacy in Britain*, p. 155. 13. Whittle, *The Plant Hunters*, p. 18. 14. Lloyd, "Vegetable Drugs Employed by American Physicians", *JAPA*, Nov. 1912, p. 15.

CHAPTER 2 Medicine in Transition
1. Talbot, *Medicine in Medieval England*, pp. 13–14. 2. Rohde, *The Old English Herbals*, pp. 8–9. 3. Cockayne, *Leechdoms, Wortcunning and Starcraft of Early England*, II, p. 265. 4. *Ibid*. 5. *Ibid*, p. 259. 6. Thompson, *Magic and Healing*, pp. 62–3. 7. Abithel, *The Physicians of Myddfai*, p. 79. 8. *Ibid*, p. 357. 9. Thompson, p. 63. 10. Maple, *Magic, Medicine and Quackery*, p. 53. 11. Talbot, p. 27. 12. *Ibid*, p. 31. 13. Sami K. Harmaneh, "The Life Sciences", in Hayes (ed.), *The Genius of Arab Civilisation*, p. 155. 14. Buchan, *Domestic Medicine*, p. xviii. 15. Gerard, *Herbal*, "To the Reader". 16. Ziegler, *The Black Death*, p. 46. 17. *Ibid*, p. 38.

CHAPTER 3 The New Disease and the New Medicine
1. Sherwood Taylor, *The Alchemists*, p. 86. 2. Packard, "The Earlier Methods Employed in the Treatment of Syphilis", *AMH* V, 1923, p. 227. 3. Ambroise Paré, *Surgery, Book XIX*, cited Samuel Lane, "A course of Lectures on Syphilis", *The Lancet*, 27 Nov. 1841, p. 285. 4. Hermannus, *An Excellent Treatise teaching how to cure the French-Pockes* (London, 1590), p. 95. 5. Benzoni, *Novae Novi Orbis Historiae*, lib. I, cap. 17, cited Lane, "Syphilis", *The Lancet*, 18 Dec. 1841, p. 393. 6. Louis, *Parallèle des Traitmens*, chap. 2, cited Lane, "Syphilis" *The Lancet*, 18 Dec. 1841, pp. 393–4. 7. Lane, "Syphilis", *The Lancet*, 18 Dec. 1841, p. 394. 8. Goldwater, *Mercury*, p. 226.

CHAPTER 4 The Revolutionary
1. La Wall, *4000 Years of Pharmacy*, p. 243. 2. Stoddart, *Life of Paracelsus*, p. 32, cited Quinby "The Influence of Paracelsus on Modern Therapy", *New England Journal of Medicine*, 19 Jan. 1933, p. 164. 3. Paracelsus, *Sämtliche Werke* (ed. Sudhoff), IV, pp. 3–4, Intimatio Theophrasti: 'The Basle Programme" 5 June, 1527. 4. Pagel *Paracelsus*, pp. 29–30. 5. Paracelsus, *Sämtliche Werke* (ed. Aschner) I, p. 937. 6. *Ibid*, p. 936. 7. Paracelsus (ed. Sudhoff), IV, p. 4. 8. Debus, *The English Paracelsians*, p. 16. 9. Paracelsus (ed. Sudhoff), VII, pp. 78–79. 10. Paracelsus (ed. Aschner), III pp. 491–4; "Introduction to the Herbarius of Theophrastus". 11. *Ibid*. 12. Paracelsus (ed. Aschner), II, pp. 584–5 "Another Fragment on the Errors of Macer". 13. *Ibid*. 14. Paracelsus (ed. Aschner), III, p. 495. 15. Kremers and Urdang, *History of Pharmacy*, p. 41. 16. Paracelsus, *Selected Writings* (ed. Jacobi), p. 169. 17. Paracelsus (ed. Aschner), III, pp. 491–4, "Introduction to the Herbarius of Theophrastus". 18. Paracelsus (ed. Aschner), III, pp. 628. "Of St John's Wort". 19. Biggs, *Mataeotechnica Medicinae Praxeos*, pp. 33–4. 20. Paracelsus (ed. Aschner), III, pp. 628–33; "Of St. John's Wort". 21. Paracelsus (ed. Aschner), III, pp. 491–4 "Introduction to the Herbarius of Theophrastus". 22. Paracelsus (ed.

Aschner), XIV, p. 516, "Of the Supreme Mysteries of Nature", cited Debus, *The English Paracelsians*, p. 22. 23. Kocher, "Paracelsan Medicine in England", *JHM*, Aut. 1947, p. 478. 24. Clowes, *A Treatise for the Artificial Cure of Struma* (1602), "Epistle to the Reader", cited Kocher, *JHM*, Aut. 1947, p. 475. 25. Paracelsus, *Selected Writings* (ed. Jacobi), p. 167.

CHAPTER 5 The Quacks' Charter
1. Sloane ms 1047 (BM), cited Blaxland Stubbs, "Henry VIII and Pharmacy: Part I", *The Chemist and Druggist*, 27 June 1931, p. 794. 2. LaWall, p. 210. 3. Sloane ms 1047, op. cit. 4. Walpole, *Correspondence with the Rev. William Cole* (ed. Lewis and Wallace), p. 332. 5. Gerard, *Herbal*, cited Grieve, p. 828. 6. *Ibid*, pp. 525–6. 7. *Preface to the Grete Herball*, printed Peter Treveris 1526, cited Rohde, pp. 68–9. 8. Gerard, *Herbal*, "To the Reader". 9. *Ibid*, p. 525–6. 10. La Wall, pp. 227–230. 11. Gerard, *Herbal*, "To the Reader". 12. Fuchs, *De Historia Stirpium*, preface, cited Arber, *Herbals*, p. 67. 13. Turner, *A New Herball*, preface. 14. *Ibid*. 15. Rosebury, *Microbes and Morals*, p. 171. 16. *Letters and Papers of the Reign of Henry VIII*, 2, pt. 11, 4450. 17. *Letters and Papers of the Reign of Henry VIII*, 2nd Ed. xvii, 1255, cited Roberts, "The Personnel and Practice of Medicine in Tudor and Stuart England: Part II, London", *MH*, 1962, VI, p. 223. 18. Statutes of the Realm, 34–35, Henry VIII, c. 8. 19. Grieve, p. 820. 20. Goodall, *An Historical Account*, etc. p. 316 ff. 21. *Ibid*, pp. 317–8. 22. *Ibid*, pp. 320–1.

CHAPTER 6 "All Manner of Minerals"
1. Roberts, "The Personnel and Practice of Medicine in Tudor and Stuart England: Part I" *MH*, Oct. 1962, 372. 2. *Ibid*, p. 373. 3. Brunschwig, *The Vertuose Boke of Distyllacion* (1527), cited Kocher, *JHM*, Aut. 1947, p. 453. 4. Gesner, *The Treasure of Euonymus* (1559), cited Kocher *JHM*, Aut. 1947, p. 458. 5. Kocher, *JHM*, Aut. 1947, p. 458. 6. Gesner, *The Newe Iewell of Health*, "George Baker to the Reader". 7. *Ibid*. 8. *Ibid*. 9. Banister, *A Storehouse of Physicall and Philosophicall Secrets*, preface. 10. Clowes, *A Brief and necessarie Treatise, touching the Cure of the Disease called Morbus Gallicus*, p. 23. 11. Banister, p. 43. 12. Multhauf, "Medical Chemistry and 'The Paracelsians' " *BHM*, XXVIII, 2, p. 108. 13. For an interesting discussion of this point see Multhauf, above. 14. *Ibid*, p. 120–121. 15. Clowes, *Approved Practise for All Young Chirurgians* (1588), cited Kocher, *JHM*, Aut. 1947, p. 469. 16. Clowes, *A Treatise for the Artificiall Cure of Struma* (1602); "Epistle to the Reader", cited Debus, p. 70. 17. Gibson, "A Sketch of the Career of Theodore Turquet de Mayerne", *AMH*, New Series, V, no. 4; July 1933, 4, p. 320. 18. *Ibid*, pp. 321 and 323. 19. *Pharmacopoeia Londonensis* (1618), preface, cited Debus, p. 152. 20. Oswald Croll, *Basilica Chymica*, p. 130, trans., and cited Urdang, "How Chemicals entered the Official Pharmacopoeias", *Archives internationales d'histoire des sciences*, xxxiii, 1954, pp. 310–11. 21. *Ibid*.

CHAPTER 7 Galen or Paracelsus?
1. Letter to William Harvey, 3 Feb. 1636, cited Gibson, *AMH*, New Series, V, no. 4, July 1933, p. 323. 2. *Journal de la santé du roi*, p. 26–9. 3. *Journal de la santé*

du roi, p. 86, cited Bernard, "Medicine at the Court of Louis XIV", *MH*, July 1962, p. 202. 4. *Journal du Marquis de Dangeau* (Paris 1854–60), IV, p. 389, cited Bernard, *MH*, July 1962, p. 202. 5. Packard, "Gui Patin and the Medical Profession in Paris in the Seventeenth Century", *AMH*, IV, no. 3, pp. 215–16. 6. *Ibid*, no. 4, p. 364. 7. *Ibid*, no. 3, p. 227. 8. *Ibid*, no. 3, p. 232. 9. *Ibid*, no. 4, p. 370. 10. Pilpoul, *La querelle de l'antimoine*, p. 58. 11. *Ibid*, pp. 40–41. 12. *Ibid*, p. 68. 13. *Ibid*, p. 72. 14. Packard, *AMH*, IV, no. 4, p. 359. 15. *Journal de la santé du roi*, cited in Deguéret, *Histoire médicale du grand roi*, p. 102. 16. Levy-Valensi, *La Médicine et les Médecins Français au XVIIe siècle*, pp. 134–157. 17. Pilpoul, p. 90.

CHAPTER 8 The Seventeenth–Century Superwoman
1. Markham *The English House-wife*, p. 4. 2. *Ibid*. 3. Howard, *Life of the Hon. Lady Anne, Countess of Arundel* (1857), p. 213, and *Home Life of English Ladies in the Seventeenth Century* (1861), p. 42, cited Guthrie, "The Lady Sedley's Receipt Book, 1686, and other Seventeenth-Century Receipt Books", *PRSM*, VI, 1913, p. 164. 4. Skelton, *A Plea for the Botanic Practice of Medicine*, pp. 60–61. 5. Ashby, *Recipe Book in the National Library of Medicine*, cited Blake, "The Compleat Housewife", *BHM*, 1975, no. 49, p. 39. 6. Markham, pp. A3–4. 7. Hole, *The English Housewife in the Seventeenth Century*, p. 86. 8. Markham, p. 50. 9. *The Queen's Closet Opened* (1657), cited Guthrie, *PRSM*, VI, 1913, p. 164. 10. Hole, p. 83. 11. Markham, p. 24. 12. *Ibid*, p. 103. 13. *Arcana Fairfaxiana*, cited Rohde, p. 177. 14. Böttcher, *Miracle Drugs*, p. 243. 15. Blunden, "The Family Physician in the 17th Century", *Elixir*, Spring 1955, p. 16. 16. *Ibid*, p. 16. 17. Mary Kettilby, *A Collection of Above Three Hundred Receipts in Cookery, Physick and Surgery* (2nd ed., 1719), cited Blake, *BHM*, 49, 1975, pp. 38–9. 18. Guthrie, *PRSM*, VI, 1913, p. 154. 19. *Culpeper's School of Physick* (1659), cited Poynter, "Nicholas Culpeper and his books", *JHM*, Jan. 1962, p. 153. 20. *Ibid*. 21. *Ibid*. 22. Culpeper, *A Physicall Directory*, "To the Reader", A1. 23. *Ibid*. 24. *Ibid*, p. 66. 25. *Ibid*. 26. Culpeper, *London Dispensatory*, 1653, p. 128. 27. *Ibid*, p. 128. 28. *Mercurius Pragmaticus*, pt. ii. no. 21, 4–9 Sept. 1649. 29. Culpeper, *Complete Herbal*, p. x. 30. *Ibid*, p. vi. 31. *Ibid*, p. 5. 32. *Ibid*, p. 6. 33. *The Works of Thomas Sydenham*, (trans. Latham), I (London, 1848–50), pp. xcii–xcvi, cited Brockbank, "Sovereign Remedies: A Critical Depreciation of the 17th-Century London Pharmacopoeia", *MH*, January 1964, p. 12.

CHAPTER 9 Indian Physic
1. Hariot, *A Briefe and True Report of the New Found Land of Virginia* (1588), cited Vogel, *American Indian Medicine*, p. 36. 2. A.C., *Tobaco, The Distinct and Severall Opinions of the Late and Best Phisitians That Have Written of the Divers Natures and Qualities Thereof*, cited Vogel, p. 382. 3. Wood, *New England's Prospect*, p.74. 4. Wassenaer, *Historisch Verhael* (1624) in Jameson (ed.), *Narratives of New Netherland* (1909), p. 72. 5. Stone, "Medicine Among the Iroquois", *AMH*, no. 56, 1934, p. 529. 6. Vogel, p. 6. 7. Stone, *AMH*, no. 56, 1934, p. 530. 8. McLuhan, *Touch the Earth*, p. 22. 9. Bradford, *History of Plymouth Plantation* 1620–1647 (Boston, 1912), cited Blake, "Diseases and

Medical Practice in Colonial America" in Marti-Ibanez, (ed.), *History of American Medicine*, p. 34. 10. Blake, Marti-Ibanez, p. 36. 11. T. Thacher, *A brief rule to guide the common people of New England how to order themselves and theirs in the small-pocks or measels*, (Boston 1677–78) cited Blake in Marti-Ibanez, p. 39. 12. Higginson, "New England's Plantation" (1630), in American Colonial Documents to 1776, *English Historical Documents*, IX, pp. 109–110. 13. "Representation of New Netherland" (1650), Jameson, cited Heaton, "Medicine in New Amsterdam", *BHM*, ix, no. 2, 1941, pp. 136–8. 14. Josselyn, *New England's Rarities Discovered*, p. 2. 15. *Ibid*, passim. 16. Governor John Winthrop in a letter written to Sir Nathaniel Rice, 1634, cited Bradley, "Medical practices of the New England Aborigines", *JAPA*, XXV, 1936, p. 144. 17. Vogel, p. 45. 18. "Receipts to cure various disorders. For my worthy friend Mr. Winthrop" (1643), *The Badger Pharmacist*, no. 15, April 1937, pp. 1–24. 19. Wendell Holmes, "The Medical Profession in Massachusetts", *Medical Essays*, pp. 332–3. 20. Locke, "A Drug List of King Philip's War", *The Badger Pharmacist*, no. 25, Feb. 1939, pp. 1–18. 21. cited Scott, "New York Doctors and London Medicines" (1677), *MH* July 1967, pp. 389–398. 22. cited Thompson, *The Quacks of Old London*, p. 94.

CHAPTER 10 "Horrid Electuaries"
1. Culpeper, *Physicall Directory*, "To the Reader" A2. 2. Stokeham, *Medela Medicorum*, p. 62. 3. Banyer, *Pharmacopoeia Pauperum, or The Hospital Dispensatory Containing the Medicines Used in the Hospitals of London* (1718), p. 58, cited Berman, "Evolution of the Printed Hospital Formulary", *The Bulletin of the American Society of Hospital Pharmacists*, vol. 13, May–June 1956. 4. Salmon, *Seplasium*, p. 514. 5. Burill, *The Marquise de Sévigné* (Paris, 1932), p. 37. 6. *Ibid*, p. 67. 7. cited Treve, *Doctor at Court*, p. 26. 8. *Ibid*, pp. 26–7. 9. *Ibid*, p. 27. 10. Dodoens, *Herbal*, cited Grieve, p. 135. 11. cited Treve, p. 27. 12. *Ibid*, p. 29. 13. Aubrey, *Brief Lives*, pp. 232–3. 14. Harvey, *The Family Physician*, pp. 2–3. 15. *Ibid*, pp. 4–6. 16. Culpeper, *School of Physick*, cited Poynter, *JHM*, Jan. 1962, p. 155. 17. Thomson, *Galeno-Pale*, p. 70. 18. *Biggs*, p. 64. 19. *Ibid*, "To the Parliament". 20. *Ibid*, p. 49. 21. Helmont, *Pharmaco & Dispensat. Nov.*, p. 458, cited Needham, *Medela Medicinae*, p. 498. 22. Biggs, p. 64. 23. Needham, p. 430. 24. "Certain Necessary Directions . . . issued by the College of Physicians" (25 May 1665), cited Thomas, "The Society of Chymical Physitians" in Underwood (ed.), *Science, Medicine and History*, pp. 55–57. 25. *An Advertisement from the Society of Chymical Physitians*, BM C120, h5, cited Thomas in Underwood, pp. 55–57. 26. Letter written by Sir Nathaniel Hodges, 8 May 1666, cited Thomas in Underwood, p. 70. 27. Packard, p. 366. 28. Cabanes, *Comment se soignaient nos pères*, pp. 429–30, cited Sulblé, *Quelques charlatans célèbres au XVIIe siècle*, p. 24. 29. Thompson, *Quacks of Old London*, p. 51. 30. *Ibid*, p. 109. 31. Greene, *Lord Rochester's Monkey*, p. 120. 32. *Ibid*, p. 124. 33. Thompson, *The Quacks of Old London*, p. 120. 34. Culpeper, *Complete Herbal*, p. 62. 35. Krieg, *Green Medicine*, p. 217. 36. *Ibid*, pp. 174–5. 37. *Ibid*, p. 178. 38. *Ibid*, p. 176.

CHAPTER 11 "Systematic Slaughter"
1. Biggs, p. 31. 2. Withering, *A Botanical Arrangement of all the Vegetables*

Naturally Growing in Great Britain, pp. iv–v. 3. Needham, pp. 496–7. 4. *Ibid*, p. 475. 5. King, *The Medical World of the Eighteenth Century*, p. 59. 6. Needham, p. 476. 7. Culpeper, *Complete Herbal*, p. 60. 8. Lind, *A Treatise of the Scurvy*, pp. 129–30. 9. Gerard, pp. 401–402. 10. Woodall, *The Surgion's Mate*, p. 185. 11. Lind, p. 41. 12. *Ibid*, p. 31. 13. *Ibid*, p. 41. 14. *Ibid*, p. 45. 15. *Ibid*, pp. 322–323. 16. *Ibid*, p. 5. 17. *Ibid*, pp. 145–148. 18. *Ibid*, p. 91. 19. *Ibid*, p. 153.

CHAPTER 12 The English Practice
1. Dr. Cadwallader Colden to Dr. John Mitchell, 7 Nov. 1745, Colden Letters and Papers, VIII, pp. 335–6. 2. Wafer, *A New Voyage and Description of the Isthmus of Panama*, p. 131, cited Vogel, p. 149. 3. Stearns, *The American Herbal or Materia Medica*, p. 15. 4. *Ibid*, p. 16. 5. *Ibid*, p. 19. 6. *Ibid*, pp. 18–19. 7. *Ibid*, p. 339. 8. *Ibid*, p. 23. 9. Colden papers, cited Vogel, p. 113. 10. *The New York Gazette Revived in the Weekely Post Boy*, 3 August 1725, New Jersey Archives, First Series, XIX, p. 175, cited Gordon, "Medicine in Colonial New Jersey and Adjacent Areas", *BHM*, XVII, 1945, p. 51. 11. Blanton, *Medicine in Virginia in the Eighteenth Century* p. 34. 12. De Warville, *New Travels in the United States of America performed in 1788*, p. 351, cited Blanton, p. 131. 13. William Douglass, *A Summary, historical and political, of the first planting, progressive improvements and present state of the British Settlements in North America.*, 2 vols. (London 1760), II, p. 352, cited Duffy, *Epidemics in Colonial America*, (Baton Rouge, 1953), p. 8, and Gill, *The Apothecary in Colonial America*, p. 33. 14. James Adair, *The History of the American Indians, Particularly those Nations Adjoining to the Mississippi*, p. 234, cited Vogel, pp. 100–101. 15. Blanton, p. 181. 16. Bassett, *Writings of Colonel Byrd*, p. 107, cited Blanton, p. 184. 17. *Ibid*, p. 211, cited Blanton, p. 183. 18. Blanton, p. 184. 19. Phillips, *Plantation and Frontier*, I, p. 109, cited Blanton, p. 156. 20. Bassett, *Writings of Colonel Byrd*, p. 113, cited Blanton, p. 184. 21. *Ibid*, p. 384, cited Blanton, p. 182. 22. Drinker, *Not So Long Ago*, p. 245. 23. Hertzer, *The Horse and Buggy Doctor*, pp. 1–2. 24. Drinker, p. 108–9. 25. Dr. James Jackson, *Letters to a Young Physician*, cited Wendell Holmes, "Scholastic and Bedside Teaching", *Medical Essays*, p. 307.

CHAPTER 13 The Foxglove Saga
1. Letter from William Withering to his parents, 1764 cited Roddis, "William Withering and the Introduction of Digitalis into Medical Practice: Part I" *AMH* New Series, VIII, March 1936, p. 93. 2. Withering, *A Botanical Arrangement*, I, p. xxiv. 3. *Ibid*, p. 528. 4. *Ibid*, p. 349. 5. *Ibid*, p. 523. 6. *Ibid*, p. 376. 7. Withering, *An Account of the Foxglove*, p. 2. 8. *Ibid*, p. 9. 9. *Ibid*, p. 3. 10. *Ibid*, pp. 1–2. 11. *Ibid*, pp. 1–2. 12. *Ibid*. 13. *Ibid*. 14. Abraham, *J. J. Lettsom, His Life, Times, Friends and Descendants* (London 1933), p. 480, cited Blanton P. Seward, "Pioneer Medicine in Virginia", *AMH*, New Series, X, 1938, p. 172. 15. Buchan, pp. xi–xii. 16. John Wesley in a letter to Ebenezer Blackwell, cited Hill, *John Wesley among the Physicians*, p. 47. 17. Good, *The History of Medicine so far as it relates to the Profession of the Apothecary* (1795), pp. 149–155. 18. Wesley, *Primitive Physic*, pp. 120–121. 19. George Berkeley, "Further Thoughts on Tar-Water", *Works*, III, p. 343, cited King, *The Medical World of the Eighteenth Century*, p. 43. 20. Wesley, p. xv. 21. *Ibid*, p. v. 22. *Ibid*. 23. "The

Lititz Pharmacopoeia", in *The Badger Pharmacist*, nos. 22–25, June–Dec. 1938. 24. Schopf, *Travels in the Confederation (1783—1784)*, ed. Morrison, I, 289, cited Vogel, p. 66. 25. *Ibid*, pp. 284–287, cited Vogel, p. 66. 26 Rush, *An Inquiry into the Natural History of Medicine among the Indians of North America*, p. 152, cited Vogel, p. 63.

CHAPTER 14 Heroic Medicine
1. Wells, *Last Illness and Death of Washington*, cited Blanton, pp. 305–6. 2. Lossing, *The Pictorial Field-Book of the Revolution*, V, p. 506, cited Blanton, pp. 206–7. 3. *The Rush Light*. The English journalist William Cobbett published several issues of a periodical under this title around 1800 in New York, in which he mercilessly attacked the medical practices of Dr. Rush. See Lasagna, *The Doctors' Dilemmas*, p. 56. 4. Rush, *Works of Thomas Sydenham*, pp. 7–9, cited Coulter, *Divided Legacy*, III, p. 29. 5. Rush, *Sixteen Introductory Lectures*, p. 147, cited Coulter, III, p. 37. 6. *Ibid*, p. 147, cited Coulter, III, p. 38. 7. Kaufman, *Homoeopathy in America*, p. 2. 8. Rush, *An Inquiry into the Functions of the Spleen, Liver, Pancreas and Thyroid Gland*, p. 27, cited Coulter, III, p. 39. 9. Rush, *Sixteen Introductory Lectures*, p. 9, cited Coulter, III, p. 62. 10. Hooker, *Rational Therapeutics*, p. 160. 11. Drinker, pp. 123–6. 12. *Western Journal of the Medical and Physical Sciences*, XI–XII (1837–1838), p. 71, cited Coulter, III, p. 63. 13. Eberle, *Materia Medica and Therapeutics*, II, p. 2, cited Coulter, III, p. 63. 14. John Duffy, *Rudolph Matas History of Medicine in Louisiana* (Baton Rouge, 1962) II, p. 5, cited Kaufman, p. 10. 15. Kelly, *Cyclopedia of American Medical Biography* (Philadelphia and London, 1912), I, pp. 199–201, cited Kaufman, p. 10. 16. Wendell Holmes, "Currents and Counter-Currents in Medical Science": an Address delivered before the Massachusetts Medical Society at the Annual Meeting, 30 May 1860, *Medical Essays*, p. 193. 17. *Southern Medical and Surgical Journal*, New Series, VI (1850) p. 257, cited Coulter, III, pp. 67–8. 18. Beach, *The British and American Reformed Practice of Medicine*, p. 89.

CHAPTER 15 Roots and Herbs
1. Thomson, *A Narrative of the Life and Medical Discoveries of Samuel Thomson*, p. 124. 2. *Ibid*, p. 124. 3. *Ibid*, p. 26–7. 4. *Ibid*, p. 25. 5. *Ibid*, pp. 22–3. 6. *Ibid*, p. 26. 7. *Ibid*, p. 31. 8. *Ibid*, p. 24. 9. *Ibid*, p. 25. 10. *Ibid*, p. 29. 11. *Ibid*, pp. 49–50. 12. *Ibid*, p. 40. 13. *Ibid*, pp. 15–6. 14. *Ibid*, p. 196. 15. *LLB*, no. 11, Series 7, 1909, p. 82. 16. Thomson, p. 196. 17. *Ibid*, p. 43. 18. *Ibid*, pp. 72–3. 19. *LLB*, p. 83. 20. *Ibid*, p. 85. 21. *Ibid*, pp. 83–4. 22. Thomson, p. 141. 23. *LLB*, no. 11, Series 7, 1909, p. 85. 24. Thomson, p. 46. 25. *Ibid*, p. 122–3. 26. Family Right issued to Joseph Chapman, 1839. Reproduced in Zeuch, *History of Medical Practice in Illinois*, (Illinois, 1927), I, p. 326, cited Berman "The Thomsonian Movement", *BHM*, XXV, Sept.–Oct. 1951, p. 416. 27. Thomson, p. 46. 28. Lasagna, p. 53. 29. Thomson, p. 123.

CHAPTER 16 Botanic Warfare
1. Curtis, *Discussions between Several Members of the Regular Medical faculty and the Thomsonian Botanic Physicians on the Comparative Merits of their Respective*

Systems, p. 36. 2. *Stethoscope and Virginia Medical Gazette*, 1851, I, pp. 16 and 20, cited Blanton, *Medicine in Virginia in the Nineteenth Century*, p. 196. 3. Peter Smith, *The Indian Doctor's Dispensatory* (Cincinnati, 1813), cited Pickard and Buley, *The Midwest Pioneer* (New York, 1946), pp. 45–6. 4. Henry, *A New and Complete American Family Herbal*, p. v. 5. Vogel, p. 132. 6. Bigelow, *American Medical Botany*, II, p. xvi. 7. *Stethoscope and Virginia Medical Gazette*, 1851, I, pp. 16 and 20, cited Blanton, p. 196. 8. *LLB*, no. II, Series 7, 1909, pp. 56–7. 9. *Ibid*, p. 61. 10. Mitchell, *Homoepathy*, p. 12. 11. Hahnemann, *Organon*, section 28, cited Coulter, III, p. 24. 12. Beach, *The Rise, Progress, and Present State of the New York Medical Institution and Reformed Medical Society of the United States*, cited Felter, *History of the Eclectic Medical Institute*, p. 81. 13. *Ibid*, p. 82. 14. *Ibid*. 15. Editorial, *The Western Medical Reformer*, III, no. 3, p. 43, March 1838, cited Berman, *BHM XXV*, Nov.–Dec. 1951, no. 5, p. 535. 16. *Thomsonian Recorder*, IV, no. 17, p. 187, cited Berman, *BHM*, op. cit. 17. The *Boston Thomsonian Medical Journal*, I, p. 69, 1845, cited Berman, "Social Roots of the 19th-century Botanico-Medical Movement in the United States", *Actes du VIIIe Congres International d'histoire des sciences*, 1956, vol. 2, p. 562. 18. Beach, *The Rise, Progess etc.*, cited Felter, p. 82. 19. Beach, *The Telescope*, IV, no. 86, 1827. Facsimile sheet reproduced in Berman, "Wooster Beach and the Early Eclectics", *University of Michigan Medical Bulletin*, XXIV, no. 7, 1958, p. 278. 20. *Ibid*. 21. Forman, "The Worthington School and Thomsonianism", *BHM*, XXI, 1947, p. 775. 22. Morrow, *Western Medical Reformer* I, 1836, p. 5, cited Felter, p. 12. 23. Report of Nathanial Magoon, *Botanico-Medical Recorder*, Nov. 1843, reprinted *LLB*, no. 11, series 7, 1909, pp. 68–88. 24. Letter Dr. Benjamin Waterhouse to Samuel Thomson, 3 March 1836, *LLB*, no. 11, Series 7, 1909, p. 63.

CHAPTER 17 The Age of Calomel

1. Chambers, *A Pocket Herbal*, dedication. 2. *Ibid*. 3. *Ibid*, passim. 4. *Ibid*, p. 307. 5. Eliot, *Middlemarch* (Penguin), p. 116. 6. Reece, *The Medical Guide*, pp. 1–4. 7. Graham, *Modern Domestic Medicine*, preface, p. vi. 8. Reece, pp. 40–41. 9. *Ibid*, p. 40. 10. Reece, *A Practical Dissertation, etc.*, p. 352. 11. *Ibid*, p. 1. 12. Reece, *Medical Guide*, p. 36. 13. Eliot, p. 175. 14. *Ibid*, p. 486. 15. Hill, *The Useful Family Herbal*, p. vii. 16. *Ibid*, pp. xii–xiii. 17. *Ibid*, p. xiii. 18. Waller, *The New British Domestic Herbal*, preface, p. 1. 19. Woodville, *Medical Botany*, I, preface, p. 3. 20. *Ibid*, p. 1. 21. Blackall on dropsies, pp. 248 ff., cited Hamilton, *Observations on the Use and Abuse of Mercurial Medicines in Various Diseases*, p. 129. 22. *Ibid*, p. 130. 23. Whitlaw, *The Scriptural Code of Health, with Observations on the Mosaic prohibitions and on the principles and benefits of the medicated vapour bath*, pp. 87–8. 24. *Ibid*, p. 133, 25. *Ibid*, p. 97. 26. *Ibid*, p. 98. 27. *Ibid*.

CHAPTER 18 "Coffinism"

1. Watmore, "Our Medical Heroes: Albert Isaiah Coffin, M.D., U.S.A." *The Medical Herbalist*, 26 May 1926, p. 190. 2. *DSBR*, 1 May 1852, p. 3. 3. *Ibid*, p. 3. 4. *Ibid*, p. 3. 5. Coffin, *Lectures on Medical Botany*, pp. 174–9. 6. The *Thomsonian Recorder*, I, 1832, p. 158. 7. Coffin, pp. 218–20. 8. *Ibid*, pp. 221–2. 9. *CBJ*, I,

2 Dec. 1848, p. 193, 10. *Ibid*, I, 4 Sept. 1847, pp. 68–9. 11. *Ibid*, I, 4 Sept. 1847, p. 72. 12. Watmore, *Medical Herbalist*, May 1926, p. 191. 13. *CBJ*, V, 19 Nov. 1853, pp. 44–7. 14. *Lancet*, 22 April 1848, p. 454. 15. Issues repeatedly aired in the *Journal* and in Coffin's lectures. 16. *DSBR*, 1 Jan. 1853, pp. 138–9. 17. *ibid*, pp. 138–9. 18. *Ibid*. 19. *CBJ*, III, 8 May 1852, pp. 328–9. 20. *Ibid*, I, 4 Aug. 1849, pp. 270–71. 21. *Ibid*, I, 6 July, 1850, p. 141. 22. Baly & Gull, *Reports on Epidemic Cholera drawn up at the desire of the Cholera Committee of the Royal College of Surgeons* (1854). 23. *CBJ*, I, 2 Sept. 1848, p. 171, and Fox, *Family Botanic Guide*, pp. 1725. 24. p.c. Frederick Fletcher Hyde. 25. *Association Medical Journal* (London), 1853, p. 1045. 26. *Morning Advertiser*, 5 Nov. 1853. 27. *Coffin's Botanical Journal*, V, 19 Nov. 1853, pp. 39–40. 28. *Ibid*, p. 45.

CHAPTER 19 Dr. Coffin v. Dr. Skelton
1. *CBJ*, III, 27 March 1852, p. 286. 2. *DSBR* 1 May 1852, pp. 3–4 and p. 21. 3. Skelton, *A Plea*, p. 50–51. 4. *DSBR*, 1 May 1852, p. 3. 5. *Ibid*, p. 4. 6. *Ibid*, pp. 4, 21, *CBJ*, II, 19 Jan. 1850, pp. 21–3. 7. *Ibid*, p. 22. 8. *DSBR*, 1 May 1852, p. 22. 9. Beach, pp. 128–9. 10. *DSBR*, op. cit., p. 5. 11. By the end of 1853 Skelton was a member of the Syracuse Eclectic Institution. 12. *DSBR*, op. cit., p. 6. 13. *DSBR*, 7 Aug. 1852, p. 59. 14. *Ibid*, pp. 49–54. 15. *DSBR*, 4 Sept. 1852, pp. 67–79. 16. *DSBR*, 1 April 1854, p. 372. 17. *Ibid*, p. 370. 18. *DSBR*, 1 Oct. 1853, p. 275. 19. *DSBR*, 2 June 1855, p. 597. 20. *Ibid*, p. 596. 21. *CBJ*, II, 17 Aug. 1850, p. 185. 22. *DSBR*, 2 June 1855, p. 597. 23. *Ibid*, 1 Oct. 1853, p. 273. 24. *Ibid*, 4 Sept. 1852, p. 65. 25. Figures arrived at by Mr. Brady after consulting the Registrar General's office and the various medical directories, see *Medical Times and Gazette*, 13 May 1854. 26. *DSBR*, 7 Jan. 1854, p. 323. 27. *CBJ*, VI, 28 July 1955, pp. 172–4, and IX, 27 Nov. 1858, p. 54. 28. *Ibid*, X, 4 Feb. 1860, p. 45–47. 29. Coffin's personal fortunes were considerable as his Will shows. Among his assets were the freehold Château de Capolle near Boulogne; the leasehold of no. 134 High Holborn, from which his business was run; the lavish household effects which impressed visitors in his rented house at 24 Montague Place; the goodwill of his wholesale herbal business and a large holding in the London & Yorkshire Railway Co. 30. Watmore, *Medical Herbalist*, May 1926, pp. 90–1. 31. Coffin's death certificate, issued 4 Aug. 1866, gives cause of death as "carcinoma of stomach". 32. *Medical Free Press*, I, 1 Oct. 1866, p. 149.

CHAPTER 20 Fruitless Medication
1. Blasingame, "The American Medical Association: from Mastodons to Modern Medicine", *The Medical Journal of Australia*, 19 May 1962, pp. 765–6. 2. Code of Ethics of the A.M.A. adopted Philadelphia, May 1847, pp. 18–19, cited Kaufman, p. 53. 3. Berman, "Wooster Beach and the Early Eclectics", *University of Michigan Medical Bulletin*, XXIV, 7, 1958, pp. 283–284. 4. *Transactions of the A.M.A.*, IV, 1851, p. 198, cited Coulter, *Homoeopathic Influences*, pp. 46–7. 5. Fishbein, *A History of the A.M.A.*, pp. 30–31. 6. Dickson Smith, *A Few Facts in Relation to the Lobelia and Pepper Practice: Its Prospects and Policy*, p. 2. 7. *Ibid*, pp. 16–17. 8. Dr. King in *The Western Medical Reformer*, 1846, p. 175, cited "The Eclectic Alkaloids", *LLB*, no. 12, Pharmacy Series 2, 1910, p. 6. 9.

"The Eclectic Alkaloids", op. cit., pp. 8–9. 10. *Ibid*, p. 9. 11. King, cited "The Eclectic Alkaloids" op. cit., p. 7. 12. Editorial by John Scudder, *EMJ*, March 1870, cited *LLB*, no. 19, Pharmacy Series 5, 1912, p. 273. 13. Scudder, "Brief History of Eclectic Medicine", *EMJ*, XXXIX, p. 305, 1879, cited Berman in *University of Michigan Medical Bulletin*, op. cit., pp. 281–2. 14. Lloyd, "Fragments from an Autobiography", A paper read at the 63rd meeting of the Ohio Eclectic Medical Association, Akron, May 1927, *EMJ*, July 1927. 15. Scudder, *EMJ*, 1877, reprinted *LLB*, no. 19, Pharmacy Series 5, 1912, p. 322. 16. Lloyd, "Fragments from an Autobiography", op. cit. pp. 9–10. 17. *Ibid*, p. 9. 18. "The Eclectic Alkaloids", *LLB*, no. 12, Pharmacy Series 2, 1910, p. 41. 19. *British and Foreign Medical and Chirurgical Review*, July 1858, p. 1, cited Dickson Smith, op. cit., pp. 4–5. 20. Dickson Smith, op. cit., p. 5. 21. Kramer, *The Beginnings of the Public Health Movement in the United States*, cited Coulter, *Divided Legacy*, III, p. 72. 22. Wendell Holmes, "Scholastic and Bedside Teaching" in *Medical Essays*, p. 294. 23. Hooker, p. 175. 24. Cook, *Women's Herbal Book of Health*, p. vi. 25. Wendell Holmes, "Currents and Counter-Currents in Medical Science" in *Medical Essays*, p. 199. 26. Kramer, cited Coulter, op. cit., p. 72. 27. Hooker, p. 185. 28. *Ibid*, pp. 172–3. 29. Wendell Holmes, "Currents and Counter-Currents", op. cit., p. 203. 30. *Buffalo Medical and Surgical Journal* X, (1870–1871), p. 133, cited Coulter, *Homoeopathic Influences*, p. 10. 31. Lloyd, "Eclectic Pharmacy", *ECM*, Nov. 1924, p. 5.

CHAPTER 21 Regulars and Rivals

1. *The New Era of Eclecticism*, I, 1870, p. 78. 2. *Ibid*, I, 1870 p. 55, and Vol II, 1871, pp. 402–404. 3. *Medical Times and Gazette*, 16 Dec. 1871, p. 755. 4. *The New Era of Eclecticism*, I, 1870, p. 21. 5. *Ibid*, IV, 1874, p. iii. 6. Chapman, *Jesse Boot*, pp. 6–7. 7. Thompson, *Lark Rise*, p. 105. 8. Boyd Mushet, "A Glance at an Obsolete Materia Medica", *Pract.* IV, 1870, pp. 141–3. 9. Lauder Brunton, *A Textbook of Pharmacology, Therapeutics and Materia Medica*, II, p. 757. 10. *Ibid*, II, p. 829. 11. NIMH. 12. *Ibid*. 13. *Ibid*. 14. Coulter, *Divided Legacy* III, p. 423. 15. *Ibid*. 16. Fishbein, p. 96. 17. *JAMA*, XXXI, 1903, p. 736. 18. Lloyd, "Eclectic Pharmacy", Ohio Transactions 1905, p. 327. 19. *Ibid*, p. 4. 20. Fishbein, p. 989. 21. Flexner, *Medical Education in the United States and Canada*, p. 227. 22. *Ibid*. 23. *Ibid*, p. 212. 24. *Ibid*, p. 213. 25. *Ibid*, p. x. 26. *Ibid*, pp. vii–ix. 27. *Ibid*, p. xvi. 28. *Ibid*, p. xvi. 29. *Ibid*, p. 162–3. 30. *Ibid*, p. 163. 31. *Ibid*, p. 156. 32. *Ibid*, pp. 156–7. 33. *Ibid*, p. 62. 34. *Ibid*, pp. 63–4. 35. *Ibid*, p. 65. 36 Kerr White, "Health Care Arrangements in the United States: A.D. 1972", *Medical Care and Medical Cure, The Milbank Memorial Fund Quarterly*, L, pt. 2, no. 4, Oct. 1972, cited Carlson, *Frontiers of Science and Medicine*, p. 38. 37. Fishbein, *Fads and Quackery*, pp. 35–6. 38. *The General Education Board Review and Final Report* 1902–62, New York, 1964, pp. 34, 37, cited Coulter, *Divided Legacy* III, pp. 449–50. 39. Griffin, *World Without Cancer*, p. 375.

CHAPTER 22 Magic Bullets

1. Inglis, *History of Medicine*, pp. 160–3. 2. Baldry, *Battle Against Bacteria*, p. 68. 3. Dennie, *A History of Syphilis*, pp. 113–8. 4. NIMH. 5. *Ibid*. 6. Pusey, *A*

Doctor of the 1870s and 80s, p. 95. 7. Adams, "Some New Drugs and Remedies", *BMJ*, 28 March 1936, p. 625. 8. McKechnie, *Strong Medicine*, p. 162. 9. Campbell, "The Last Fifty Years of Medicine", *Manchester Medical Gazette*, L, 1971, pp. 50–51. 10. Linnell, "Further Examples of the Misuse of Common Remedies", *Pract.*, 1936, p. 212. 11. Lloyd, "Back to the People", a paper read at the National Eclectic Medical Association in 1914, *EMJ*, May 1925, pp. 4–6. 12. *Ibid*, pp. 4–6. 13. Adams, op. cit, p. 627. 14. Campbell, op. cit., p. 51. 15. Moreau, "Medicine 1916–1976", *Vogue,* London, 15 Oct. 1976, pp. 147, 154, 156. 16. Kraemer, "Medicinal Plants: Present and Future Supplies", *American Journal of Pharmacy*, 18 June 1918, p. 407. 17. *Ibid*, p. 414. 18. Haag, "Rafinesque's Interests a Century Later: Medicinal Plants", *Science*, XCIV, no. 2444, 31 Oct. 1941, p. 404. 19. Minchin, "The Germicidal and Therapeutic Action of Garlic", *Pract.*, 1918, p. 145. 20. *Ibid*, pp. 145–54. 21. Fishbein, *Fads and Quackery*, p. 37. 22. *Ibid*, p. 37–8. 23. *Ibid*. 24. *Ibid*, pp. 38–9.

CHAPTER 23 Return to Nature.
1. Monardes, *Joyfull Newes out of the Newe Found World*, introduction by S. Gaselee, p. xviii. 2. Albutt, "On the Use of Sarsaparilla in Syphilis", *Pract.* May 1970, pp. 258–9. 3. *Potter's Bulletin*, Aut. 1938, p. 20. 4. *Sunday Dispatch*, 22 March 1936, cited *Potter's Bulletin*, Sprin 1936. 5. Teetgen, *Profitable Herb Growing and Collecting*, p. 9. 6. Grieve, "Grow Herbs!", *Weekly Dispatch,* 11 June 1916, reprinted in "Raspberry", *Herbs Go to War* series, 1914–18. 7. "Medical Herbs in Wartime", *BMJ*, 14 June 1941, p. 901. 8. Production of Drugs at Home and Within the Empire", *BMJ*, 14 June 1941, p. 568. 9. Grieve, pamphlet on Foxglove, Lily of the Valley, Solomon's Seal, in *Herbs Go to War* op. cit. 10. Grieve, Sphagnum Moss in *Herbs Go to War*, op. cit. 11. "Physic–Gardeners" *Pall Mall Gazette*, 15 Sept. 1915, reprinted "Marigold" in *Herbs Go to War*, op. cit. 12. Leyel, introduction to Grieve, *Modern Herbal*, p. xiv. 13. NIMH. 14. *Ibid*. 15. *Ibid*. 16. *Ibid*. 17. *Sunday Dispatch*, 22 March 1936, op. cit. 18. Weiss, "Gegenwartsaufgaben einer wissenschaftlichen Pflanzenheilkunde", *Deutsche Medizinische Wochenschrift*, 24 June 1938, pp. 922–4. 19. Fletcher Hyde, Presidential Address at 11th Annual Conference of the NIMH, *New Herbal Practitioner*, II, no. 1, p.3. 20. NIMH. 21. Haggard, *The Doctor in History*, p. 99. 22. Fairbarn, "Some Recent Advances in the Knowledge of the Constituents of Vegetable Drugs", *Journal of Pharmacy and Pharmacology*, no. 5, 1953, p. 281. 23. Farnsworth, "The Plant Kingdom – Supplier of Steroids", *Tile and Till*, LIII, no. 55, September 1967. 24. *Ibid*. 25. Farnsworth & Bingel, "Problems and Prospects of Discovering New Drugs from Higher Plants by Pharmacological Screening", in Wagner and Wolff (eds.), *New Natural Products and Plant Drugs with Pharmacological, Biological or Therapeutical Activity*, pp. 1–22. 26. *Ibid*. 27. Scheindlin, "New Developments in Plant Drugs", *AMJ*, CXXXVI, Sept.–Oct. 1964.

CHAPTER 24 The Price of Miracles
1. Dubos, "On the Present Limitations of Drug Research", in Talalay (ed.), *Drugs in Our Society*, p. 41. 2. p.c. 3. Richards, "A Clinician's View of Advances in Therapeutics", in Talalay, op. cit., p. 33–4. 4. *Ibid*. 5. Illich,

Medical Nemesis, p. 1. 6. Task Force on the Preparation of Drugs: Final Report, U.S. Department of Health, Education and Welfare, cited Davies, *Modern Medicine*, p. 35. 7. London *Evening Standard*, 1 April 1977. 8. Public statement of 17 drug scientists after Meeting on the Rational Regulation of the Development of New Medicines, *European Journal of Clinical Pharmacology*, II, 233, (1977), cited Laurence and Black, *The Medicine You Take*, pp. 136–7. 9. Doyle, "How Doctors missed Heart Drug's Dangers", London *Observer*, 5 Sept. 1976. 10. "The Medicines You Take – A Shock Report", *Woman's Own*, London, 20 May 1978. 11. Fisher & Christie, *A Dictionary of Drugs*, p. 10. 12. "Drugs in Pregnancy", *Medical Letter*, XIV, 94, 8 Dec. 1972, cited Silverman & Lee, *Pills, Profits and Politics*, p. 268. 13. "The Medicines You Take", *Woman's Own*, op. cit. 14. London *Sunday Times*, 2 March 1980. 15. Silverman, *The Drugging of the Americas*, pp. 7–13. 16. Report by Neville Hodgkinson, London *Daily Mail*, 5 May 1979. 17. London *Evening Standard*, 1 June 1979. 18. Bonnet & Villeneuve, "La Folie des Medicaments", *L'Express*, no. 1245, 19–25 May 1975, pp. 80–84. 19. London *Sunday Times*, 5 Dec. 1976. 20. *Sunday Times*, 7 Dec. 1975. 21. London *Daily Express*, 28 June 1977, 22. Carlson, *The Frontiers of Science and Medicine*, p. 40. 23. Okute, or Shooter, Sioux Indian quoted in McLuhan, p. 18. 24. Skelton, *A Plea for the Botanic Practice of Medicine*, p. 256. 25. Fletcher Hyde, "Therapeutic Use of Herbal Remedies" A lecture delivered at a symposium on herbal remedies in Europe, arranged by the Pharmaceutical Society of Great Britain at the School of Pharmacy, Bradford University, 22 May 1974. Printed in *New Herbal Practitioner*, I, 1974, p. 19. 26. Forbes, *Try Being Healthy*, p. 54. 27. Tompkins & Bird, *The Secret Life of Plants*, p. 273. 28. Forbes, "New Approaches to Cancer Therapy" in W.H.O.: Consultation on Potentials for Use of Plants indicated by Traditional Medicine in Cancer Therapy, Geneva, 13–17 Nov. 1978. WHO CAN/TRM/79. 1. 29. Holmes, "Borderlines in Medical Science". Introductory lecture delivered before the Medical Class of Harvard University, 6 Nov. 1861, in *Medical Essays*, p. 255.

CHAPTER 25 Herbs and the Law
1. Frank Power of Messrs Potter's, "Herbal Medicine and the Medicine Bill", unpublished report. 2. *Ibid.* 3. Fletcher Hyde, Presidential address to the 111th Annual Conference of the NIMH, in *New Herbal Practitioner*, II, no. 1, p. 4. 4. p.c. from Fletcher Hyde. 5. *New Herbal Practitioner*, editorial, IV, no. 3, April 1978. 6. Defares, Kema & van der Werff, "The Effect of Bio-Strath consumption on some psychological variables in a group of retarded children", unpublished report, p.c. F. Pestalozzi. 7. Michel & Fritz-Niggli, "Die Beeinflüssung der Fertilität der weissen Maus durch kleine Strahlenmengen und ein Hefepreparat (Bio-Strath)", *Radiologica Clinica et Biologica*, XLII, no. 3, 1973. 8. "Auswertung von 1140 ärztlichen Erfahrungsberichten über die Wirkung von 11 Präparaten der Bio-Strath" – Reihe *Pharma*, Switzerland, I, 1979, pp. 1–2. 9. Van Straten, London *Observer*, 2 Jan. 1977. 10. Brunner & Schwarzenbach, "Die Wirkung eines standardisierten Hefeextractes (Bio-Strath Elizier) auf den Allgemeinzustand therapeutisch bestrahlter Tumorpatienten", unpublished paper, 10 June 1962. 11. Van Straten, "Recent Studies of the

Therapeutic Value of Herbs", paper presented at the 2nd World Congress of Natural Medicine, Bienne, Switzerland, August 1976, p. 9. 12. Oliver Gillie, London *Sunday Times*, 23 April 1978. 13. *National Health Federation Bulletin*, April 1974, cover, cited Griffin, p. 453. 14. "The F.D.A. on Herbs: Where do they sand?", *The Natural Foods Merchandiser*, Feb. 1979, p. 43. 15. p.c. Farnsworth. 16. *Ibid*. 17. Kourennoff, p. 176. 18. Kourennoff, preface by Krauer. 19. Segelman and others "Sassafras and Herb Tea: Potential Health Hazards", *JAMA*, CCXXXVI, no. 5, 2 Aug. 1976, p. 477. 20. "Toxic Reactions to Plant Products sold in health-food stores", *Medical Letter*, XXI, 1979, pp. 29–31, cited Farnsworth, *The Nature and Validity of Adverse Publicity and the Future of Herb Teas in the United States*, pp. 2–3. 21. p.c. Farnsworth. 22. *Ibid*.

CHAPTER 26 East and West
1. Farnsworth, "Pharmacy Practice and Pharmaceutical Education in the People's Republic of China", *American Journal of Pharmaceutical Education*, XL, May 1976, p. 115. 2. *Ibid*, pp. 115–20. 3. Li Ching-Wei, "Creating a new Chinese Medicine", *Herbal Review*, III, no. 2, Spring 1978, pp. 13–14. 4. The Revolutionary Health Committee of Hunan Province, *A Barefoot Doctor's Manual*, pp. 338–9, and Thompson, *Herbs that Heal*, p. 138. 5. Chang Jung-Lieh "Anti-tumour Experiments and Clinical Observations of '757' – an Extract from Zhu-ling (*Polyporus Umbellata*)", WHO report, Nov. 1978, op. cit. 6. Silverman & Lee, p. 265. 7. Davies, *Modern Medicine*, p. 116. 8. p.c. Dr. Percy Brown. 9. Coleman, *Paper Doctors*, pp. 13–14. 10. *To the Point* (South Africa), 14 March 1980, p. 28. 11. *Time* Magazine, 1 Dec. 1975. 12. *The Soil Association Quarterly Review* IV, no. 4, Dec. 1978. 13. Farnsworth, "The Development of Pharmacological and Chemical Research for Application to Traditional Medicine in Developing Countries", paper presented at symposium, Plants in Traditional Medicine, Rome, 3–5 April 1979, p. 3. 14. Soejarto & others, "Fertility Regulating Agents from Plants", *Bulletin of the World Health Organization*, 56 (3): 343–352, 1978. 15. Glasser, *The Greatest Battle*, preface, p. viii. 16. WHO report, Nov. 1978, op. cit. 17. *International Herald-Tribune*, 16 Sept. 1977. 18. *International Herald-Tribune*, 2 Oct. 1980. 19. "Indigenous Systems of Medicine in India", *BMJ*, 15 Sept. 1923, pp. 479–480. 20. Elliott, "The Madras Government and Indigenous Systems of Medicine", letter in *BMJ*, 25 Oct. 1924, pp. 786–8. 21. p.c. Gladys Tantaquidgeon. 22. p.c. David Besaw. 23. p.c. Nora Thompson Dean. 24. Kokwaro, *Medicinal Plants of East Africa*, preface. 25. *Ibid*, p. 1. 26. London *Daily Mail*, 14 April 1977. 27. London *Evening Standard*, 13 April 1977. 28. Withering, *A Botanical Arrangement*, pp. iv–v.

CHAPTER 27 The Green Sweep
1. Penso, "Present-day Problems Relating to the Use of Medical Plants Throughout the World", WHO:DPM/77. 1, p. 9. 2. p.c. Directors Biohorma. 3. Statistics published 1980 by the Statistical Bureau Lagendijk and Report of the National Secretary from Holland to the AGM of the International Federation of Natural Therapeutics, Brussels, 4 June 1978. 4. *Sofia News*, 20 July 1977. 5. *Trud*, Sofia, 29 July 1980, p.c. Dr. Dimiter

Pamukov and his wife Dr. Lilia Tomova-Pamukova. 6. Gonzalez, "The Scourge of German Medicine", *World Medicine*, 3 May 1980, pp. 29–31. 7. Farnsworth & Bingel, "Problems and prospects of discovering new drugs from higher plants by pharmacological screening", in Wagner & Wolff (eds.), *New Natural Products and Plant Drugs with Pharmacological, Biological and Therapeutic Activity*, pp. 1–22. 8. Newton-Fenbow, *A Time to Heal*, pp. 133–4. 9. Warren-Davis, "The Theory and Practice of Herbalism", lecture given to Wrekin Trust Open Conference on Health and Healing, Loughborough University, 15 July 1977, *New Herbal Practitioner*, IV, no. 1, 1977, pp. 18–9. 10. *Ibid*, pp. 19–20. 11. Farnsworth, "Rational Approaches Applicable to the Search for and Discovery of New Drugs from Plants", lecture at the First Latin-American and Caribbean Symposium on Naturally Occurring Pharmacological Agents, Havana, Cuba, 23–28 June 1980, p. 4. 12. *Ibid*, p. 5. 13. Farnsworth and others, "The Current Status of the Use of *Eleutherococcus senticosus* in the USA and its Potential Value in the American Health Care System", paper to First International Congress on Eleutherococcus, Hamburg, West Germany, 29 May 1980. 14. Fulder, passim. 15. Hill, *The Useful Family Herbal*, preface pp. ix–x. 16. Skelton, *A Plea for the Botanic Practice of Medicine*, p. 57.

Tailpiece: Unattributed Latin tag quoted Lind, *A Treatise on Scurvy*. Translation: "Chemistry makes an excellent handmaid but is the worst possible mistress'.

Index